Childhood Obsessive-Compulsive and Related Disorders

This book is a comprehensive evidence-based guide for clinicians and trainees on the assessment and treatment of youth with obsessive-compulsive and related disorders (OCRDs).

OCRDs typically begin in childhood or adolescence and can be highly prevalent and impairing, though there has been minimal clinical guidance on treatment of such disorders in youth. This go-to handbook on OCRDs in childhood has an international range of expert contributors providing evidence-based guidance on assessment and treatment of these conditions including adapting treatment for very young children, digital mental health interventions, and family-based, parent-based, and intensive treatment formats. Chapters also review other areas in the field such as clinical presentation, causal and maintaining factors, and features and transdiagnostic psychological dimensions of ORCDs. The concluding chapters discuss future directions for the field and emphasize the need for diversity, dissemination, and implementation in childhood OCRD research.

This book is essential for clinicians specializing in OCD and related disorders in children and adolescents. It is also applicable to clinicians, trainees, and students across a wide range of mental health disciplines.

Eric A. Storch is professor and McIngvale presidential endowed chair in the Department of Psychiatry and Behavioral Sciences at Baylor College of Medicine, Houston, TX. He serves as vice chair of psychology and specializes in the nature and treatment of childhood and adult obsessive-compulsive disorder, anxiety disorders, PTSD, and anxiety among youth with autism.

Andrew G. Guzick is a clinical psychologist and assistant professor in the Department of Psychiatry at the University of Pennsylvania, Philadelphia, PA. Through his position in the Center for the Treatment and Study of Anxiety, his clinical and research focus is on children and adults with anxiety, obsessive-compulsive, and related disorders.

"Storch and Guzick, themselves authorities in the assessment and treatment of OCD and related disorders in children and adolescents, coordinated a set of perceptive chapters/reviews that are fully referenced and with applied relevance. The worldly collection provides updated and useful information on the range of empirically supported treatments (CBT, medication), various treatment modalities (youth, family, parent), and pressing issues (diversity, dissemination). OCD is not a singular problem, and this scholarly and practical book exemplifies the several mental health disorders that are relevant to OCD. Readers will benefit from the recent treatment innovations, suggestions for developmental adjustments, and future directions."

Philip C. Kendall, *University Professor, Temple University*

"Expertly edited by leaders in the field, this comprehensive text is an indispensable resource for anyone in the field of pediatric OCD. It skillfully combines the latest research, treatment innovations, and clinical insights. With a focus on both well-established and emerging approaches, including digital and parent-led interventions, it addresses critical issues like treatment access and diversity in OCRD research. Essential for professionals, it's a must-have for advancing knowledge and improving outcomes."

Jonathan S. Abramowitz, *Professor and Director of Clinical Training, University of North Carolina at Chapel Hill*

"Drs. Storch and Guzick have compiled the most up-to-date information on the assessment and treatment of OCRDs in youth and topped it off with recommendations of where we as a field are still lacking and need to improve. As such, this book should serve as an indispensable guide for both clinicians looking to treat and clinical researchers looking to better understand the OCRDs."

Caleb W. Lack, *Professor, University of Central Oklahoma*

"Storch and Guzick have assembled an impressive collection of experts on the topic of childhood obsessive-compulsive and related disorders. The chapters are thoughtful and comprehensive and written with both researchers and clinicians in mind. The volume is a much-needed contribution to the field. Add it to your bookshelves. You'll refer to it often and each time you'll discover answers to some of the most complex and intriguing questions on this important topic."

Michael A. Tompkins, *Co-director, San Francisco Bay Area Center for Cognitive Therapy, University of California at Berkeley*

"Clinicians devoted to helping youth with OCD and related disorders rightly pride themselves on using 'evidence-based' treatments. Paradoxically, non-researchers like myself spend so much time face-to-face with our patients and their families providing psychotherapy (or supervising new clinicians) that we rarely have time to dive deeply into the evolving evidentiary studies. Should I keep using this rating scale or is there a more effective one? Is the CBT/ERP approach I'm using tried and true or are there adjustments to be made that improve outcomes? This book is a reliable resource for establishing the fundamentals and keeping us up to date."

Jon Hershfield, *LCMFT, Director of the Center for OCD and Anxiety at Sheppard Pratt*

"An exceptional and comprehensive guide to the most recent advances in assessment and treatment in the complex arena of childhood OCD and related disorders. Skillfully compiled by top experts in OCD, it brings timely clarity to a rapidly evolving field and provides empirically driven guidance for practice. A valuable, must-read resource that will be frequently referenced by treatment providers."

Aureen P. Wagner, *The Anxiety Wellness Center, Cary, NC; author of* What to Do When Your Child has OCD *and* Up and Down the Worry Hill.

"This book has everything you need to build a state-of-the-art OCD spectrum disorder program! Truly comprehensive in scope, the volume is a collection of expert-authored chapters spanning the pediatric OCD landscape, including crucial but often overlooked aspects of care. Each topic achieves both breadth and depth, including supporting studies, case examples, and concrete developmentally tailored skills. Providers trained to treat youth with OCRDs are critically needed. Whether new to specialized behavioral approaches or honing your skills and keeping up with the evidence base, you can't find a more complete guide to treating OCD and related disorders."

Erika Nurmi, *Associate professor, University of California, Los Angeles*

Childhood Obsessive-Compulsive and Related Disorders

Assessment and Treatment

Edited by Eric A. Storch and
Andrew G. Guzick

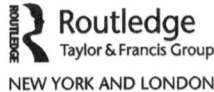
Routledge
Taylor & Francis Group

NEW YORK AND LONDON

Designed cover image: © Getty Images

First published 2025
by Routledge
605 Third Avenue, New York, NY 10158

and by Routledge
4 Park Square, Milton Park, Abingdon, Oxon, OX14 4RN

Routledge is an imprint of the Taylor & Francis Group, an informa business

Library of Congress Cataloging-in-Publication Data
Names: Storch, Eric A., editor. | Guzick, Andrew G., editor.
Title: Childhood obsessive-compulsive and related disorders : assessment and treatment / edited by Eric A. Storch and Andrew G. Guzick.
Description: New York, NY : Routledge, 2025. | Includes bibliographical references and index.
Identifiers: LCCN 2024027929 (print) | LCCN 2024027930 (ebook) | ISBN 9781032478630 (hbk) | ISBN 9781032478623 (pbk) | ISBN 9781003386278 (ebk)
Subjects: MESH: Obsessive-Compulsive Disorder—diagnosis | Obsessive-Compulsive Disorder—therapy | Child
Classification: LCC RJ506.O25 C485 2025 (print) | LCC RJ506. O25 (ebook) | NLM WM 176 | DDC 616.85/22700835—dc23/ eng/20240909
LC record available at https://lccn.loc.gov/2024027929
LC ebook record available at https://lccn.loc.gov/2024027930

ISBN: 978-1-032-47863-0 (hbk)
ISBN: 978-1-032-47862-3 (pbk)
ISBN: 978-1-003-38627-8 (ebk)

DOI: 10.4324/9781003386278

Typeset in Sabon
by Apex CoVantage, LLC

Dedicated with love to the people, the animals, and the distant shores in my heart. Thank you all for everything. Namaste.

Contents

Contributors

Editors

Eric A. Storch, PhD, is professor and McIngvale presidential endowed chair in the Department of Psychiatry and Behavioral Sciences at Baylor College of Medicine (BCM), Houston, TX. He serves as vice chair and head of psychology and co-directs the Obsessive-Compulsive and Related Disorders program at BCM. Dr. Storch specializes in the nature and treatment of childhood and adult obsessive-compulsive disorder, anxiety disorders, post-traumatic stress disorder (PTSD), and anxiety among youth with autism. In addition to over 850 published articles and chapters and 22 books, he has received multiple federal grants to investigate treatment efficacy, mechanisms of action, genetics, bioethics, innovative approaches to phenotyping, and how to enhance outcomes for those struggling with obsessive-compulsive disorder (OCD) and related conditions.

Andrew G. Guzick, PhD, is a clinical psychologist and assistant professor in the Department of Psychiatry at the University of Pennsylvania, Philadelphia, PA. His research and clinical interests are in the assessment and treatment of children and adults with anxiety, obsessive-compulsive, mood, and related disorders. His research has resulted in over 80 peer-reviewed publications and grant support from state, federal, and foundation funders. He also provides cognitive behavioral therapy (CBT) and supervises trainees within the Center for the Treatment and Study for Anxiety at the University of Pennsylvania, Philadelphia, PA.

Contributors

Ana I. Rosa-Alcázar is professor of the Department of Personality, Evaluation and Psychological Treatment at the University of Murcia, Murcia, Spain. She is the coordinator of the Master's in general health psychology, and a member of the Unit of Behavior Therapy, Service of Applied

Psychology, in the Department of Psychology at the university. She is author of numerous publications in the field of clinical and health psychology, and has extensive experience working with parents, children, and adolescents. Her research interests focus on OCRD in children and adolescents and borderline personality disorder.

Ángel Rosa-Alcázar has a doctorate in psychology, a Master's degree in clinical and health psychology, a Master's degree in general health psychology, and is professor of the Department of Personality, Evaluation and Psychological Treatment at the University of Murcia, Murcia, Spain. He has extensive experience as a researcher and health psychologist.

Amanda Balkhi, PhD, is director of the Balkhi Foundation, West Palm Beach, FL. Amanda's research interests include barriers to adherence and treatment augmentation strategies for pediatric populations, with a special interest in utilizing technology.

Megan A. Barthle-Herrera, PhD, completed her doctoral degree in counseling psychology. She has completed an American Psychological Association (APA)-approved pre-doctoral internship in clinical and health psychology and a postdoctoral fellowship in psychology. Dr. Barthle's research interests include treatment outcomes for CBT/exposure and response prevention (ERP) and parent-child interaction therapy (PCIT) treatment interventions, as well as topics associated with OCD and related disorders.

Dr Cristina Bernal-Ruiz is on faculty at the University of Murcia in the Department of Personality, Assessment, and Psychological Treatment located in Murcia, Spain. She is an expert in childhood OCD and related treatments.

Andreas Bezahler is currently a graduate student at Fordham University, New York, NY. His main research interests are in the intersection of OCD and sexual minority health. Specifically, how minority stress may exacerbate and maintain obsessive-compulsive symptoms.

Elizabeth S. Bocanegra received her BA in psychology and sociology with a minor in art from the University of Miami, Coral Gables, FL. After graduating, she was selected to participate in the Minority Health and Health Disparities International Research Training Program (MHIRT) in Mexico City, Mexico, where she studied the incidence and prevalence of depression in Mexican youth. She is currently a fourth-year graduate student in the CALMA Lab, Los Angeles, CA, with interests in anxiety and depression in the Latin/x community and how to develop new ways to deliver treatment to low-income individuals.

Abigail Candelari, PhD, is assistant professor of psychology at Baylor College of Medicine, Houston, TX, and program director of the Maternal

Perinatal Addiction Treatment (MPAT) Clinic at Ben Taub Hospital, Houston, TX. Dr. Candelari has co-authored over 20 peer-reviewed journal articles, and has co-authored five book chapters. Dr. Candelari's research interests lie in developmental psychopathology, and specifically focus on interventions for parents, temperamental and parental risk/resilience factors, and how these traits influence psychopathology throughout development.

Molly J. Church, PsyD, is currently a clinical psychology post-doctoral fellow at the OCD and Related Disorders Program at Menninger Department of Psychiatry and Behavioral Sciences, Baylor College of Medicine, Houston, TX. Her research interests include the treatment of anxiety, OCD, and related disorders, including comorbidities such as eating disorders, as well as the connection between individual factors and experiences of OCD. Clinically, she provides treatment to youth and adults with anxiety, OCD, and related disorders.

Fanny A. Dietel is a postdoctoral fellow working with Dr. Silja Voc at Osnabrück University, Osnabrück, Germany. Her research focus includes anxiety disorders, obsessive-compulsive disorder, and body dysmorphic disorder.

Nicholas R. Farrell is a licensed clinical psychologist and regional clinical director at NOCD, Chicago, IL, where he provides clinical leadership and direction for teletherapy services. He is a recognized expert in researching and treating OCD and other related conditions. Dr. Farrell has published numerous scholarly works, including peer-review journal articles, book chapters, and books, and he frequently gives presentations at international conferences on maximizing the effectiveness of treatment for OCD and related conditions. He also has experience designing and overseeing several successful training programs that have enhanced the dissemination of evidence-based treatment for OCD.

Dr Jamie D. Feusner is chief medical officer at NOCD, Chicago, IL, where he designs, manages, and advances treatment protocols and oversees clinical outcomes. He is also professor of psychiatry at the University of Toronto, Ontario, Canada, clinician scientist at the Centre for Addiction & Mental Health, Toronto, Ontario, Canada, and adjunct professor at the Karolinska Institute, Solna, Sweden. Dr. Feusner has 18 years clinical and research experience with OCD and BDD, has published over 130 peer-reviewed papers and book chapters, and lectures nationally and internationally on the topics of OCD, BDD, and eating disorders. Dr. Feusner's research program seeks to understand perceptual and emotional processing phenotypes across conditions involving body image and obsessions/compulsions, including BDD, eating disorders, and OCD.

Dr Daniel A. Geller is director of the Pediatric OCD and Tic Disorder Program and founded the Pediatric Obsessive Compulsive Disorder Program in 1992. At Massachusetts General Hospital, Boston, MA, he has collected and characterized a large sample of children and adolescents with OCD and tic disorders. Among his research efforts is collaborative work with other leading universities and the National Institute of Mental Health for the study of genetics of psychiatric disorders. Dr. Geller is a founding member of the International OCD Genetics Consortium, collaborating with senior scientists from many countries, with the goal of identifying genes responsible for OCD and delineating mechanisms by which genetic vulnerabilities are translated into clinical symptoms.

Wayne K. Goodman, MD, is professor and D.C. and Irene Ellwood chair in psychiatry in the Department of Psychiatry and Behavioral Sciences at Baylor College of Medicine, Houston, TX. He specializes in obsessive-compulsive disorder and deep brain stimulation (DBS) for intractable psychiatric illnesses. He is the principal developer of the Yale-Brown Obsessive Compulsive Scale (Y-BOCS), the gold standard for assessing OCD, and co-founder of the International OCD Foundation.

Dr Sisi Guo is director of the Pediatric OCD Intensive Outpatient Program at the Resnick Neuropsychiatric Hospital, University of California, Los Angeles (UCLA), Los Angeles, CA, assistant health sciences professor of Child Psychiatry at UCLA Semel Institute, UCLA, and assistant clinical professor in the Department of Psychology at UCLA. Dr. Guo's clinical and research interests are in the training and delivery of evidence-based treatments for youth and families, with a particular focus on anxiety and OCD-related disorders.

Davíð R. M. A. Højgaard is a clinical psychologist and senior researcher at the Department of Child and Adolescent Psychiatry, Aarhus University Hospital Psychiatry in Aarhus, Denmark and an external lector at the Department of Psychology and Behavioral Sciences at Aarhus University. He earned his PhD from Aarhus University, Denmark and psychology degree from the University of Iceland. His research focus has been child and adolescent psychopathology, particularly obsessive-compulsive and related disorders and cognitive behavioral therapy for children and adolescents.

Cate W. MacDonald is a senior at Harvard College in Cambridge, Massachusetts. As a psychology concentrator, she has conducted comprehensive research working in the Nock Lab at Harvard with a focus on childhood trauma and suicidal thoughts and behaviors. As a clinical intern at NOCD for the past two years, she has played a significant role in developing and launching a variety of educational programs as well as enhancing the resources available for mental health professionals who are treating anxiety and mood disorders.

Katie H. Mangen, PhD, is a postdoctoral fellow at Menninger Department of Psychiatry and Behavioral Sciences at Baylor College of Medicine, Houston, TX. Her research interests include factors related to the development, maintenance, and treatment of obsessive-compulsive and related disorders and anxiety disorders. She has worked with patients with these disorders across a variety of settings in individual and group therapy.

Dr Patrick B. McGrath serves as the chief clinical officer for NOCD, Chicago, IL, where he oversees the company's clinical protocols and team of OCD specialists.

Dr Joseph F. McGuire is associate professor in the Department of Psychiatry and Behavioral Sciences at Johns Hopkins University School of Medicine, Baltimore, MD. He is director of research for the Division of Child and Adolescent Psychiatry, serves as director of psychology in the Center for Developmental Behavioral Health at the Kennedy Krieger Institute, Baltimore, MD, and co-directs the Tourette Syndrome Center of Excellence at Johns Hopkins Medicine, Baltimore, MD. His research focuses on investigating the learning processes and mechanisms that underlie the etiology and treatment of OCD, anxiety, Tourette syndrome, and related disorders in children, adolescents, and young adults, using clinical rating scales, physiological markers, and innovative technologies. His work seeks to improve evidence-based treatments to help patients and families achieve optimal outcomes. Dr. McGuire has received numerous national and international awards. He has co-edited three books with Elsevier, published over 140 peer-reviewed journal articles, and has given dozens of conference presentations. Dr. McGuire's research has been supported by the National Institute Health, Tourette Association of America, Hilda and Preston Davis Foundation, Misophonia Research Fund, and the American Academy of Neurology.

Dr Joseph P.H. McNamara is a licensed psychologist and associate professor in the College of Medicine at the University of Florida, Gainesville, FL. Dr. McNamara is the chief of the Psychology Division in the Department of Psychiatry, director of the OCD Treatment Program, and co-director of the Center for OCD, Anxiety, and Related Disorders (COARD).

Dr Michelle Miller is currently completing her general psychiatry residency at Johns Hopkins University School of Medicine, Baltimore, MD. She will continue her training at Johns Hopkins when she begins her fellowship in child and adolescent psychiatry in summer of 2024. Her research interests include understanding the underlying processes, such as intolerance of uncertainty, that contribute to the development and maintenance of OCD, anxiety, and eating disorders. Clinically, she is interested in treating children and adolescents struggling with anxiety-related disorders and eating disorders.

Tannaz MirHosseini is a fourth-year graduate student primarily mentored by Dr. McNamara in the Florida Exposure and Anxiety Research (FEAR) Lab, University of Florida, Gainesville, FL. Tannaz graduated from the University of Florida in 2017 with a BSc in psychology. After graduation, she worked in the Language and Cognitive Development Lab, University of Florida, under Dr. Jeff Farrar researching Theory of Mind in pre-schoolers, and in the FEAR Lab under Dr. Joseph McNamara, working with adolescents with OCD, anxiety, and related disorders. She then continued her research at the Mood and Emotion Regulation Lab in Cleveland, OH, examining the role of emotion regulation in the transmission of depression risk between parents and their offspring. Her research interests include the effects of parent involvement and practices on OCD and anxiety treatment outcome as well as the impact on quality of life from psychological symptoms.

Melissa Munson, PhD, is an assistant professor. She completed her postdoctoral work with the Division of Medical Psychology within the Department of Psychiatry at the University of Florida, Gainesville, FL. Her responsibilities include the evaluation and treatment of child and adult psychological problems, with a specialization in obsessive-compulsive disorder, and their anxiety concerns.

Dr Mia C. Nuñez is a licensed clinical psychologist and clinical director for the West Region of NOCD, Chicago, IL. Dr. Nuñez earned her degrees from UCLA and Northwestern University, Evanston, IL, and completed her pre-doctoral internship at Rogers Behavioral Health. Dr. Nuñez served as supervising psychologist for several inpatient and residential programs specializing in treatment of OCD and related disorders.

Cynthia Onyeka, PhD is a postdoctoral associate in the OCD Program in the Department of Psychiatry and Behavioral Sciences at Baylor College of Medicine, Houston, TX. Her research and clinical interests center on understanding risk and resilience factors for youth of color experiencing internalizing symptoms (anxiety, trauma, OCD), critical consciousness, and positive youth development. She embraces a Community-Based Participatory Action Research (CBPAR) approach to involve community members in her research, aiming to leverage research to support the communities and populations they serve.

Ashley Ordway, MEd, EdS, LMHC, earned her Master's of education and education specialist degrees from the nationally recognized Counselor

Education program, University of Florida, Gainesville, FL, in 2016. She is the founder and co-owner of Magnolia Behavioral Health. She is a certified Parent-Child Interaction Therapy clinician recognized by Parent Child Interaction Therapy International.

Ainsley K. Patrick is a PhD student in the Clinical Child Psychology Program at the University of Kansas, Lawrence, KS. Her research focuses on the intersection of emotion regulation, attention biases, and intergenerational anxiety within anxiety disorders. Her work utilizes multi-informant, multimodal data sources to understand comprehensively the mechanisms underlying childhood anxiety disorders.

Dr Aditya Kumar Singh Pawar is a graduate of Lala Lajpat Rai Medical college in Meerut, India. He completed his first psychiatry residency in India at All India Institute of Medical Sciences, Jodhpur, India, and then pursued residency training in the USA in adult psychiatry at The Drexel University College of Medicine, Philadelphia, PA, followed by child and adolescent psychiatry training at the Harvard Medical School's Massachusetts General Hospital, Boston, MA, and McLean Hospital, Belmont, MA, where he also served as chief fellow. Dr. Pawar's clinical interests include adolescent substance use, attention deficit hyperactivity disorder, and autism spectrum disorder. He has been actively engaged in research on early intervention for psychosis, substance use disorders, and the use of technology in childhood disruptive behavior disorders.

Dr Tara S. Peris is professor of psychiatry and biobehavioral sciences. She is currently vice chair for research and associate director of the Division of Child and Adolescent Psychiatry, UCLA, Los Angeles, California. In addition, she is program director of the UCLA Achievement, Behavior, and Cognition (ABC) Partial Hospitalization Program and co-director of the UCLA Child OCD, Anxiety, and Tic Disorders Program. Dr. Peris's research and clinical interests are in developmental psychopathology, with a particular focus on anxiety, OCD, and related disorders. Her research examines developmental trajectories of these conditions as well as strategies for optimizing treatment outcome.

Caitlin M. Pinciotti, PhD, is a licensed clinical psychologist and assistant professor in the Menninger Department of Psychiatry and Behavioral Sciences at Baylor College of Medicine. Houston, TX. Her research interests include obsessive-compulsive disorder, trauma, and post-traumatic stress disorder, particularly the intersections and implications of these conditions and experiences when they co-occur. She has a secondary interest in identifying and addressing mental health inequities in sexual and gender minority individuals.

Dr Aarya Krishnan Rajalakshmi completed medical school from Sri P S Govindasamy Naidu (PSG) Institute of Medical Sciences and Research in Coimbatore, India followed by general psychiatry residency training at the Postgraduate Institute of Medical Science and Research, Chandigarh, India. She spent three years at the All India Institute of Medical Sciences, Jodhpur, India, as a senior resident doctor in the Department of Psychiatry after which she moved to the USA and worked as a research scholar at the Division of Child and Adolescent Psychiatry at the Zucker Hillside Hospital, Glen Oaks, NY. Dr. Rajalakshmi nurtures a special interest in treating children and adolescents with obsessive-compulsive disorder as well as anxiety and mood disorders.

Kesley A. Ramsey, PhD is a licensed clinical psychologist at Johns Hopkins University School of Medicine in the Department of Psychiatry and Behavioral Sciences, Baltimore, MD. She currently conducts clinical research at the Center for OCD, Anxiety, and related disorders for Children (COACH). Her research centers on investigating the mechanisms that underlie the etiology, maintenance, and treatment of neuropsychiatric conditions, specifically Tourette syndrome, obsessive-compulsive disorder and obsessive-compulsive and related disorders, and anxiety disorders. Dr. Ramsey has received national recognition for her innovative research, including the Tourette Association of America's Young Investigator Award and the American Psychological Association's Society for Clinical Child and Adolescent Psychology (Division 53) Future Directions Launch Award.

Gudmundur Skarphedinsson is clinical child psychologist and professor at the Faculty of Psychology, University of Iceland, Reykjavik, Iceland. He earned his PhD from the University of Oslo, Oslo, Norway, and his MSc in clinical psychology from the University of Iceland. His research is dedicated to the evidence-based assessment and treatment of psychological disorders. Gudmundur's work notably focuses on evaluating and enhancing clinical assessments and treatments for obsessive-compulsive disorder, anxiety disorders, and related conditions in children and adolescents.

Orri Smárason, PhD, is a clinical child and adolescent psychologist and researcher at the Department of Child and Adolescent Psychiatry, Landspitali National University Hospital, Iceland. His research interests include the assessment and treatment of obsessive-compulsive and related disorders, anxiety disorders, emotional dysregulation, and other psychiatric conditions in children and adolescents.

Dr Elizabeth R. Steuber is currently a child and adolescent psychiatry fellow within the Department of Psychiatry at Boston Children's Hospital, Boston, MA. Prior to fellowship training, she completed her medical school education at Harvard Medical School, Boston, MA, and adult psychiatry residency at Johns Hopkins Hospital, Baltimore, MD. Her research interests center on the aberrant fear leaning processes that drive disorders, including anxiety spectrum disorders, OCD, and PTSD.

Berta J. Summers, PhD is assistant professor at the University of North Carolina Wilmington (UNCW). Her clinical and research expertise center around OCRDs such as OCD and body dysmorphic disorder (BDD). Specifically, her work focuses on cognitive bias modification, problematic safety behaviors, "not just right" experiences, and broad factors influencing etiology and treatment outcome across these illnesses.

Erika S. Trent, MA, LPA, is a doctoral candidate in clinical psychology at the University of Houston, Houston, TX. She is currently completing her pre-doctoral internship at Baylor College of Medicine, Houston, TX, in the obsessive-compulsive and related disorders (OCRDs) track. Her research interests include anxiety disorders and OCRDs, with a focus on parenting and affective factors that contribute to the development and maintenance of childhood anxiety disorders. Clinically, she has worked with youth and adults with anxiety disorders and OCRDs in outpatient clinics and clinical trials.

Dr Andres G. Viana is associate professor of psychology, a licensed clinical child psychologist, and director of the Child Temperament, Thoughts, and Emotions Laboratory at the University of Houston, Houston, TX. He also serves as associate director of the Sleep and Anxiety Center of Houston, TX. Dr. Viana received his MS and PhD in clinical child psychology from Penn State University. Camp Hill, PA, and completed his psychology residency training at the University of Mississippi Medical Center (UMMC), Jackson, MS, where he remained as a tenure-track member of the Psychiatry Department until 2015. Dr. Viana's program of research is grounded in the developmental psychopathology perspective of psychological functioning and focuses on the study and assessment of risk factors for childhood psychopathologies, with an emphasis on temperamental, emotional, cognitive, and parenting factors that may exacerbate anxiety, as well as the nature of the co-variation among these processes. A growing aspect of his research program involves cognitive and emotion-related factors associated with risk behaviors in children with internalizing difficulties.

1 Introduction

Eric A. Storch[1] and Andrew G. Guzick[2]

[1] Baylor College of Medicine, Menninger Department of Psychiatry & Behavioral Sciences, Houston, TX

[2] Department of Psychiatry, University of Pennsylvania, Philadelphia, PA

Over the past several decades, there has been a tremendous expansion of research in childhood obsessive-compulsive disorder (OCD), given the recognition of its frequency and associated impairment and disability. Indeed, prior to the 1990s, OCD among children was inaccurately believed to be quite uncommon, which was partially due to limited/problematic assessment options, knowledge of the condition, beliefs about mental illness in children, and stigma. With knowledge of the disabling nature of OCD as well as its relative frequent occurrence, development of behavioral and pharmacological interventions took place. While these interventions are not perfect, nearly 75–80 percent of youth respond to first-line interventions (McGuire et al., 2015; Öst et al., 2016; Torp et al., 2015) and as many as 90 percent of youth with OCD significantly improve three years after starting treatment (Melin et al., 2020).

During this time, there has also been increased recognition of other conditions proposed to be related to OCD with potentially shared underlying mechanisms and phenotypic presentations. Obsessive-compulsive and related disorders (OCRD) classification within the *Diagnostic and Statistical Manual of Mental Disorders* (5th edition, DSM-5) (American Psychiatric Association, 2013) has come to include conditions such as body dysmorphic disorder (BDD), hoarding disorder, excoriation or skin-picking disorder, and trichotillomania or hair-pulling disorder. While not listed in this DSM-5 OCRD classification, chronic tic disorders such as Tourette disorder is typically included in this grouping given a close relationship with OCD, and has been cross-listed with OCRDs in the *International Classification of Diseases* (11th revision) (World Health Organisation, 2019). Although all these diagnoses have been reported to most often onset during childhood or adolescence, the majority of treatment and assessment research has focused on youth with OCD and chronic tic disorders. For these conditions, advances in assessment have yielded clarity on evidence-based approaches to measurement at initial presentation

DOI: 10.4324/9781003386278-1

as well as throughout treatment. Extant behavioral and pharmacological interventions have a sound supporting evidence base (but more limited dissemination). In contrast, the "related disorders," including body-focused repetitive behavior disorders, body dysmorphic disorder, and hoarding disorder, lag behind. These conditions have received relatively less attention in the childhood treatment and assessment literature, perhaps due to their later onset, which typically occurs in adolescence, and as, in the case of hoarding, symptoms may not lead to considerable functional impairment for years or decades. Regardless, as these conditions do most often onset during the adolescence, there is a critical window for early intervention, and recent years have seen a substantially growing literature on promising clinical practices in these areas as well.

It was our belief that the literature had sufficiently matured to necessitate a comprehensive text detailing the state of the field in assessment and treatment of OCRDs in childhood and adolescence. The goal of bringing together experts in the field to compile such a text is to further propel knowledge in this space to support the 10 percent of youth who are not doing well after several years, as well as address disparities in treatment access, which remains a massive problem, particularly for the "related disorders." To this end, much remains to be done. The text concludes with a discussion of two key areas in need of attention, namely dissemination/implementation and improving diversity in OCRD work.

This book is broken into two main sections. The first section is focused on assessment and treatment, with chapters providing overviews of a specific form of cognitive behavioral therapy (CBT) for OCD-termed exposure and response prevention (ERP), CBT as it is applied to adolescents with BDD, as well as habit reversal training for tic disorders and body-focused repetitive behavior disorders. Chapters will also focus on recent treatment innovations and developmental modifications, particularly as they apply to childhood OCD, including family-based and parent-led treatments, intensive treatment approaches, the treatment of young children with OCD, digital modifications, and psychopharmacology.

The second section of the book discusses considerations of future directions in OCRD research, with a particular focus on dissemination and implementation of evidence-based treatments and improving diversity in childhood OCRD research.

This text offers a group of leading experts in the field the opportunity to speak on the current state of assessment and treatment of childhood OCRDs – as well as areas in need of attention and growth. Long-standing treatments for OCRDs are discussed (e.g., medications, ERP, comprehensive behavioral intervention for tics (CBIT)), but so are newer areas like parent-led and digital interventions. The goal of this volume was to summarize the ongoing work comprehensively in order to continuously edge our field forward and ethically evaluate our progress – and hence we include chapters discussing the need for improving diversity in OCRD research as well as reducing health disparities related to treatment access. In the end, the goal is to summarize how we might best take what we know about assessment and treatment of these conditions and advance toward expanding access further while improving outcomes for affected youth and their families.

References

American Psychiatric Association. (2013). *Diagnostic and statistical manual of mental disorders* (5th ed.). https://doi.org/10.1176/appi.books.9780890425596.

McGuire, J.F., Piacentini, J., Lewin, A.B., Brennan, E.A., Murphy, T.K., & Storch, E.A. (2015). A meta-analysis of cognitive behavior therapy and medication for child obsessive-compulsive disorder: Moderators of treatment efficacy, response, and remission. Research article. Treatment outcomes and moderators in pediatric OCD. *Depression and Anxiety*, *32*(8), 580–593. https://doi.org/10.1002/da.22389.

Melin, K., Skarphedinsson, G., Thomsen, P.H., Weidle, B., Torp, N.C., Valderhaug, R., Højgaard, D.R.M.A., Hybel, K.A., Nissen, J.B., Jensen, S., Dahl, K., Skärsäter, I., Haugland, B.S., & Ivarsson, T. (2020). Treatment gains are sustainable in pediatric obsessive-compulsive disorder: Three-year follow-up from the NordLOTS. *Journal of the American Academy of Child & Adolescent Psychiatry*, *59*(2), 244–253. https://doi.org/10.1016/j.jaac.2019.01.010.

Öst, L.-G., Riise, E.N., Wergeland, G.J., Hansen, B., & Kvale, G. (2016). Cognitive behavioral and pharmacological treatments of OCD in children: A systematic review and meta-analysis. *Journal of Anxiety Disorders*, *43*, 58–69. https://doi.org/10.1016/j.janxdis.2016.08.003.

Torp, N.C., Dahl, K., Skarphedinsson, G., Thomsen, P.H., Valderhaug, R., Weidle, B., Melin, K.H., Hybel, K., Nissen, J.B., Lenhard, F., Wentzel-Larsen, T., Franklin, M.E., & Ivarsson, T. (2015). Effectiveness of cognitive behavior treatment for pediatric obsessive-compulsive disorder: Acute outcomes from the Nordic Long-term OCD Treatment Study (NordLOTS). *Behaviour Research and Therapy*, *64*, 15–23. https://doi.org/10.1016/j.brat.2014.11.005.

World Health Organisation. (2019). *International classification of diseases and related health problems (11th ed.).* https://icd.who.int/browse11.

2 Evidence-based Assessment of Childhood Obsessive-Compulsive and Related Disorders

Elizabeth R. Steuber,[1] *Michelle Miller,*[1] *and Joseph F. McGuire*[1]

[1] *Department of Psychiatry and Behavioral Sciences, Johns Hopkins University School of Medicine, Baltimore, MD*

Introduction

Across mental health fields (e.g., psychiatry, psychology, social work), greater emphasis has been placed on the evidence-based assessment of psychiatric conditions to achieve diagnostic accuracy, characterize symptom severity, and monitor therapeutic response to interventions. Indeed, the standardization of measurement approaches across clinicians allows for the comparison of patients across time and minimizes the variability seen in the absence of clear objective markers of disease presence and severity. Psychometrically sound rating scales are a critical component of clinical care and treatment research that have provided clinicians with reliable, valid, and quantifiable metrics for disease presence and severity.

The use of evidence-based assessments for the diagnosis and treatment of obsessive-compulsive and related disorders (OCRDs) is of particular importance for several reasons. These conditions have considerable overlap with one another, and they also share characteristics with other psychiatric and medical disorders – which necessitates careful and thorough clinical evaluations to differentiate conditions. As with many psychiatric disorders, accurate diagnosis and severity classification is informed by a combination of child-, parent-, and clinician-reports. This is especially important for pediatric patients, as the ability to engage in behaviors associated with OCRDs (e.g., compulsions and/or avoidance behavior) can be influenced by external factors (e.g., caregivers may discard hoarded items, hand-washing compulsions may be limited by accessibility of hand soap). Additionally, insight into symptoms may be affected (on either side of the caregiver or child dyad). Thus, it is critical to characterize insight level as it is diagnostic specifier and also informs treatment recommendations. Finally, as treatment recommendations are

DOI: 10.4324/9781003386278-2

often informed by the specific OCRD and severity of symptoms (M.H. Bloch & Storch, 2015; Essoe et al., 2019), it is essential to comprehensively characterize symptoms and their severity to ensure appropriate treatment recommendations and implementation.

In this chapter, we present common rating scales for childhood OCRDs. We have used the following conventions to characterize descriptively the reliability, validity, and treatment sensitivity of these rating scales. Reliability was characterized using internal consistency, test-retest reliability, and inter-rater reliability. Internal consistency was typically reported using Cronbach's alpha, in which a desired value is typically greater than 0.70 (Cicchetti, 1994). Meanwhile, test-retest reliability was typically evaluated using correlation coefficients, with the strength of the desired associations varying by test-retest window. Finally, inter-rater reliability was often assessed using intra-class correlation (ICC), Spearman's rank correlation, or Cohen's kappa statistic. Conventions suggest that inter-rater reliability of <0.40 is poor, 0.40–0.59 is fair, 0.60–0.74 is good and 0.75–1.00 is excellent (Cicchetti, 1994). Alongside reliability, we also considered the validity of rating scales. Broadly, validity can be separated into two main categories: convergent and discriminant validity. Convergent validity evaluates whether scores from the scale in question correlate with metrics known to measure the same construct. Convergent validity is important because it provides a check to confirm that the measure is truly measuring its intended construct. Meanwhile, discriminant validity assesses the relationship between the intended construct and unrelated constructs. This ensures that the identified scale appropriately distinguishes between related constructs that may present together (e.g., anxiety, depression, obsessive-compulsive severity). Lastly, we also sought to identify whether a rating scale is sensitive to treatment effects. This is evidenced by anticipated changes in rating-scale scores in an appropriate direction following a course of treatment (i.e., significant reductions in a rating-scale score following evidence-based treatment, whereas minimal changes would be anticipated following a waitlist condition).

In this chapter, we review the current available measures to assess common OCRDs (e.g., obsessive-compulsive disorder (OCD), Tourette's disorder, trichotillomania (hair-pulling disorder), excoriation disorder (skin-picking disorder), hoarding disorder, body dysmorphic disorder). This includes clinician-administered scales, parent-reported scales, and child-reported scales. We briefly review the psychometric properties of these rating scales – where this information is available – and identify the limitations of extant scales to help guide clinicians' selection of these tools. Finally, we provide guidance on rating-scale selection that comprises an evidence-based assessment informed by the available evidence.

Childhood Obsessive-Compulsive Disorder

Obsessive-compulsive disorder (OCD) is a debilitating condition that pre-dominantly onsets in childhood and is defined by unwanted, intrusive, and upsetting thoughts and associated compulsive behaviors that cause signifi-cant distress and functional impairment and also diminish quality of life. Fortunately, there are several clinician-rated scales, parent-report scales, and child-report scales that can be used to identify OCD symptoms, char-acterize symptom severity, and monitor response to therapeutic interven-tions (Patrick et al., 2022; Rapp et al., 2016).

Clinician-Administered Scales

OCD is a heterogeneous condition that can present differently across patients, which can complicate an accurate diagnosis. Consequently, struc-tured and semi-structured interviews have the benefit of decreased vari-ability among clinician interviewers and tend to be more reliable (Mueller & Segal, 2015). Common diagnostic interviews that have been validated in youth include: the Mini International Neuropsychiatric Interview for Children and Adolescents (MINI-KID) (Sheehan et al., 2010); the Sched-ule for Affective Disorders and Schizophrenia for School-Aged Children (K-SADS-PL) (Kaufman et al., 1997); the Anxiety Disorder Interview Schedule – Child and Parent Report (ADIS-C/P), (Silverman & Albano, 1996); and the Diagnostic Interview for DSM-5 Anxiety, Mood, and Obsessive-Compulsive and Related Disorders (DIAMOND) (Tolin et al., 2018b). While helpful to administer to differentiate specific psychiatric con-ditions, it is also important to note that the administration of these scales is often time intensive.

The gold-standard and most common clinician-administered rat-ing scale is the Children's Yale-Brown Obsessive-Compulsive Scale (CY-BOCS) (Scahill et al., 1997). The CY-BOCS consists of two main components, a symptom checklist and a 10-item severity scale. The symp-tom checklist inquires about common obsessions and compulsions that are experienced by youth with OCD. Parent and child responses on the symptom checklist are used to inform the severity scale rating over a period of the past week. The severity scale consists of five questions that focus on obsessions and compulsions (e.g., time, resistance, control, dis-tress, and interference), with each question rated on a five-point Likert scale (range: 0–4). The five obsession items are summed to produce a total obsession severity score (range: 0–20), and the five compulsion items are summed to produce a total compulsion severity score (range: 0–20), with the obsession and compulsion severity scores summed to produce a total OCD severity score (range: 0–40). In general, symptom ratings have shown that mild severity (or less) corresponds to a score of 0–13, moderate severity to a score of 14–24, moderate–severe severity to a score of 25–30, and severe scores 30 and higher (Lewin et al., 2014). The CY-BOCS total score has excellent internal consistency, good test-retest reliability, and excellent inter-rater reliability (Scahill et al., 1997; Storch et al., 2004a; Yucelen et al., 2006). In regard to validity, the CY-BOCS has been shown to have both convergent validity with other measures of OCD severity and adequate discriminant validity from related constructs such as anxiety, depression, and externalizing symptoms (Scahill et al., 1997; Storch et al., 2004a). Finally, in regard to treatment sensitivity, the CY-BOCS has been shown to demonstrate treatment sensitivity across clinical trials (Piacentini et al., 2011; Skarphedinsson et al., 2017; Storch et al., 2010a; Storch et al., 2016).

Given advances in the phenomenology of pediatric OCD, the CY-BOCS scale was updated to create the Children's Yale-Brown Obsessive-Compulsive Scale – II (CY-BOCS-II) (Storch et al., 2019; Storch et al., 2010b). The modifications include: (1) the incorporation of avoidance in severity ratings; (2) increase in severity scale range to increase sensitivity; (3) removal of the resistance to obsession item; and (4) expansion and refinement of the symptom checklist to increase the utility and precision of administration (McGuire et al., 2012b; Storch et al., 2019; Storch et al., 2010b). The CY-BOCS-II continues to demonstrate good psychometric properties of reliability and validity (Storch et al., 2019).

Self-Reported and/or Parent-Report Measures of Obsessive-Compulsive Disorder Severity

There are several self-report and/or parent-report measures of OCD severity. The Children's Yale-Brown Obsessive-Compulsive Scale Child-Report and/or Parent-Report (CY-BOCS-CR/CY-BOCS-PR) is a child-and/or parent-reported version of the CY-BOCS. The child and/or parent complete ten items to assess the severity of obsessions and compulsions. Psychometric evaluations have found that the CY-BOCS-CR and CY-BOCS-PR have good internal consistency and good validity (Storch et al., 2006a). The Obsessive-Compulsive Inventory – Child Version (OCI-CV) is a 21-item child-report scale that assesses the frequency of common obsessive-compulsive symptoms (Foa et al., 2010; Jones et al., 2013). There are six subscales that include checking, obsessions, hoarding, washing, ordering, and neutralizing. Items are summed across scales to produce a total score. The OCI-CV has good reliability (i.e., internal consistency, test-retest reliability) and validity (i.e., convergent and divergent validity) (Aspvall et al., 2020; Foa et al., 2010; Jones et al., 2013; Martínez-González et al., 2015). The OCI-CV has shown treatment sensitivity as well (McGuire et al., 2019). Despite its good psychometric properties in smaller samples, the OCI-CV was revised, based on improved phenomenological understanding of the scale in larger samples (Abramovitch et al., 2022a). The Obsessive-Compulsive Inventory – Child Version – Revised (OCI-CV-R) removed the hoarding subscale, which resulted in an 18-item scale (Abramovitch et al., 2022a). Psychometric examinations have shown the revised measure to have improved reliability and validity (Abramovitch et al., 2022a) and identified five items that have shown promise as a screening measure (i.e., the Obsessive-Compulsive Inventory – Child Version – Five [OCI-CV-5]) (Abramovitch et al., 2022b).

The Children's Florida Obsessive-Compulsive Inventory (C-FOCI) is a child-report measure that includes a brief 20-item symptom checklist of common obsessions and compulsions (Storch et al., 2009). These symptoms are rated on a five-item severity scale that parallels the CY-BOCS severity scale. Psychometric evaluations have shown the C-FOCI to have fair reliability (i.e., internal consistency and test-retest reliability) and good validity (i.e., convergent and divergent validity) (Piqueras et al., 2017; Storch et al., 2009). The C-FOCI has shown treatment sensitivity as well (Piqueras et al., 2017). The Children's Obsessive-Compulsive Inventory-Revised (ChOCI-R) is a 32-item scale with two subscales of 16 items each, assessing the presence and severity of obsessions and compulsions in youth (Uher et al., 2008). There are both child- and parent-report versions of the ChOCI-R. Psychometric evaluations have found the ChOCI-R to have good reliability (i.e., internal consistency) and good validity (i.e., convergent and divergent validity) (Uher et al., 2008). Lastly, the Obsessive-Compulsive Subscale of the Child Behavior Checklist (CBCL-OCS) is a parent-rated screening tool that consists of eight questions on the CBCL (Storch et al., 2006b). Overall, the psychometric properties of the CBCL-OCS have been generally favorable with good sensitivity and specificity for an OCD diagnosis (Hudziak et al., 2006) and generally good reliability and validity (Geller et al., 2006; Storch et al., 2006b).

There are other OCD rating scales used in youth that have relatively limited evaluation and/or limited demonstration of adequate psychometric properties. These include the Leyton Obsessional Inventory – Child Version Survey Form (LOI-CV Survey Form) and the Short Leyton Obsessional Inventory – Child Version Survey Form (Short LOI-CV Survey Form) (Storch et al., 2011c). Additionally, the Short OCD Screener (SOCS) is a seven-item self-report screening tool that has an excellent sensitivity to detect OCD in youth, but lacks specificity in a psychiatric sample, limiting its utility outside of general pediatrician's offices (Uher et al., 2008).

Important Related Constructs in Obsessive-Compulsive Disorder: Impairment, Accommodation, and Insight

Impairment

As OCD can cause impairment in across-life domains (e.g., academic, social, family), it is important to characterize youth's level of impairment. A more generalized report of impairment is the Child Sheehan Disability Scale – Parent Report and Child Report (CSDS-P/C). The CSDS-PC is based on the adult version, but modified to assess parent and child responses to disability across school, home, and social life (Soler et al., 2021; Whiteside, 2009). More specific to OCD, the Child Obsessive-Compulsive Impact Scale – Revised (COIS-R) are parent- and child-report scales that assess impairments in school, home, and social functioning due to OCD symptoms (Piacentini et al., 2007; Skarphedinsson et al., 2015). Studies show that the COIS-R has good psychometric properties of reliability, validity, and treatment sensitivity (Garcia et al., 2010; Lewin et al., 2011; Piacentini et al., 2007, 2011; Skarphedinsson et al., 2015).

Family Accommodation

Given the importance of familial involvement in both OCD symptoms and its treatment (Wu et al., 2016), it is important to assess family accommodation among youth with OCD. Several measures exist to assess family accommodation; they include clinician-rated scales such as the Family Accommodation Scale – Interview Report (FAS-IR) (Calvocoressi et al., 1995), as well as parent-reported scales of family accommodation such as the Family Accommodation Scale for OCD (Flessner et al., 2011; Lebowitz, Scharfstein, & Jones, 2014). Across these scales, parents are asked to reflect upon ways in which they might accommodate their child's OCD symptoms in daily life.

Insight

Insight is an important prognostic factor for the treatment of OCD (Selles et al., 2018). The CY-BOCS and CY-BOCS-II each have one item assessing insight, but this single item may not encompass the construct in totality. Clinicians may also consider utilizing the Brown Assessment of Beliefs Scale (BABS), a semi-structured interview assessing insight performed by the clinician (Eisen et al., 1998).

Tourette's Disorder and Other Tic Disorders

Tourette's disorder and other persistent tic disorders (collectively TS) that is characterized by the presence of tics that onset in childhood, cause impairment (Hanks et al., 2016; McGuire et al., 2013a; Storch et al., 2007a), and can diminish quality of life (Storch et al., 2007a; Storch et al., 2007b)). Tics often present alongside other repetitive behaviors (e.g., hyperactivity/impulsivity, obsessive-compulsive symptoms, stereotypies), which have different evidence-based pharmacological and behavioral treatments (Essoe et al., 2019). Thus, an accurate and timeline diagnosis is essential. Fortunately, there are several clinician-rated scales, parent-report scales, and child-report scales that can be used to identify TS symptoms, characterize symptom severity, and monitor response to therapeutic interventions (McGuire et al., 2012a; Szejko et al., 2022).

Clinician-Reported Measures

TS is a heterogeneous condition in which tic symptoms can present differently across patients. The most commonly used and gold-standard clinician-administered assessment is the Yale Global Tic Severity Scale (YGTSS) (Leckman et al., 1989). The YGTSS consists of three main components: a symptom checklist, a severity scale, and an impairment scale. The symptom checklist inquires about the presence of the most common motor and vocal tics in the past week. These tics are used to inform the ratings on the severity scale, which assesses the number, frequency, intensity, complexity, and interference of tics. Scores across the five domains are summed to produce a total motor tic score (range: 0–25), total phonic tic score (range: 0–25), and a total tic score (range: 0–50). The impairment scale helps clinicians assess overall impairment due to tics across life domains (range: 0–50). The YGTSS has demonstrated excellent reliability (i.e., internal consistency, inter-rater reliability) and validity (Leckman et al., 1989; Storch et al., 2005). The YGTSS total tic score has shown treatment sensitivity, with a 25–35 percent reduction corresponding with a clinically meaningful response to treatment (Jeon et al., 2013; Storch et al., 2011a).

Given advances in the phenomenology of TS, the YGTSS was revised to create the Yale Global Tic Severity Scale – Revised Version (YGTSS-R) (McGuire et al., 2018). The conceptual framework of the YGTSS-R has remained the same as the original version (i.e., symptom checklist, severity scale, and impairment scale). However, based on a multi-site psychometric evaluation and a modified-Delphi process, several minor modifications were proposed to optimize scale administration and promote full use of ratings on severity scale dimensions (McGuire et al., 2018).

These revisions included: (1) increasing the number of examples of simple phonic tics on the symptom checklist; and (2) refinement of anchor-point descriptions for three domains on the severity scale – tic frequency, tic complexity, and tic interference. These minor revisions were not considered to influence the reliability, validity, and/or treatment sensitivity of the instrument (McGuire et al., 2018)

The Hopkins Motor and Vocal Tic Scale (HM/VTS) is a clinician-administered measure that assesses the most bothersome motor and vocal tics, which is personalized to the individual with TS. For each bothersome tic, a clinician inquires about the frequency, forcefulness, interference, and subjective distress in the past week. This information is used to guide clinician ratings on a five-point scale (range 0–4). The HM/VTS produces a total bothersome motor tic score and a total bothersome vocal tic score, which can be summed to produce a total bothersome tic score. The HM/VTS has shown good reliability (i.e., inter-rater reliability) and validity (Walkup et al., 1992). It has also shown to be sensitivity to treatment (Bergin et al., 1998; McGuire et al., 2015; McGuire et al., 2020a).

Two other clinician-rated scales are also available to assess tic severity, but they are less commonly used for several reasons (e.g., do not separately assess motor and vocal tics, measurement times are uncertain, assess co-occurring conditions such as OCD and attention deficit hyperactivity disorder (ADHD) alongside TS). These included the Shapiro Tourette Syndrome Severity Scale (STSS) (Shapiro & Shapiro, 1984) and the Tourette Disorder Scale – Clinician Report (TODS-CR) (Shytle et al., 2003).

Parent and Self-Reported Measures

While the YGTSS/YGTSS-R are the most common clinician-administered measure, there has been less consensus about the parent- and/or self-reported scales. The Parent Tic Questionnaire (PTQ) (Chang et al., 2009) and Adult Tic Questionnaire (ATQ) (Abramovitch et al., 2015) are parallel parent- and self-report scales that assess tic severity. These scales consist of a checklist of 14 common motor tics and 14 common vocal tics, which are rated as being absent or present over the past week. Tics that have presented in the past week are rated according to frequency (range: 0–4) and intensity (range: 0–4). Items are summed to produce a total motor tic severity score, total vocal tic severity score, and a total tic severity score. The total tic severity score has shown good reliability (i.e., internal consistency, test-retest reliability) and validity (i.e., convergent and divergent validity) (Abramovitch et al., 2015; Chang et al., 2009; Ricketts et al., 2018). The PTQ and ATQ have shown treatment sensitivity (Piacentini et al., 2010; Ricketts et al., 2018; Wilhelm et al., 2012).

Aside from the PTQ and ATQ, several other self-report and/or parent-report measures of tic symptoms exist. These include the Tourette Syndrome Symptom List (TSSL) and the Tic Symptom Self Report (TSSR). The TSSL asks respondents to rate the frequency of 35 different tics or related behaviors over the past week on a 0–5 scale, with items summed to produce a total score (Cohen et al., 1980; Cohen, Leckman, & Shaywitz, 1985). While the TSSL has demonstrated treatment sensitivity (Cohen et al., 1980), aspects of its reliability (i.e., internal consistency, test-retest reliability) and validity (i.e., convergent and discriminant validity) have not been examined. The TSSL was later revised to create the Tic Symptom Self Report, a parent- and/or self-report measure that inquires about the frequency of 20 common motor tics and 20 common vocal tics over the past week (Scahill et al., 2003). Similar to the TSSL, the TSSR has shown treatment sensitivity (Allen et al., 2005; Scahill et al., 2003), but aspects of its reliability (i.e., internal consistency, test-retest reliability) and validity (i.e., convergent and discriminant validity) have yet to be examined.

Whilst previously mentioned rating scales have exclusively focused on rating tic symptoms, some parent- and/or self-report rating scales also include tics alongside common co-occurring conditions. The Tourette Disorder Scale – Parent Report (TODS-PR) is a parent-report version that includes 15 items that assess the overall severity and impairment of tics and common comorbid symptoms (e.g., hyperactivity, aggression, OCD) (Shytle et al., 2003). The TODS-PR has a total severity score (i.e., the summation of all 15 items) and a two-item tic subscale (Shytle et al., 2003). The TODS-PR has shown excellent internal consistency for its total score, but low specificity for its tic subscale score (Shytle et al., 2003; Storch et al., 2004b; Storch et al., 2007a) and no examination of test-retest reliability. The TODS-PR tic subscale has demonstrated good convergent and discriminant validity (Shytle et al., 2003; Storch et al., 2007a). The Motor Tic, Obsessions and Compulsions, Vocal Tic Evaluation Survey (MOVES) is a parent- and/or self-report measure that consists of 20 items that assess the frequency of motor and phonic tics, alongside other common co-occurring symptoms such as compulsions (Gaffney Sieg, & Hellings, 1994). Items are summed to produce a total score as well as a tic subscale score. The tic subscale has shown low test-retest reliability (Gaffney, Sieg, & Hellings, 1994), but has shown convergent validity (Harcherik et al., 1984) and treatment sensitivity (Gaffney, Sieg, & Hellings, 1994).

Important Related Constructs in Tic Disorders: Premonitory Urges, Impairment, and Accommodation

Premonitory Urges

Premonitory urges are aversive somatosensory phenomena that are proceed tic symptoms (Leckman, Walker, & Cohen, 1993). There are at least two scales to assess premonitory urges. The Premonitory Urge for Tic Scale (PUTS) is nine-item self-report scale that assesses the presence and severity of premonitory urges (Woods et al., 2005). Items are summed to produce a total premonitory urge severity score. The PUTS total score has shown good psychometric properties and treatment sensitivity (Houghton et al., 2017; Reese et al., 2014; Woods et al., 2005). The Individualized Premonitory Urge to Tic Scale (I-PUTS) is a clinician-administered measure that assesses the presence, frequency, and intensity of each tic identified on the YGTSS. Similar to the PUTS, the I-PUTS has also shown good psychometric properties (i.e., reliability and validity) (McGuire et al., 2016)

Tic-Related Impairment

Whilst the YGTSS has a clinician-rated impairment scale, there are also other measures to assess tic-related impairment across life domains. This includes the Child Tourette Syndrome Impairment Scale (CTIM), which is a 37-item parent-report scale that assesses impairment related to tic and non-tic symptoms (e.g., anxiety, OCD symptoms, oppositional behaviors) across home, school, and social activities (Storch et al., 2007a). Items are summed to create separate scores for tic-related impairment and non-tic-related impairment. The CTIM has shown good psychometric properties (Storch et al., 2007a), and abbreviated versions of the scale have also shown good psychometric properties (Barfell et al., 2017; Cloes et al., 2017; Garris et al., 2021).

Accommodation and Reaction

In order to evaluate accommodations and reactions in response to tic symptoms, there are at least two options. The Tic Family Accommodation Scale (T-FAS) is a 13-item scale based on the Family Accommodation Scale for OCD, which assesses family accommodations related to tic and tic-related impairment (Storch et al., 2017). Similarly, the Tic Accommodation and Reaction Scale (TARS) is a 35-item scale that assesses common reactions, accommodations, and responses from tics (Capriotti et al., 2015). These two scales have shown good initial psychometric properties (Capriotti et al., 2015; Storch et al., 2017).

Trichotillomania (Hair-Pulling Disorder)

Trichotillomania (TTM) (sometimes called hair-pulling disorder, HPD) is characterized by repetitive hair pulling that results in hair loss. Symptoms typically onset in childhood or adolescence and affect around 5 percent of the population. Hair-pulling behaviors can be automatic (i.e., outside of one's awareness) and/or focused pulling (i.e., within one's awareness) in nature. Hair pulling is associated with significant impairment and a poor quality of life. Given that TTM commonly presents alongside other co-occurring conditions (e.g., anxiety, depression, OCD), an accurate and precise assessment is important to characterize the severity of symptoms and monitor response to therapeutic interventions.

Clinician Reported Measures

Several clinician-administered assessments of TTM exist to characterize the severity of hair-pulling behaviors. These include the Psychiatric Institute Trichotillomania Scale (PITS), the Yale-Brown Obsessive Compulsive Scale – Trichotillomania (Y-BOCS-TM), and the National Institute of Mental Health's Trichotillomania Severity Scale and Impairment Scale (NIMH-TSS/TIS). The Psychiatric Institute Trichotillomania Scale is a six-item clinician-rated scale that assesses the number of body sites affected by hair pulling, severity of hair loss, duration of hair pulling, resistance, negative affect associated with hair pulling, and interference with daily functioning (Winchel et al., 1992). The six items are summed to create a PITS total score. The PITS has demonstrated reliability (i.e., inter-rater reliability), validity (i.e., convergent validity), and treatment sensitivity (Diefenbach et al., 2005; Grant, Odlaug, & Kim., 2009; Stanley et al., 1997; Stanley et al., 1999; Winchel et al., 1992). However, aspects of its reliability (i.e., internal consistency, test-retest reliability) and validity remain unexamined.

Similar to the PITS, the National Institute of Mental Health's (NIMH) Trichotillomania Severity Scale (TSS) is a six-item clinician-rated scale that assesses time spent hair pulling, distress related to hair pulling, resistance to hair pulling, and related interference in a person's daily life (Swedo et al., 1989). Items are summed to produce a total TTM severity score. The NIMH-TSS has shown reliability (i.e., test-retest reliability) and treatment sensitivity (Franklin et al., 2011; Swedo et al., 1989). Alongside the NIMH-TSS, the National Institute of Mental Health's Trichotillomania Impairment Scale (NIMH-TIS) consists of a single clinician-rated item that captures the impairment attributed to TTM on an individual's life. Scores range from no impairment (0), minimal impairment (1–3), mild impairment (4–6), or moderate to greater impairment (7–10) (Swedo et al., 1989). Each level of impairment is associated with a behavioral description of pulling rate, control over pulling, worry about pulling, and impairment related to pulling. The NIMH-TIS has shown inter-rater reliability in adults (Stanley et al., 1999) and convergent validity (Diefenbach et al., 2005), but there is little examination of its psychometric properties in youth.

The Yale-Brown Obsessive Compulsive-Scale – Trichotillomania evaluates thoughts and behaviors associated with TTM. It is comprised of 10 items that produce subscales related to thoughts/urges associated with hair pulling, and a subscale relating to hair-pulling behaviors, with the two summed to produce a total severity score (Stanley et al., 1993; Stanley et al., 1999). In adults, the Y-BOCS-TM total severity score has shown adequate reliability (i.e., inter-rater reliability, test-retest reliability), validity (i.e., convergent validity), and treatment sensitivity (Grant et al., 2009; Stanley et al., 1993; Stanley et al., 1997; Van Ameringen et al., 2010).

Parent- and Self-Reported Measures

There are at least two child- and/or parent-report measures of TTM severity. The Massachusetts General Hospital – Hair Pulling Scale (MGH-HPS) is one of the most widely used self-report measures of TTM severity. On this scale, individuals rate 7 items about urges to hair pull, actual hair pulling, perceived control over hair pulling, and distress associated with hair pulling over the past week (Keuthen et al., 1995; O'Sullivan et al., 1995). These items are rated on a 0 to 5 scale, and summed to produce a total score. The MGH-HPS has demonstrated good reliability (i.e., internal consistency, test-retest reliability), validity (i.e., convergent and discriminant validity), and sensitivity to treatment (Diefenbach et al., 2005; Farhat et al., 2019; Keuthen et al., 1995; Rahman et al., 2017; van Minnen et al., 2003).

The Trichotillomania Scale for Children (TSC) is comprised of parallel child (TSC-C) and parent (TSC-P) versions. On the TSC, parents and children complete 12 items assessing the severity, distress, and impairment of TTM symptoms over the past week (Tolin et al., 2008a). Whilst five items are summed to produce a hair-pulling severity subscale score, the remaining seven items are summed to produce a distress/impairment subscale score, with all 12 items summed for a total severity score (Tolin et al., 2008a). The TSC-C and TSC-P have shown good reliability (i.e., internal consistency, test-retest reliability), validity (i.e., convergent and discriminant validity), and treatment sensitivity (Farhat et al., 2019; Tolin et al., 2008a).

Important Related Constructs in Trichotillomania: Subtype of Hair-Pulling Behavior

In addition to the severity of hair pulling behaviors, it can also be important to assess the subtype of hair pulling behaviors that are present as different subtypes may be more or less responsive to evidence-based interventions (McGuire et al., 2014; McGuire et al., 2020b). The Milwaukee

Inventory for Styles of Trichotillomania for Children (MIST-C) is a self-report rating scale consisting of 25 items that inquire about whether automatic (i.e., hair pulling without conscious awareness) or focused (i.e., hair pulling with conscious awareness) is present (Flessner et al., 2007). The MIST-C and its two subscale scores (automatic pulling behaviors, focused pulling behaviors) have demonstrated good reliability (i.e., internal consistency) and validity (i.e., convergent and discriminant validity) (Flessner et al., 2007). Whilst its treatment sensitivity was found in one trial of behavior therapy (McGuire et al., 2020b), its test-retest reliability has not been examined.

Excoriation Disorder (Skin-Picking Disorder)

Excoriation disorder (also known as skin-picking disorder (SPD) or dermatillomania) is characterized by the repetitive act of picking at one's skin. Despite efforts to disengage from the behavior, skin picking results in damage to the skin (e.g., skin lesions), causes significant distress, and contributes to impairment across life domains. Prevalence estimates suggest that excoriation behaviors are relatively common among youth, but not all behaviors may reach clinical levels of impairment (Selles et al., 2015). The most common sites for picking include the face, hands, and arms, and other areas are less common, perhaps because of reduced access due to clothing (Tucker et al., 2011). Similar to TTM, skin-picking behaviors may be more automatic or focused in nature. Given that excoriation behaviors often present alongside many other body-focused repetitive behaviors (BFRBs) (Ricketts et al., 2022), an accurate assessment is essential to characterize severity and monitor response to therapeutic interventions (Selles et al., 2016). There are relatively few psychometrically validated measures to characterize skin-picking behaviors, and even fewer that have been examined specifically among youth.

Clinician-Report Measures

Given that skin picking behaviors may be caused secondarily by other medical and/or psychiatric conditions, several clinician-administered scales exist to help arrive at an accurate diagnosis. These include structured diagnostic interviews previously mentioned (e.g., MINI-KID, ADIS-C/P, K-SADS-PL, and DIAMOND), but also include a skin-picking specific diagnostic supplement called the Keuthen Diagnostic Inventory for Skin Picking (K-DISP) (Keuthen, n.d.). The K-DISP is a clinician-rated measure can be used to help determine whether criteria are met for the diagnosis of excoriation disorder based on the DSM-5 criteria. Although this brief interview is helpful for determining whether an excoriation diagnosis is present, it does not provide information about the severity of the condition.

The only available clinician-administered measure is the Yale-Brown Obsessive Compulsive Scale Modified for Neurotic Excoriation (YBOCS-NE). This 10-item clinician-administered scale assesses the severity of skin-picking behaviors over the past week. Similar to other adaptations of the Y-BOCS, items are rated on a five-point scale (range: 0–4) and summed to produce a total severity score. The Y-BOCS-NE has been shown to have good reliability (i.e., test-retest reliability) and treatment sensitivity (M.R. Bloch et al., 2001; Grant et al., 2010). However, many other psychometric aspects of the measure remain unexamined.

Self-Report and/or Parent-Report Measures

Several brief self-report metrics exist to quantify the severity of skin-picking behaviors, but few have received full psychometric validation in children and adolescents. Across studies, the Skin Picking Scale (SPS) and the Skin Picking Scale – Revised (SPS-R) are the two most common scales. The SPS and SPS-R are six-item self-report scales in which respondents rate the frequency and intensity of picking urges, time spent picking, interference of other activities secondary to picking, and associated distress and avoidance (Keuthen et al., 2001b). Items are rated on a five-point scale (range: 0–4) and summed to produce a total score. The questions are rated from 0 to 4 and are summed to give a total score. The measure has shown good reliability and validity in adults and adolescents (Gallinat et al., 2017; Keuthen et al., 2001b). The Skin Picking Impact Scale (SPIS) is regularly administered alongside the SPS and the SPS-R. The SPIS is a 10-item self-report questionnaire that assesses the influence of picking on the individual over the past week (Keuthen et al., 2001a). Items are rated on a six-point scale (range: 0–5) and summed to produce a total impact score. The SPIS has shown excellent reliability (i.e., internal consistency) and good convergent validity (Keuthen et al., 2001a). However, the strong correlations with depression and anxiety suggest some overlap with these constructs, and indicate relatively modest divergent validity (Keuthen et al., 2001a).

Important Related Constructs in Excoriation: Subtype of Picking Behavior

Unfortunately, there is no specific scale for youth to assess the subtypes of picking behavior. The closest available measure is the Milwaukee Inventory for the Dimensions of Adult Skin Picking (MIDAS) (Walther et al., 2009). The MIDAS is a 12-item self-report scale, with six items assessing automatic picking behavior and six items assessing focused picking behavior. Items are rated on a six-point scale (range: 0–5) and summed to produce a total score for each subscale (Walther et al., 2009). In adults, the MIDAS has shown good reliability (i.e., internal consistency) and validity (i.e., discriminant validity) (Walther et al., 2009).

Another approach to subtyping picking behaviors focuses on differences in "wanting" and "liking" these behaviors. The Skin Picking Reward Scale (SPRS) is a 12-item self-report measure that is comprised of six items focused on "wanting" to skin pick and six items focused on "liking" to skin pick (Snorrason et al., 2015). Items are rated on a five-point Likert scale and summed to produce two separate subscale scores. Psychometric evaluations have yielded adequate results for internal consistency and test-retest reliability for the SPRS (Snorrason et al., 2015).

Hoarding Disorder

Hoarding disorder (HD) is characterized by difficulty with disposing of one's possessions, while often excessively acquiring other items, leading to an extreme accumulation of belongings. Hoarding behavior is different from collecting – which can have similar behaviors – especially among children who have specific interests. While there is often a strong emotional attachment to hoarded items, these items may have very little practical value (e.g., mail, newspapers, clothing). Whilst symptoms are reported to begin earlier in life, when left untreated symptoms often worsen over time – with older adults facing financial difficulty and experiencing a reduced quality of life (McGuire et al., 2013b; Ong et al., 2015). Hoarding behaviors in children can be limited by caregiver interventions or exacerbated by caregiver accommodations. As such, the accurate assessment of hoarding behaviors in children can sometimes prove challenging – particularly as it can manifest alongside other common psychiatric conditions such as anxiety, depression, ADHD, trauma, and autism spectrum disorder (ASD) – as well as may also manifest within OCD. As we outline evidence-based approaches to assess OCD symptoms above, here we will specifically focus on assessment measures of hoarding behaviors.

Clinician-Reported Measures

Given that hoarding behaviors often present alongside other psychiatric conditions, several clinician-administered interviews exist to help guide accurate diagnoses. These include previously mentioned diagnostic interviews (e.g., MINI-KID, ADIS-C/P, K-SADS-PL, and DIAMOND). In addition to these general interviews, the Structured Interview for Hoarding Disorder (SIHD) is a semi-structured interview that inquires about the presence of DSM-5 diagnostic criteria (Nordsletten et al., 2013). Initial evidence suggests that this brief interview has good reliability and validity for identifying hoarding disorder (Nordsletten et al., 2013).

The most commonly used clinician rating scale to assess the severity of hoarding behaviors is the Hoarding Rating Scale – Interview (HRS-I) (Tolin, Frost, & Steketee, 2010). The HRS-I consists of five questions assessing clinical features of hoarding. These items inquire about the severity of clutter, difficulty discarding, excessive acquisition, distress, and interference. The HRS-I demonstrates good psychometric properties of reliability and validity (Tolin et al., 2018a).

Self-Reported and/or Parent-Report Measures

Given that hoarding behaviors can be influenced by parental responses (e.g., parental discarding of hoarded items), reliance on hoarding disorder scales for adults would not yield accurate information regarding the presence and/or severity of the condition. To date, the only validated measure of hoarding behavior in children is the Child Saving Inventory (CSI) (Storch et al., 2011b). The CSI is based on the Saving Inventory – Revised (SI-R), which is a validated adult measure of hoarding tendencies (Frost, Steketee, & Grisham, 2004). The CSI measure relies on parent ratings of their children's hoarding behaviors over the past week. The items on the CSI are summed to produce a total severity score of hoarding behaviors (Soreni et al., 2018; Storch et al., 2011b). The CSI has shown good reliability (i.e., internal consistency, test-retest reliability), validity, and treatment sensitivity (Hacker et al., 2016; Ong et al., 2021; Soreni et al., 2018; Storch et al., 2011b; Storch et al., 2016a).

Several self-report measures of hoarding behaviors exist, including the Saving Inventory – Revised, the Hoarding Rating Scale-Self Report, UCLA (University of California) Hoarding Severity Scale, and Hoarding Assessment Scale (Frost, Steketee, & Grisham, 2004; Saxena et al., 2015; A. F. Schneider et al., 2008; Tolin et al., 2008b). However, these scales have not been psychometrically evaluated in children and/or adolescents at this time.

Body Dysmorphic Disorder

Body dysmorphic disorder (BDD) is a condition characterized by an individual's persistent preoccupation with an imagined or slight flaw in physical appearance. Individuals with BDD are typically concerned with perceived defects related to body areas (e.g., bumps on skin are visible, nose is too large, stomach is not "flat enough"). Given the distressing nature of these preoccupations, individuals with BDD feel compelled to perform repetitive behaviors (e.g., mirror checking, skin picking, covering up perceived flaws) and/or mental acts (e.g., self-comparison) to alleviate distress and dissatisfaction elicited by these concerns. Individuals with BDD may also engage in avoidance behaviors to minimize contact with anything that might trigger cognitive preoccupations (e.g., remove all mirrors around the house). While some preoccupation with physical appearance can be developmentally normative in adolescence, BDD is distinctive in that it leads individuals to experience marked distress and impairment in daily life.

Prevalence estimates suggest that about 2 percent of the general population meet the criteria for BDD, with symptoms first emerging during adolescence (Bjornsson et al., 2013; Phillips et al., 2005). Given the developmentally normative preoccupations with physical appearance in adolescence, an accurate assessment is essential to appropriately differentiate BDD symptoms from normative behaviors and monitor responses to therapeutic interventions.

Clinician-Reported Measures

The gold-standard assessment is the Yale Brown Obsessive Compulsive Scale Modified for Body Dysmorphic Disorder (BDD-YBOCS) (Phillips et al., 1997a). The BDD-YBOCS is a clinician-administered scale that assesses the severity of BDD symptoms during the past week. In this semi-structured interview, clinicians inquire about common BDD-related symptoms that the individual currently experiences. Afterward, clinicians rate the severity of BDD preoccupations and compulsive behaviors according to the duration, interference, distress, resistance, and control over symptoms experienced by the individual in the past week. The BDD-YBOCS also has two separate ratings to assess the individual's insight and avoidance related to BDD. These 12 items are summed to produce a total severity score. The BDD-YBOCS has demonstrated good reliability (i.e., internal consistency, test-retest reliability, inter-rater reliability) and validity (i.e., convergent and discriminant validity) (Phillips et al., 1997b). Meanwhile, the Yale-Brown Obsessive Compulsive Scale Modified for BDD-Adolescent Version (BDD-YBOCS-A) is nearly identical to the BDD-YBOCS, but uses more developmentally appropriate wording and prompts (Monzani et al., 2022). Initial examinations of the BDD-YBOCS-A have found it to have good reliability (i.e., internal consistency), validity (i.e., convergent and divergent validity), and treatment sensitivity (Monzani et al., 2022; Rautio et al., 2022).

In addition to the BDD-YBOCS, there are at least two other clinician-rated scale to assess the severity of BDD. The Body Dysmorphic

Disorder Examination (BDDE) is also a semi-structured clinical interview that assesses preoccupation with negative appearance, negative evaluation of appearance, self-consciousness, excessive importance attributed to appearance in self-evaluation, avoidance of activities, body camouflaging, and body checking (Rosen & Reiter, 1996). The BDDE has shown reliability (i.e., internal consistency, inter-rater reliability, test-retest reliability), validity (i.e., convergent and discriminant validity), and treatment sensitivity (Rosen & Reiter, 1996). Despite its promising characteristics, the BDDE was initially designed to measure dysmorphic concerns among individuals with eating disorders, and it does not assess compulsive behaviors often observed in BDD. The Psychiatric Status Rating Scale for Body Dysmorphic Disorder (BDD-PSR) is a clinician-rated seven-item measure of BDD symptom severity (Phillips et al., 2006). The BDD-PSR has demonstrated good reliability (i.e., inter-rater and test-retest reliability) and validity (i.e., convergent validity) (Phillips et al., 2006).

Parent-Report and Self-Reported Measures

There are few measures specifically designed to assess BDD in children and adolescents. The adolescent version of the Body Dysmorphic Questionnaire – Adolescents (BDDQ-A) is an adaptation of the BDDQ for adults. It consists of four self-report items that ask yes/no questions regarding concerns about physical appearance and the impact any concerns have on functioning, with follow-up open-ended free-text questions for certain responses. It has been used to screen adolescents for BDD in both psychiatric (Grant, Kim, & Crow, 2001) and community settings (S.C. Schneider et al., 2017). Although its psychometric properties in adolescents remain largely undetermined, the BDDQ has shown good concurrent validity with clinical assessment in an adult female community sample (Brohede et al., 2013) and in adults and adolescents presenting for psychiatric inpatient admission (Grant, Kim, & Crow, 2001).

Two other scales specific to youth include the Multidimensional Youth Body Dysmorphic Inventory (MY BODI) and the Body Dysmorphic Disorder Scale for Youth (BDDSY). The MY BODI is a 21-item self-report measure of BDD symptom severity across three factors: impairment/avoidance, preoccupation/repetitive behaviors, and insight/distress (Roberts, Zimmer-Gembeck, & Farrell, 2019). It is designed to reduce socially desirable responding and has good reliability (i.e., internal consistency) and validity (i.e., convergent and divergent validity) (Roberts, Zimmer-Gembeck, & Farrell, 2019). The BDDSY consists of a five-item brief screening tool alongside a 15-item severity scale to assess common BDD cognitions and behaviors. BDDSY has demonstrated good reliability (i.e., internal consistency) and validity (i.e., concurrent, convergent, and divergent validity) (Hanley, Bhullar, & Wootton, 2020).

Although mostly used in adults, the Body Dysmorphic Symptom Scale (BDD-SS) may also be useful for some adolescents. The BDD-SS is a self-report measure that assesses the presence of 54 BDD-related symptoms over the past week, which are categorized into seven groups (e.g., checking rituals, grooming rituals, shape-/weight-related rituals, hair-pulling/skin-picking rituals, surgery-/dermatology-seeking rituals, avoidance, and BDD-related cognitions) (Wilhelm et al., 2016). If an individual endorses the presence of at least one symptom in any one of the seven symptom groups, they are asked to rate the overall severity of symptoms within that group on a 0–10 scale (Wilhelm et al., 2016). In adults, the BDD-SS has demonstrated good reliability and validity (i.e., convergent and discriminant validity) (Wilhelm et al., 2016).

Conclusion

This chapter has reviewed the evidence-based assessment of pediatric OCD and related conditions. Given the lack of biomarkers and/or objective testing to diagnose and assess symptom severity, the utilization of psychometrically validated measures is of utmost importance. While there are existing rating scales to aid clinicians and guide research protocols, many of the existing measures are inferred to be of use in children (rather than having demonstrated psychometric evidence). As a result, future research into scale validation is needed, along with the development of child-specific clinician- and self-report scales.

References

Abramovitch, A., Abramowitz, J.S., McKay, D., Cham, H., Anderson, K.S., Farrell, L., Geller, D.A., Hanna, G.L., Mathieu, S., McGuire, J.F., Rosenberg, D.R., Stewart, S.E., Storch, E.A., & Wilhelm, S. (2022a). The OCI-CV-R: A revision of the Obsessive-Compulsive Inventory – Child Version. *Journal of Anxiety Disorders*, *86*, 102532. https://doi.org/10.1016/j.janxdis.2022.102532.

Abramovitch, A., Abramowitz, J.S., McKay, D., Cham, H., Anderson, K.S., Farrell, L.J., Geller, D.A., Hanna, G.L., Mathieu, S., McGuire, J.F., Rosenberg, D.R., Stewart, S.E., Storch, E.A., & Wilhelm, S. (2022b). An ultra-brief screening scale for pediatric obsessive-compulsive disorder: The OCI-CV-5. *Journal of Affective Disorders*, *312*, 208–216. https://doi.org/10.1016/j.jad.2022.06.009.

Abramovitch, A., Reese, H., Woods, D.W., Peterson, A., Deckersbach, T., Piacentini, J., Scahill, L., & Wilhelm, S. (2015). Psychometric properties of a self-report instrument for the assessment of tic severity in adults with tic disorders. *Behavior Therapy*, *46*(6), 786–796.

Allen, A.J., Kurlan, R.M., Gilbert, D.L., Coffey, B.J., Linder, S.L., Lewis, D.W., Winner, P.K., Dunn, D.W., Dure, L.S., Sallee, F.R., Milton, D.R., Mintz, M.I.,

Ricardi, R.K., Erenberg, G., Layton, L.L., Feldman, P.D., Kelsey, D.K., & Spencer, T.J. (2005). Atomoxetine treatment in children and adolescents with ADHD and comorbid tic disorders. *Neurology*, 65(12), 1941–1949. https://doi. org/10.1212/01.wnl.0000188869.58300.a7.

Aspvall, K., Cervin, M., Andrén, P., Perrin, S., Mataix-Cols, D., & Andersson, E. (2020). Validity and clinical utility of the obsessive compulsive inventory – child version: Further evaluation in clinical samples. *BMC Psychiatry*, 20(1), 42. https://doi.org/10.1186/s12888-020-2450-7.

Barfell, K.S.F., Snyder, R.R., Isaacs-Cloes, K.M., Garris, J.F., Roeckner, A.R., Horn, P.S., Guthrie, M.D., Wu, S.W., & Gilbert, D.L. (2017). Parent and patient perceptions of functional impairment due to Tourette syndrome: Development of a shortened version of the Child Tourette Syndrome Impairment Scale. *Journal of Child Neurology*, 32(8), 725–730. https://doi. org/10.1177/0883073817702782.

Bergin, A., Waranch, H.R., Brown, J., Carson, K., & Singer, H.S. (1998). Relaxation therapy in Tourette syndrome: A pilot study. *Pediatric Neurology*, 18(2), 136–142. https://doi.org/10.1016/S0887-8994(97)00200-2.

Bjornsson, A.S., Didie, E.R., Grant, J.E., Menard, W., Stalker, E., & Phillips, K.A. (2013). Age at onset and clinical correlates in body dysmorphic disorder. *Comprehensive Psychiatry*, 54(7), 893–903. https://doi.org/10.1016/j. comppsych.2013.03.019.

Bloch, M.H., & Storch, E.A. (2015). Assessment and management of treatment-refractory obsessive-compulsive disorder in children. *Journal of the American Academy of Child & Adolescent Psychiatry*, 54(4), 251–262. https://doi. org/10.1016/j.jaac.2015.01.011.

Bloch, M.R., Elliott, M., Thompson, H., & Koran, L.M. (2001). Fluoxetine in pathologic skin-picking: Open-label and double-blind results. *Psychosomatics*, 42(4), 314–319. https://doi.org/10.1176/appi.psy.42.4.314.

Brohede, S., Wingren, G., Wijma, B., & Wijma, K. (2013). Validation of the Body Dysmorphic Disorder Questionnaire in a community sample of Swedish women. *Psychiatry Research*, 210(2), 647–652. https://doi.org/10.1016/j. psychres.2013.07.019.

Calvocoressi, L., Lewis, B., Harris, M., Trufan, S., Goodman, W., McDougle, C., & Price, L. (1995). Family accommodation in obsessive compulsive disorder. *American Journal of Psychiatry*, 152, 441–443.

Capriotti, M.R., Piacentini, J.C., Himle, M.B., Ricketts, E.J., Espil, F.M., Lee, H J., Turkel, J.E., & Woods, D.W. (2015). Assessing environmental consequences of ticcing in youth with chronic tic disorders: The Tic Accommodation and Reactions Scale. *Children's Health Care*, 44(3), 205–220. https://doi.org/10.1080/02 739615.2014.948164.

Chang, S., Himle, M.B., Tucker, B.T., Woods, D.W., & Piacentini, J. (2009). Initial psychometric properties of a brief parent-report instrument for assessing tic severity in children with chronic tic disorders. *Child & Family Behavior Therapy*, 31(3), 181–191.

Cicchetti, D.V. (1994). Guidelines, criteria, and rules of thumb for evaluating normed and standardized assessment instruments in psychology. *Psychological Assessment*, 6(4), 284–290.

Cloes, K.I., Barfell, K.S.F., Horn, P.S., Wu, S.W., Jacobson, S.E., Hart, K.J., & Gilbert, D.L. (2017). Preliminary evaluation of child self-rating using the Child Tourette Syndrome Impairment Scale. *Developmental Medicine & Child Neurology*, 59(3), 284–290.

Cohen, D.J., Detlor, J., Young, J.G., & Shaywitz, B.A. (1980). Clonidine amelio-rates Gilles de la Tourette syndrome. *Archives of General Psychiatry, 37*(12), 1350–1357.

Cohen, D.J., Leckman, J.F., & Shaywitz, B.A. (1985). The Tourette syndrome and other tics. *The Clinical Guide to Child Psychiatry*, 3–28.

Diefenbach, G.J., Tolin, D.F., Crocetto, J., Maltby, N., & Hannan, S. (2005). Assessment of trichotillomania: A psychometric evaluation of hair-pulling scales. *Journal of Psychopathology and Behavioral Assessment, 27*(3), 169–178. https://doi.org/10.1007/s10862-005-0633-7.

Eisen, J.L., Phillips, K.A., Baer, L., Beer, D.A., Atala, K.D., & Rasmussen, S.A. (1998). The Brown Assessment of Beliefs Scale: Reliability and validity. *American Journal of Psychiatry, 155*(1), 102–108. https://doi.org/10.1176/ajp.155.1.102.

Essoe, J.K.-Y., Grados, M.A., Singer, H.S., Myers, N S., & McGuire, J.F. (2019). Evidence-based treatment of Tourette's disorder and chronic tic disorders. *Expert Review of Neurotherapeutics, 19*(11), 1103–1115.

Farhat, L.C., Olfson, E., Levine, J.L., Li, F., Franklin, M.E., Lee, H.-J., Lewin, A.B., McGuire, J.F, Rahman, O., & Storch, E.A. (2019). Measuring treatment response in pediatric trichotillomania: A meta-analysis of clinical trials. *Journal of Child and Adolescent Psychopharmacology.*

Flessner, C.A., Sapyta, J., Garcia, A., Freeman, J.B., Franklin, M.E., Foa, E., & March, J. (2011). Examining the psychometric properties of the Family Accommodation Scale – Parent-Report (FAS-PR). *Journal of Psychopathology and Behavioral Assessment, 33*(1), 38–46. https://doi.org/10.1007/s10862-010-9196-3.

Flessner, C.A., Woods, D.W., Franklin, M.E., Keuthen, N.J., Piacentini, J., Cashin, S.E., & Moore, P.S. (2007). The Milwaukee Inventory for Styles of Trichotillomania – Child Version (MIST-C): Initial development and psychometric properties. *Behavior Modification, 31*(6), 896–918. https://doi.org/10.1177/0145445507302521.

Foa, E.B., Coles, M., Huppert, J.D., Pasupuleti, R.V., Franklin, M.E., & March, J. (2010). Development and validation of a child version of the Obsessive Compulsive Inventory. *Behavior Therapy, 41*(1), 121–132. https://doi.org/10.1016/j.beth.2009.02.001.

Franklin, M.E., Edson, A.L., Ledley, D.A., & Cahill, S.P. (2011). Behavior therapy for pediatric trichotillomania: A randomized controlled trial. *Journal of the American Academy of Child and Adolescent Psychiatry, 50*(8), 763–771. https://doi.org/10.1016/j.jaac.2011.05.009.

Frost, R.O., Steketee, G., & Grisham, J. (2004). Measurement of compulsive hoarding: Saving Inventory – Revised. *Behaviour Research and Therapy, 42*(10), 1163–1182. https://doi.org/10.1016/j.brat.2003.07.006.

Gaffney, G.R., Sieg, K., & Hellings, J. (1994). The MOVES: A self-rating scale for Tourette's syndrome. *Journal of Child and Adolescent Psychopharmacology, 4*(4), 269–280. https://doi.org/10.1089/cap.1994.4.269.

Gallinat, C., Keuthen, N.J., Stefini, A., & Backenstrass, M. (2017). The assessment of skin picking in adolescence: Psychometric properties of the Skin Picking Scale – Revised (German version). *Nordic Journal of Psychiatry, 71*(2), 145–150. https://doi.org/10.1080/08039488.2016.1259427.

Garcia, A.M., Sapyta, J.J., Moore, P.S., Freeman, J.B., Franklin, M.E., March, J.S., & Foa, E.B. (2010). Predictors and moderators of treatment outcome in the Pediatric Obsessive Compulsive Treatment Study (POTS I). *Journal of the American Academy of Child & Adolescent Psychiatry, 49*(10), 1024–1033. https://doi.org/10.1016/j.jaac.2010.06.013.

Garris, J.F., Huddleston, D.A., Jackson, H.S., Horn, P.S., & Gilbert, D.L. (2021). Implementation of the Mini-Child Tourette Syndrome Impairment Scale: Relationships to symptom severity and treatment decisions. *Journal of Child Neurology*, 36(4), 288–295. https://doi.org/10.1177/0883073820967518.

Geller, D.A., Doyle, R., Shaw, D., Mullin, B., Coffey, B., Petty, C., Vivas, F., & Biederman, J. (2006). A quick and reliable screening measure for OCD in youth: Reliability and validity of the obsessive compulsive scale of the Child Behavior Checklist. *Comprehensive Psychiatry*, 47(3), 234–240. https://doi.org/10.1016/j.comppsych.2005.08.005.

Grant, J.E., Kim, S.W., & Crow, S.J. (2001). Prevalence and clinical features of body dysmorphic disorder in adolescent and adult psychiatric inpatients. *The Journal of Clinical Psychiatry*, 62(7), 517–522. https://doi.org/10.4088/jcp.v62n07a03.

Grant, J.E., Odlaug, B.L., Chamberlain, S.R., & Kim, S.W. (2010). A double-blind, placebo-controlled trial of Lamotrigine for pathologic skin picking: Treatment efficacy and neurocognitive predictors of response. *Journal of Clinical Psychopharmacology*, 30(4), 396–403. https://doi.org/10.1097/JCP.0b013e3181e617a1.

Grant, J.E., Odlaug, B.L., & Kim, S.W. (2009). N-acetylcysteine, a glutamate modulator, in the treatment of trichotillomania: A double-blind, placebo-controlled study. *Archives of General Psychiatry*, 66(7), 756–763. https://doi.org/10.1001/archgenpsychiatry.2009.60.

Hacker, L.E., Park, J.M., Timpano, K.R., Cavitt, M.A., Alvaro, J.L., Lewin, A.B., Murphy, T.K., & Storch, E.A. (2016). Hoarding in children with ADHD. *Journal of Attention Disorders*, 20(7), 617–626. https://doi.org/10.1177/1087054712455845.

Hanks, C.E., McGuire, J.F., Lewin, A.B., Storch, E.A., & Murphy, T.K. (2016). Clinical correlates and mediators of self-concept in youth with chronic tic disorders. *Child Psychiatry & Human Development*, 47(1), 64–74. https://doi.org/10.1007/s10578-015-0544-0.

Hanley, S.M., Bhullar, N., & Wootton, B.M. (2020). Development and initial validation of the Body Dysmorphic Disorder Scale for Youth. *Clinical Psychologist*, 24(3), 254–266. https://doi.org/10.1111/cp.12225.

Harcherik, D.F., Leckman, J.F., Detlor, J., & Cohen, D.J. (1984). A new instrument for clinical studies of Tourette's syndrome. *Journal of the American Academy of Child Psychiatry*, 23(2), 153–160. https://doi.org/10.1097/00004583-198403000-00006.

Houghton, D.C., Capriotti, M., Franklin, M.R., Scahill, L., Wilhelm, S., Peterson, A.L., Walkup, J.T., Piacentini, J., & Woods, D.W. (2017). Investigating habituation to premonitory urges in behavior therapy for tic disorders: Evidence from a randomized controlled trial. *Behavior Therapy*, 48(6), 834–846.

Hudziak, J.J., Althoff, R.R., Stanger, C., Beijsterveldt, C.E.M., Nelson, E.C., Hanna, G.L., Boomsma, D.I., & Todd, R.D. (2006). The Obsessive Compulsive Scale of the Child Behavior Checklist predicts obsessive-compulsive disorder: A receiver operating characteristic curve analysis. *Journal of Child Psychology and Psychiatry*, 47(2), 160–166. https://doi.org/10.1111/j.1469-7610.2005.01465.x.

Jeon, S., Walkup, J.T., Woods, D.W., Peterson, A., Piacentini, J., Wilhelm, S., Katsovich, L., McGuire, J.F., Dziura, J., & Scahill, L. (2013). Detecting a clinically meaningful change in tic severity in Tourette syndrome: A comparison of three methods. *Contemporary Clinical Trials*, 36(2), 414–420. https://doi.org/10.1016/j.cct.2013.08.012.

Jones, A.M., De Nadai, A.S., Arnold, E.B., McGuire, J.F., Lewin, A.B., Murphy, T.K., & Storch, E.A. (2013). Psychometric properties of the Obsessive Compulsive Inventory: Child version in children and adolescents with obsessive-compulsive disorder. *Child Psychiatry & Human Development*, 44(1), 137–151. https://doi.org/10.1007/s10578-012-0315-0.

Kaufman, J., Birmaher, B., Brent, D., Rao, U., Flynn, C., Moreci, P., Williamson, D., & Ryan, N. (1997). Schedule for affective disorders and schizophrenia for School-Age Children-Present and Lifetime Version (K-SADS-PL): Initial reliability and validity data. *Journal of the American Academy of Child & Adolescent Psychiatry*, 36(7), 980–988. https://doi.org/10.1097/00004583-199707000-00021.

Keuthen, N. (n.d.). *The Keuthen Diagnostic Inventory for Skin Picking (K-DISP)*. Unpublished inventory.

Keuthen, N.J., Deckersbach, T., Wilhelm, S., Engelhard, I., Forker, A., O'Sullivan, R.L., Jenike, M.A., & Baer, L. (2001a). The Skin Picking Impact Scale (SPIS): Scale development and psychometric analyses. *Psychosomatics*, 42(5), 397–403. https://doi.org/10.1176/appi.psy.42.5.397.

Keuthen, N.J., O'Sullivan, R.L., Ricciardi, J.N., Shera, D., Savage, C.R., Borgmann, A.S., Jenike, M.A., & Baer, L. (1995). The Massachusetts General Hospital (MGH) Hairpulling Scale: 1. Development and factor analyses. *Psychotherapy and Psychosomatics*, 64(3–4), 141–145. https://doi.org/10.1159/000289003.

Keuthen, N.J., Wilhelm, S., Deckersbach, T., Engelhard, I.M., Forker, A.E., Baer, L., & Jenike, M.A. (2001b). The Skin Picking Scale: Scale construction and psychometric analyses. *Journal of Psychosomatic Research*.

Lebowitz, E.R., Scharfstein, L.A., & Jones, J. (2014). Comparing family accommodation in pediatric obsessive-compulsive disorder, anxiety disorders, and non-anxious children. *Depression and Anxiety*, 31(12), 1018–1025. https://doi.org/10.1002/da.22251.

Leckman, J.F., Riddle, M.A., Hardin, M.T., Ort, S.I., Swartz, K.L., Stevenson, J., & Cohen, D.J. (1989). The Yale Global Tic Severity Scale: Initial testing of a clinician-rated scale of tic severity. *Journal of the American Academy of Child & Adolescent Psychiatry*, 28(4), 566–573. https://doi.org/10.1097/00004583-198907000-00015.

Leckman, J.F., Walker, D.E., & Cohen, D.J. (1993). Premonitory urges in Tourette's syndrome. *The American Journal of Psychiatry*.

Lewin, A.B., Piacentini, J., De Nadai, A.S., Jones, A.M., Peris, T.S., Geffken, G.R., Geller, D.A., Nadeau, J.M., Murphy, T.K., & Storch, E.A. (2014). Defining clinical severity in pediatric obsessive-compulsive disorder. *Psychological Assessment*, 26(2), 679–684. https://doi.org/10.1037/a0035174.

Lewin, A.B., Wood, J.J., Gunderson, S., Murphy, T.K., & Storch, E.A. (2011). Phenomenology of comorbid autism spectrum and obsessive-compulsive disorders among children. *Journal of Developmental and Physical Disabilities*, 23(6), 543–553. https://doi.org/10.1007/s10882-011-9247-z.

Martínez-González, A.E., Rodríguez-Jiménez, T., Piqueras, J.A., Vera-Villarroel, P., & Godoy, A. (2015). Psychometric properties of the Obsessive-Compulsive Inventory – Child Version (OCI-CV) in Chilean children and adolescents. *PLOS ONE*, 10(8), e0136842. https://doi.org/10.1371/journal.pone.0136842.

McGuire, J.F., Geller, D.A., Murphy, T.K., Small, B.J., Unger, A., Wilhelm, S., & Storch, E.A. (2019). Defining treatment outcomes in pediatric obsessive-compulsive disorder using a self-report scale. *Behavior Therapy*, 50(2), 314–324. https://doi.org/10.1016/j.beth.2018.06.003.

McGuire, J.F., Ginder, N., Ramsey, K., Essoe, J.K.-Y., Ricketts, E.J., McCracken, J.T., & Piacentini, J. (2020a). Optimizing behavior therapy for youth with Tourette's disorder. *Neuropsychopharmacology, 45*(12), 2114–2119.

McGuire, J.F., Hanks, C., Lewin, A.B., Storch, E.A., & Murphy, T.K. (2013a). Social deficits in children with chronic tic disorders: Phenomenology, clinical correlates and quality of life. *Comprehensive Psychiatry, 54*(7), 1023–1031.

McGuire, J.F., Kaercher, L., Park, J.M., & Storch, E.A. (2013b). Hoarding in the community: A code enforcement and social service perspective. *Journal of Social Service Research, 39*(3), 335–344. https://doi.org/10.1080/01488376.2013.770813.

McGuire, J.F., Kugler, B.B., Park, J.M., Horng, B., Lewin, A.B., Murphy, T.K., & Storch, E.A. (2012a). Evidence-based assessment of compulsive skin picking, chronic tic disorders and trichotillomania in children. *Child Psychiatry & Human Development, 43*(6), 855–883. https://doi.org/10.1007/s10578-012-0300-7.

McGuire, J.F., McBride, N., Piacentini, J., Johnco, C., Lewin, A.B., Murphy, T.K., & Storch, E.A. (2016). The premonitory urge revisited: An individualized premonitory urge for tics scale. *Journal of Psychiatric Research, 83*, 176–183. https://doi.org/10.1016/j.jpsychires.2016.09.007.

McGuire, J.F., Myers, N.S., Lewin, A.B., Storch, E.A., & Rahman, O. (2020b). The influence of hair pulling styles in the treatment of trichotillomania. *Behavior Therapy, 51*(6), 895–904. https://doi.org/10.1016/j.beth.2019.12.003.

McGuire, J.F., Piacentini, J., Scahill, L., Woods, D.W., Villarreal, R., Wilhelm, S., Walkup, J.T., & Peterson, A.L. (2015). Bothersome tics in patients with chronic tic disorders: Characteristics and individualized treatment response to behavior therapy. *Behaviour Research and Therapy, 70*, 56–63. https://doi.org/10.1016/j.brat.2015.05.006.

McGuire, J.F., Piacentini, J., Storch, E.A., Murphy, T.K., Ricketts, E.J., Woods, D.W., Walkup, J.W., Peterson, A.L., Wilhelm, S., Lewin, A.B., McCracken, J.T., Leckman, J.F., & Scahill, L. (2018). A multicenter examination and strategic revisions of the Yale Global Tic Severity Scale. *Neurology, 90*(19), e1711–e1719. https://doi.org/10.1212/WNL.0000000000005474.

McGuire, J.F., Storch, E.A., Lewin, A.B., Price, L.H., Rasmussen, S.A., & Goodman, W.K. (2012b). The role of avoidance in the phenomenology of obsessive-compulsive disorder. *Comprehensive Psychiatry, 53*(2), 187–194. https://doi.org/10.1016/j.comppsych.2011.03.002.

McGuire, J.F., Ung, D., Selles, R.R., Rahman, O., Lewin, A.B., Murphy, T.K., & Storch, E.A. (2014). Treating trichotillomania: A meta-analysis of treatment effects and moderators for behavior therapy and serotonin reuptake inhibitors. *Journal of Psychiatric Research, 58*, 76–83. https://doi.org/10.1016/j.jpsychires.2014.07.015.

Monzani, B., Fallah, D., Rautio, D., Gumpert, M., Jassi, A., Fernández de la Cruz, L., Mataix-Cols, D., & Krebs, G. (2022). Psychometric evaluation of the Yale-Brown Obsessive-Compulsive Scale Modified for Body Dysmorphic Disorder for Adolescents (BDD-YBOCS-A). *Child Psychiatry and Human Development.* https://doi.org/10.1007/s10578-022-01376-x.

Mueller, A.E., & Segal, D.L. (2015). Structured versus semistructured versus unstructured interviews. In R.L. Cautin & S.O. Lilienfeld (Eds.), *The Encyclopedia of Clinical Psychology* (pp. 1–7). John Wiley & Sons. https://doi.org/10.1002/9781118625392.wbecp069.

Nordsletten, A.E., Fernández de la Cruz, L., Pertusa, A., Reichenberg, A., Hatch, S.L., & Mataix-Cols, D. (2013). The Structured Interview for

Hoarding Disorder (SIHD): Development, usage and further validation. *Journal of Obsessive-Compulsive and Related Disorders*, 2(3), 346–350. https://doi.org/10.1016/j.jocrd.2013.06.003.

Ong, C., Pang, S., Sagayadevan, V., Chong, S.A., & Subramaniam, M. (2015). Functioning and quality of life in hoarding: A systematic review. *Journal of Anxiety Disorders*, 32, 17–30. https://doi.org/10.1016/j.janxdis.2014.12.003.

Ong, C.W., Krafft, J., Levin, M.E., & Twohig, M.P. (2021). A systematic review and psychometric evaluation of self-report measures for hoarding disorder. *Journal of Affective Disorders*, 290, 136–148. https://doi.org/10.1016/j.jad.2021.04.082.

O'Sullivan, R.L., Keuthen, N.J., Hayday, C.F., Ricciardi, J.N., Buttolph, M.L., Jenike, M.A., & Baer, L. (1995). The Massachusetts General Hospital (MGH) Hairpulling Scale: 2. Reliability and validity. *Psychotherapy and Psychosomatics*, 64(3–4), 146–148. https://doi.org/10.1159/000289004.

Patrick, A.K., Ramsey, K.A., Essoe, J.K.-Y., & McGuire, J.F. (2022). Clinical considerations for an evidence-based assessment for obsessive-compulsive disorder. *Psychiatric Clinics*.

Phillips, K.A., Hollander, E., Rasmussen, S.A., Aronowitz, B.R., DeCaria, C., & Goodman, W.K. (1997a). A severity rating scale for body dysmorphic disorder: Development, reliability, and validity of a modified version of the Yale-Brown Obsessive Compulsive Scale. *Psychopharmacology Bulletin*, 33(1), 17–22.

Phillips, K.A., Hollander, E., Rasmussen, S.A., Aronowitz, B.R., DeCaria, C., & Goodman, W.K. (1997b). A severity rating scale for body dysmorphic disorder: Development, reliability, and validity of a modified version of the Yale-Brown Obsessive Compulsive Scale. *Psychopharmacology Bulletin*, 33(1), 17–22.

Phillips, K.A., Menard, W., Fay, C., & Weisberg, R. (2005). Demographic characteristics, phenomenology, comorbidity, and family history in 200 individuals with body dysmorphic disorder. *Psychosomatics*, 46(4), 317–325. https://doi.org/10.1176/appi.psy.46.4.317.

Phillips, K.A., Pagano, M.E., Menard, W., & Stout, R.L. (2006). A 12-month follow-up study of the course of body dysmorphic disorder. *American Journal of Psychiatry*, 163(5), 907–912. https://doi.org/10.1176/ajp.2006.163.5.907.

Piacentini, J., Bergman, R.L., Chang, S., Langley, A., Peris, T., Wood, J.J., & McCracken, J. (2011). Controlled comparison of family cognitive behavioral therapy and psychoeducation/relaxation training for child obsessive-compulsive disorder. *Journal of the American Academy of Child & Adolescent Psychiatry*, 50(11), 1149–1161. https://doi.org/10.1016/j.jaac.2011.08.003.

Piacentini, J., Peris, T.S., Bergman, R.L., Chang, S., & Jaffer, M. (2007). Brief report: Functional impairment in childhood OCD: Development and psychometrics properties of the Child Obsessive-Compulsive Impact Scale – Revised (COIS-R). *Journal of Clinical Child & Adolescent Psychology*, 36(4), 645–653. https://doi.org/10.1080/15374410701662790.

Piacentini, J., Woods, D.W., Scahill, L., Wilhelm, S., Peterson, A.L., Chang, S., Ginsburg, G.S., Deckersbach, T., Dziura, J., Levi-Pearl, S., & Walkup, J.T. (2010). Behavior therapy for children with Tourette disorder: A randomized controlled trial. *JAMA*, 303(19), 1929–1937. https://doi.org/10.1001/jama.2010.607.

Piqueras, J.A., Rodríguez-Jiménez, T., Ortiz, A.G., Moreno, E., Lázaro, L., & Storch, E.A. (2017). Factor structure, reliability, and validity of the Spanish version of the Children's Florida Obsessive Compulsive Inventory (C-FOCI). *Child Psychiatry & Human Development*, 48(1), 166–179. https://doi.org/10.1007/s10578-016-0661-4.

Rahman, O., McGuire, J., Storch, E.A., & Lewin, A.B. (2017). Preliminary randomized controlled trial of habit reversal training for treatment of hair pulling in youth. *Journal of Child and Adolescent Psychopharmacology, 27*(2), 132–139.

Rapp, A.M., Bergman, R.L., Piacentini, J., & McGuire, J.F. (2016). Evidence-based assessment of obsessive-compulsive disorder. *Journal of Central Nervous System Disease, 8*, JCNSD-S38359.

Rautio, D., Gumpert, M., Jassi, A., Krebs, G., Flygare, O., Andrén, P., Monzani, B., Peile, L., Jansson-Fröjmark, M., Lundgren, T., Hillborg, M., Silverberg-Mörse, M., Clark, B., Fernández de la Cruz, L., & Mataix-Cols, D. (2022). Effectiveness of multimodal treatment for young people with body dysmorphic disorder in two specialist clinics. *Behavior Therapy, 53*(5), 1037–1049. https://doi.org/10.1016/j.beth.2022.04.010.

Reese, H.E., Scahill, L., Peterson, A.L., Crowe, K., Woods, D.W., Piacentini, J., Walkup, J.T., & Wilhelm, S. (2014). The premonitory urge to tic: Measurement, characteristics, and correlates in older adolescents and adults. *Behavior Therapy, 45*(2), 177–186.

Ricketts, E.J., McGuire, J.F., Chang, S., Bose, D., Rasch, M.M., Woods, D.W., Specht, M.W., Walkup, J.T., Scahill, L., Wilhelm, S., Peterson, A. L., & Piacentini, J. (2018). Benchmarking treatment response in Tourette's disorder: A Psychometric evaluation and signal detection analysis of the Parent Tic Questionnaire. *Behavior Therapy, 49*(1), 46–56. https://doi.org/10.1016/j.beth.2017.05.006.

Ricketts, E.J., Peris, T.S., Grant, J.E., Valle, S., Cavic, E., Lerner, J.E., Lochner, C., Stein, D.J., Dougherty, D.D., O'Neill, J., Woods, D.W., Keuthen, N.J., & Piacentini, J. (2022). Clinical characteristics of youth with trichotillomania (hair-pulling disorder) and excoriation (skin-picking) disorder. *Child Psychiatry & Human Development.* https://doi.org/10.1007/s10578-022-01458-w.

Roberts, C., Zimmer-Gembeck, M.J., & Farrell, L.J. (2019). The multidimensional youth body dysmorphic inventory: Development and preliminary validation. *Child Psychiatry & Human Development, 50*(6), 927–939. https://doi.org/10.1007/s10578-019-00893-6.

Rosen, J.C., & Reiter, J. (1996). Development of the Body Dysmorphic Disorder Examination. *Behaviour Research and Therapy, 34*(9), 755–766. https://doi.org/10.1016/0005-7967(96)00024-1.

Saxena, S., Ayers, C.R., Dozier, M.E., & Maidment, K.M. (2015). The UCLA Hoarding Severity Scale: Development and validation. *Journal of Affective Disorders, 175,* 488–493. https://doi.org/10.1016/j.jad.2015.01.030.

Scahill, L., Leckman, J.F., Schultz, R.T., Katsovich, L., & Peterson, B.S. (2003). A placebo-controlled trial of risperidone in Tourette syndrome. *Neurology, 60*(7), 1130–1135. https://doi.org/10.1212/01.WNL.0000055434.39968.67.

Scahill, L., Riddle, M.A., McSwiggin-Hardin, M., Ort, S.I., King, R.A., Goodman, W.K., Cicchetti, D., & Leckman, J.F. (1997). Children's Yale-Brown Obsessive Compulsive Scale: Reliability and validity. *Journal of the American Academy of Child & Adolescent Psychiatry, 36*(6), 844–852. https://doi.org/10.1097/00004583-199706000-00023.

Schneider, A.F., Storch, E.A., Geffken, G.R., Lack, C.W., & Shytle, R.D. (2008). Psychometric properties of the Hoarding Assessment Scale in college students. *Illness, Crisis & Loss, 16*(3), 227–236. https://doi.org/10.2190/IL.16.3.c.

Schneider, S.C., Turner, C.M., Mond, J., & Hudson, J.L. (2017). Prevalence and correlates of body dysmorphic disorder in a community sample of adolescents. *The Australian and New Zealand Journal of Psychiatry, 51*(6), 595–603. https://doi.org/10.1177/0004867416665483.

Selles, R.R., Højgaard, D.R.M.A., Ivarsson, T., Thomsen, P.H., McBride, N., Storch, E.A., Geller, D., Wilhelm, S., Farrell, L.J., Waters, A.M., Mathieu, S., Lebowitz, E., Elgie, M., Soreni, N., & Stewart, S.E. (2018). Symptom insight in pediatric obsessive-compulsive disorder: Outcomes of an international aggregated cross-sectional sample. *Journal of the American Academy of Child & Adolescent Psychiatry, 57*(8), 615–619.e5. https://doi.org/10.1016/j.jaac.2018.04.012.

Selles, R.R., McGuire, J.F., Small, B.J., & Storch, E.A. (2016). A systematic review and meta-analysis of psychiatric treatments for excoriation (skin-picking) disorder. *General Hospital Psychiatry, 41*, 29–37. https://doi.org/10.1016/j.genhosppsych.2016.04.001.

Selles, R.R., Nelson, R., Zepeda, R., Dane, B.F., Wu, M.S., Carlos Novoa, J., Guttfreund, D., & Storch, E.A. (2015). Body focused repetitive behaviors among Salvadorian youth: Incidence and clinical correlates. *Journal of Obsessive-Compulsive and Related Disorders, 5*, 49–54. https://doi.org/10.1016/j.jocrd.2015.01.008.

Shapiro, A.K., & Shapiro, E. (1984). Controlled study of pimozide vs. placebo in Tourette's syndrome. *Journal of the American Academy of Child Psychiatry, 23*(2), 161–173. https://doi.org/10.1097/00004583-198403000-00007.

Sheehan, D.V., Sheehan, K.H., Shytle, R.D., Janavs, J., Bannon, Y., Rogers, J.E., Milo, K.M., Stock, S.L., & Wilkinson, B. (2010). Reliability and validity of the Mini International Neuropsychiatric Interview for Children and Adolescents (MINI-KID). *The Journal of Clinical Psychiatry, 71*(03), 313–326. https://doi.org/10.4088/JCP.09m05305whi.

Shytle, R.D., Silver, A.A., Sheehan, K.H., Wilkinson, B.J., Newman, M., Sanberg, P.R., & Sheehan, D. (2003). The Tourette's Disorder Scale (TODS): Development, reliability, and validity. *Assessment, 10*(3), 273–287. https://doi.org/10.1177/1073191103255497.

Silverman, W.K., & Albano, A.M. (1996). *The Anxiety Disorders Interview Schedule for DSM-IV – Child and Parent Versions.* Graywinds Publications.

Skarphedinsson, G., De Nadai, A.S., Storch, E.A., Lewin, A.B., & Ivarsson, T. (2017). Defining cognitive-behavior therapy response and remission in pediatric OCD: A signal detection analysis of the Children's Yale-Brown Obsessive Compulsive Scale. *European Child & Adolescent Psychiatry, 26*(1), 47–55.

Skarphedinsson, G., Melin, K.H., Valderhaug, R., Wentzel-Larsen, T., Højgaard, D.R.M.A., Thomsen, P.H., & Ivarsson, T. (2015). Evaluation of the factor structure of the Child Obsessive-Compulsive Impact Scale – Revised (COIS-R) in Scandinavia with confirmatory factor analysis. *Journal of Obsessive-Compulsive and Related Disorders, 7*, 65–72. https://doi.org/10.1016/j.jocrd.2015.03.005.

Snorrason, I., Olafsson, R.P., Houghton, D.C., Woods, D.W., & Lee, H.-J. (2015). "Wanting" and "liking" skin picking: A validation of the Skin Picking Reward Scale. *Journal of Behavioral Addictions, 4*(4), 250–260. https://doi.org/10.1556/2006.4.2015.033.

Soler, C.T., Vadlin, S., Olofsdotter, S., Ramklint, M., Sonnby, K., & Nilsson, K. (2021). Psychometric evaluation of the Swedish Child Sheehan Disability Scale in adolescent psychiatric patients. *Scandinavian Journal of Child and Adolescent Psychiatry and Psychology, 9*(1), 137–146. https://doi.org/10.21307/sjcapp-2021-015.

Soreni, N., Cameron, D., Vorstenbosch, V., Duku, E., Rowa, K., Swinson, R., Bullard, C., & McCabe, R. (2018). Psychometric evaluation of a revised scoring approach for the Children's Saving Inventory in a Canadian sample of youth with obsessive-compulsive disorder. *Child Psychiatry & Human Development, 49*(6), 966–973. https://doi.org/10.1007/s10578-018-0811-y.

Stanley, M.A., Breckenridge, J.K., Snyder, A.G., & Novy, D.M. (1999). Clinician-rated measures of hair pulling: A preliminary psychometric evaluation. *Journal of Psychopathology and Behavioral Assessment*, 21(2), 157–170. https://doi.org/10.1023/A:1022160522908.

Stanley, M.A., Breckenridge, J.K., Swann, A.C., Freeman, E.B., & Reich, L. (1997). Fluvoxamine treatment of trichotillomania. *Journal of Clinical Psychopharmacology*, 17(4), 278–283. https://doi.org/10.1097/00004714-199708000-00007.

Stanley, M.A., Prather, R.C., Wagner, A.L., Davis, M.L., & Swann, A.C. (1993). Can the Yale-Brown Obsessive Compulsive Scale be used to assess trichotillomania? A preliminary report. *Behaviour Research and Therapy*, 31(2), 171–177. https://doi.org/10.1016/0005-7967(93)90068-6.

Storch, E.A., De Nadai, A.S., Lewin, A.B., McGuire, J.F., Jones, A.M., Mutch, P.J., Shytle, R.D., & Murphy, T.K. (2011a). Defining Treatment response in pediatric tic disorders: A signal detection analysis of the Yale Global Tic Severity Scale. *Journal of Child and Adolescent Psychopharmacology*, 21(6), 621–627. https://doi.org/10.1089/cap.2010.0149.

Storch, E.A., Johnco, C., McGuire, J.F., Wu, M.S., McBride, N.M., Lewin, A.B., & Murphy, T.K. (2017). An initial study of family accommodation in children and adolescents with chronic tic disorders. *European Child & Adolescent Psychiatry*, 26(1), 99–109.

Storch, E.A., Khanna, M., Merlo, L.J., Loew, B.A., Franklin, M., Reid, J.M., Goodman, W.K., & Murphy, T.K. (2009). Children's Florida Obsessive Compulsive Inventory: Psychometric properties and feasibility of a self-report measure of obsessive-compulsive symptoms in youth. *Child Psychiatry and Human Development*, 40(3), 467–483. https://doi.org/10.1007/s10578-009-0138-9.

Storch, E.A., Lack, C.W., Simons, L.E., Goodman, W.K., Murphy, T.K., & Geffken, G.R. (2007a). A measure of functional impairment in youth with Tourette's syndrome. *Journal of Pediatric Psychology*, 32(8), 950–959. https://doi.org/10.1093/jpepsy/jsm034

Storch, E.A., Lewin, A.B., De Nadai, A.S., & Murphy, T.K. (2010a). Defining treatment response and remission in obsessive-compulsive disorder: A signal detection analysis of the Children's Yale-Brown Obsessive Compulsive Scale. *Journal of the American Academy of Child & Adolescent Psychiatry*, 49(7), 708–717. https://doi.org/10.1016/j.jaac.2010.04.005.

Storch, E.A., McGuire, J.F., Wu, M.S., Hamblin, R., McIngvale, E., Cepeda, S.L., Schneider, S.C., Rufino, K.A., Rasmussen, S.A., Price, L.H., & Goodman, W.K. (2019). Development and psychometric evaluation of the Children's Yale-Brown Obsessive-Compulsive Scale, 2nd ed. *Journal of the American Academy of Child & Adolescent Psychiatry*, 58(1), 92–98. https://doi.org/10.1016/j.jaac.2018.05.029.

Storch, E.A., Merlo, L.J., Lack, C., Milsom, V.A., Geffken, G.R., Goodman, W.K., & Murphy, T.K. (2007b). Quality of life in youth with Tourette's syndrome and chronic tic disorder. *Journal of Clinical Child & Adolescent Psychology*, 36(2), 217–227. https://doi.org/10.1080/15374410701279545.

Storch, E.A., Merlo, L.J., Lehmkuhl, H., Grabill, K.M., Geffken, G.R., Goodman, W.K., & Murphy, T.K. (2007c). Further psychometric examination of the Tourette's disorder scales. *Child Psychiatry and Human Development*, 38(2), 89–98. https://doi.org/10.1007/s10578-006-0043-4.

Storch, E.A., Muroff, J., Lewin, A.B., Geller, D., Ross, A., McCarthy, K., Morgan, J., Murphy, T.K., Frost, R., & Steketee, G. (2011b). Development and preliminary psychometric evaluation of the Children's Saving Inventory. *Child*

Psychiatry & Human Development, 42(2), 166–182. https://doi.org/10.1007/s10578-010-0207-0.

Storch, E.A., Murphy, T.K., Adkins, J.W., Lewin, A.B., Geffken, G R., Johns, N.B., Jann, K.E., & Goodman, W.K. (2006a). The Children's Yale-Brown Obsessive-Compulsive Scale: Psychometric properties of child- and parent-report formats. *Journal of Anxiety Disorders*, 20(8), 1055–1070. https://doi.org/10.1016/j.janxdis.2006.01.006.

Storch, E.A., Murphy, T.K., Bagner, D.M., Johns, N.B., Baumeister, A.L., Goodman, W.K., & Geffken, G.R. (2006b). Reliability and validity of the Child Behavior Checklist Obsessive-Compulsive Scale. *Journal of Anxiety Disorders*, 20(4), 473–485. https://doi.org/10.1016/j.janxdis.2005.06.002.

Storch, E.A., Murphy, T.K., Geffken, G.R., Sajid, M., Allen, P., Roberti, J.W., & Goodman, W.K. (2005). Reliability and validity of the Yale Global Tic Severity Scale. *Psychological Assessment*, 17(4), 486–491. https://doi.org/10.1037/1040-3590.17.4.486.

Storch, E.A., Murphy, T K., Geffken, G.R., Soto, O., Sajid, M., Allen, P., Roberti, J.W., Killiany, E.M., & Goodman, W.K. (2004a). Psychometric evaluation of the Children's Yale-Brown Obsessive-Compulsive Scale. *Psychiatry Research*, 129(1), 91–98. https://doi.org/10.1016/j.psychres.2004.06.009.

Storch, E.A., Murphy, T.K., Geffken, G.R., Soto, O., Sajid, M., Allen, P., Roberti, J.W., Killiany, E.M., & Goodman, W.K. (2004b). Further psychometric properties of the Tourette's Disorder Scale – Parent Rated Version (TODS-PR). *Child Psychiatry and Human Development*, 35(2), 107–120. https://doi.org/10.1007/s10578-004-1880-7.

Storch, E.A., Nadeau, J.M., Johnco, C., Timpano, K., McBride, N., Jane Mutch, P., Lewin, A.B., & Murphy, T.K. (2016a). Hoarding in youth with autism spectrum disorders and anxiety: incidence, clinical correlates, and behavioral treatment response. *Journal of Autism and Developmental Disorders*, 46(5), 1602–1612. https://doi.org/10.1007/s10803-015-2687-z.

Storch, E.A., Park, J.M., Lewin, A.B., Morgan, J.R., Jones, A.M., & Murphy, T.K. (2011c). The Leyton Obsessional Inventory – Child Version Survey Form does not demonstrate adequate psychometric properties in American youth with pediatric obsessive-compulsive disorder. *Journal of Anxiety Disorders*, 25(4), 574–578. https://doi.org/10.1016/j.janxdis.2011.01.005.

Storch, E.A., Rasmussen, S.A., Price, L.H., Larson, M.J., Murphy, T.K., & Goodman, W.K. (2010b). Development and psychometric evaluation of the Yale-Brown Obsessive-Compulsive Scale – Second edition. *Psychological Assessment*, 22(2), 223–232. https://doi.org/10.1037/a0018492.

Storch, E.A., Wilhelm, S., Sprich, S., Henin, A., Micco, J., Small, B.J., McGuire, J., Mutch, P.J., Lewin, A.B., Murphy, T.K., & Geller, D.A. (2016). Efficacy of augmentation of cognitive behavior therapy with weight-adjusted d-cycloserine vs placebo in pediatric obsessive-compulsive disorder: A randomized clinical trial. *JAMA Psychiatry*, 73(8), 779–788. https://doi.org/10.1001/jamapsychiatry.2016.1128.

Swedo, S.E., Leonard, H.L., Rapoport, J.L., Lenane, M.C., Goldberger, E.L., & Cheslow, D.L. (1989). A double-blind comparison of clomipramine and desipramine in the treatment of trichotillomania (hair pulling). *New England Journal of Medicine*, 321(8), 497–501. https://doi.org/10.1056/NEJM198908243210803.

Szejko, N., Robinson, S., Hartmann, A., Ganos, C., Debes, N.M., Skov, L., Haas, M., Rizzo, R., Stern, J., Münchau, A., Czernecki, V., Dietrich, A., Murphy, T.L.,

Martino, D., Tarnok, Z., Hedderly, T., Müller-Vahl, K.R., & Cath, D.C. (2022). European clinical guidelines for Tourette syndrome and other tic disorders – Version 2.0. Part I: Assessment. *European Child & Adolescent Psychiatry, 31*(3), 383–402. https://doi.org/10.1007/s00787-021-01842-2.

Tolin, D.F., Diefenbach, G.J., Flessner, C.A., Franklin, M.E., Keuthen, N.J., Moore, P., Piacentini, J., Stein, D.J., Woods, D.W., & Trichotillomania Learning Center Scientific Advisory Board. (2008a). The trichotillomania scale for children: Development and validation. *Child Psychiatry and Human Development, 39*(3), 331–349. https://doi.org/10.1007/s10578-007-0092-3.

Tolin, D.F., Frost, R.O., & Steketee, G. (2010). A brief interview for assessing compulsive hoarding: The Hoarding Rating Scale – Interview. *Psychiatry Research, 178*(1), 147–152. https://doi.org/10.1016/j.psychres.2009.05.001.

Tolin, D.F., Frost, R.O., Steketee, G., & Fitch, K.E. (2008b). Family burden of compulsive hoarding: Results of an internet survey. *Behaviour Research and Therapy, 46*(3), 334–344. https://doi.org/10.1016/j.brat.2007.12.008.

Tolin, D.F., Gilliam, C.M., Davis, E., Springer, K., Levy, H C., Frost, R.O., Steketee, G., & Stevens, M.C. (2018a). Psychometric properties of the Hoarding Rating Scale – Interview. *Journal of Obsessive-Compulsive and Related Disorders, 16*, 76–80. https://doi.org/10.1016/j.jocrd.2018.01.003.

Tolin, D.F., Gilliam, C., Wootton, B.M., Bowe, W., Bragdon, L.B., Davis, E., Hannan, S.E., Steinman, S.A., Worden, B., & Hallion, L.S. (2018b). Psychometric Properties of a structured diagnostic interview for DSM-5 anxiety, mood, and obsessive-compulsive and related disorders. *Assessment, 25*(1), 3–13. https://doi.org/10.1177/1073191116638410.

Tucker, B.T.P., Woods, D.W., Flessner, C.A., Franklin, S.A., & Franklin, M.E. (2011). The skin picking impact project: Phenomenology, interference, and treatment utilization of pathological skin picking in a population-based sample. *Journal of Anxiety Disorders, 25*(1), 88–95. https://doi.org/10.1016/j.janxdis.2010.08.007.

Uher, R., Heyman, I., Turner, C.M., & Shafran, R. (2008). Self-, parent-report and interview measures of obsessive-compulsive disorder in children and adolescents. *Journal of Anxiety Disorders, 22*(6), 979–990. https://doi.org/10.1016/j.janxdis.2007.10.001.

Van Ameringen, M., Mancini, C., Patterson, B., Bennett, M., & Oakman, J. (2010). A randomized, double-blind, placebo-controlled trial of olanzapine in the treatment of trichotillomania. *The Journal of Clinical Psychiatry, 71*(10), 1336–1343. https://doi.org/10.4088/JCP.09m05114gre.

van Minnen, A., Hoogduin, K.A.L., Keijsers, G.P.J., Hellenbrand, I., & Hendriks, G.-J. (2003). Treatment of trichotillomania with behavioral therapy or fluoxetine: A randomized, waiting-list controlled study. *Archives of General Psychiatry, 60*(5), 517–522. https://doi.org/10.1001/archpsyc.60.5.517.

Walkup, J.T., Rosenberg, L.A., Brown, J., & Singer, H.S. (1992). The validity of instruments measuring tic severity in Tourette's syndrome. *Journal of the American Academy of Child & Adolescent Psychiatry, 31*(3), 472–477. https://doi.org/10.1097/00004583-199205000-00013.

Walther, M.R., Flessner, C.A., Conelea, C.A., & Woods, D.W. (2009). The Milwaukee Inventory for the Dimensions of Adult Skin Picking (MIDAS): Initial development and psychometric properties. *Journal of Behavior Therapy and Experimental Psychiatry, 40*(1), 127–135. https://doi.org/10.1016/j.jbtep.2008.07.002.

Whiteside, S.P. (2009). Adapting the Sheehan Disability Scale to assess child and parent impairment related to childhood anxiety disorders. *Journal of Clinical*

Child & Adolescent Psychology, 38(5), 721–730. https://doi.org/10.1080/15374410903103551.

Wilhelm, S., Greenberg, J.L., Rosenfield, E., Kasarskis, I., & Blashill, A.J. (2016). The Body Dysmorphic Disorder Symptom Scale: Development and preliminary validation of a self-report scale of symptom specific dysfunction. *Body Image*, 17, 82–87. https://doi.org/10.1016/j.bodyim.2016.02.006.

Wilhelm, S., Peterson, A.L., Piacentini, J., Woods, D.W., Deckersbach, T., Sukhodolsky, D.G., Chang, S., Liu, H., Dziura, J., Walkup, J.T., & Scahill, L. (2012). Randomized trial of behavior therapy for adults with Tourette syndrome. *Archives of General Psychiatry*, 69(8), 795–803. https://doi.org/10.1001/archgenpsychiatry.2011.1528.

Winchel, R.M., Jones, J.S., Molcho, A., Parsons, B., Stanley, B., & Stanley, M. (1992). The Psychiatric Institute Trichotillomania Scale (PITS). *Psychopharmacology Bulletin*, 28(4), 463–476.

Woods, D.W., Piacentini, J., Himle, M.B., & Chang, S. (2005). Premonitory Urge for Tics Scale (PUTS): Initial psychometric results and examination of the premonitory urge phenomenon in youths with tic disorders. *Journal of Developmental & Behavioral Pediatrics*, 26(6), 397–403.

Wu, M.S., McGuire, J.F., Martino, C., Phares, V., Selles, R.R., & Storch, E.A. (2016). A meta-analysis of family accommodation and OCD symptom severity. *Clinical Psychology Review*, 45, 34–44. https://doi.org/10.1016/j.cpr.2016.03.003.

Yucelen, A.G., Rodopman-Arman, A., Topcuoglu, V., Yazgan, M.Y., & Fisek, G. (2006). Interrater reliability and clinical efficacy of Children's Yale-Brown Obsessive-Compulsive Scale in an outpatient setting. *Comprehensive Psychiatry*, 47(1), 48–53. https://doi.org/10.1016/j.comppsych.2005.04.005.

3 Cognitive Behavioral Therapy with Exposure and Response Prevention for Childhood Obsessive-Compulsive Disorder

Erika S. Trent,[1,2] *Molly J. Church,*[2,3] *Andres G. Viana,*[1,4] *Wayne K. Goodman,*[2] *Andrew G. Guzick,*[2] *and Eric A. Storch*[2]

[1] *University of Houston, Department of Psychology, Houston, TX*

[2] *Baylor College of Medicine, Menninger Department of Psychiatry and Behavioral Sciences, Houston, TX*

[3] *William James College, Clinical Psychology Department, Newton, MA*

[4] *Texas Institute of Measurement, Evaluation, and Statistics, Houston, TX*

Obsessive-compulsive disorder (OCD) impacts one to 2 percent of children and adolescents, with often debilitating consequences (Geller et al., 2012). Advances in research and practice in the past several decades have improved the identification and treatment of childhood OCD (Freeman et al., 2018; Schuyler & Geller, 2023). Cognitive behavioral therapy (CBT) with exposure and response/ritual prevention (ERP) is the gold-standard psychosocial intervention for childhood OCD (McGuire et al., 2015). CBT monotherapy (i.e., without medication) with ERP is recommended as a first-line intervention for mild to moderate childhood OCD, due to its efficacy, safety, and relative durability of effects (Geller et al., 2012), with a much stronger evidence base than other psychosocial interventions (Freeman et al., 2018).

Although initially developed to treat adult OCD, CBT with ERP (hereafter "ERP") has been adapted for use in children and adolescents with OCD. While the core principles are the same, ERP for childhood OCD places a greater emphasis on family involvement, use of age-appropriate metaphors and language, and use of reward systems, among other developmental considerations. In this chapter, we describe the theoretical foundations of ERP, core treatment elements of ERP for childhood OCD, common barriers to successful treatment outcomes, and empirical evidence supporting its efficacy.

DOI: 10.4324/9781003386278-3

Theoretical Foundations of Exposure and Response Prevention

ERP for OCD is derived from cognitive and behavioral models of OCD. These theoretical models inform what is targeted in treatment and explain the mechanisms of change (i.e., why treatment works). Empirical support for cognitive and behavioral models of OCD originates primarily from studies of adult OCD. Although further research is needed to translate many of these findings among youth, some adult findings have been replicated among youth and this theoretical foundation is considered relevant to childhood OCD (Kircanski, Peris, & Piacentini, 2011).

Behavioral Theory

The behavioral model conceptualizes OCD as a disorder that is developed through classical conditioning and maintained through operant learning. When an individual experiences an obsession (i.e., intrusive or unwanted thoughts, images, or impulses that cause significant distress or anxiety), their distress or anxiety increases rapidly; subsequently, when they perform a compulsion (i.e., overt or covert behaviors intended to reduce this distress or anxiety), the distress or anxiety is reduced (Mowrer, 1960; Rachman, 1998). Because compulsions bring temporary relief from the obsession-induced distress, they are negatively reinforced over time. The repeated process of experiencing obsessions and performing compulsions strengthens this operant learning. For example, a child with contamination-related OCD touches a door handle, which triggers fears of passing germs to their mother (obsession) and making her ill (feared outcome); the child uses hand sanitizer to decontaminate (compulsion), which alleviates these fears. Because the use of hand sanitizer brings relief and prevents the child from learning that the feared outcome would not happen (or would not be so bad if it did), the child is more likely to repeat this compulsion the next time they encounter a similar situation (negative reinforcement). Avoidance of OCD triggers, which allow individuals to circumvent the possibility of triggering obsession-related anxiety in the first place (e.g., said child using their sleeve to avoid touching a door handle), is also negatively reinforcing.

ERP is informed by the behavioral model of OCD. ERP involves an individual, under the guidance of a therapist, facing a situation that triggers obsessions (exposure) and resisting performing compulsions that would alleviate the associated anxiety or distress (response/ritual prevention). The mechanism of change in ERP has traditionally been explained in terms of *habituation*: when an individual faces a feared stimulus that triggers obsessions without carrying out the compulsion, their anxiety will naturally decrease during the encounter with the stimulus (within-trial habituation) and their anxiety will be lower at the next encounter with the same stimulus (across-trial habituation). Repeatedly achieving habituation to a feared stimulus through ERP extinguishes the fear response and weakens negative reinforcement of the compulsion.

In light of studies that found inconsistent associations between habituation and treatment outcomes (e.g., Kircanski & Peris, 2015), the *inhibitory model of learning* was put forward as an alternative framework to explain the process of change during ERP (Craske et al., 2014). This model proposes that during ERP an individual sees that their feared outcome does not occur even in the absence of a compulsion, which violates their originally held expectation. Therefore, rather than unlearning one's fear, the individual learns new information (e.g., "My dad didn't die even though I didn't repeat my prayer three times," "That felt uncomfortable but I got used to it," "I can't know if I'm going to get sick, and even if I do, I'll get through it") that inhibits the original fear (e.g., "My dad will definitely die if I don't repeat my prayer three times," "I'm not going to be able to handle my shoes being tied unevenly," "I'm going to get sick if I use my school's bathrooms"). This process is referred to as inhibitory learning. For exposure to be effective, an individual may not necessarily need to achieve habituation; rather, the experience of expectancy violation may be sufficient, which might be related to expectations of a feared outcome, a child's ability to handle distress, or how distressing facing a situation will be (Guzick et al., 2020). The inhibitory model is empirically supported in children and adolescents, and informs treatment approaches towards ERP that may generalize across different situations more effectively than habituation-based approaches (McGuire & Storch, 2019).

Cognitive Theory

The cognitive model proposes that OCD is caused by maladaptive beliefs about intrusive thoughts (Rachman, 1998). Adults with OCD tend to endorse dysfunctional beliefs about intrusive thoughts, such as overestimation of threat, inflated responsibility, over-importance of thoughts, need to control thoughts, perfectionism, and intolerance of uncertainty (Obsessive Compulsive Cognitions Working Group, 2005). CBT targets such cognitive distortions by teaching adults to replace these biases with more adaptive interpretations, making them less likely to engage in maladaptive behaviors that maintain OCD.

Whether these cognitive processes are central to childhood OCD, however, is not as clear. In a clinical sample of children diagnosed with OCD, OCD symptom severity was associated with overestimation of threat, inflated responsibility, over-importance of thoughts, and the need to control thoughts, but not with perfectionism or intolerance of uncertainty (Coles et al., 2010). In a different sample of youth with OCD, perfectionism was associated with both OCD symptom severity and depressive symptom severity; however, youth with OCD did not score significantly higher on perfectionism than a non-clinical sample of children (Ye, Rice, & Storch, 2008). While children with OCD endorse significantly higher overestimation of threat and inflated responsibility than non-anxious children, they were indistinguishable from children with other anxiety disorders (Barrett & Healy, 2003). Taken together, cognitive factors may not be specific to OCD, but may rather be a transdiagnostic process that underlies anxiety disorders including OCD.

Many forms of CBT for childhood OCD include components of cognitive therapy and incorporate cognitive factors into case conceptualization. Indeed, children with OCD endorse fewer dysfunctional beliefs after receiving CBT (Wolters et al., 2019). However, research has found that this decrease in dysfunctional beliefs does not serve as a mechanism of change, but rather is a result of improvements in OCD symptoms (Wolters et al., 2019). Moreover, treatment studies consistently find that ERP (i.e., the behavioral component of CBT) is the active ingredient that predicts OCD symptom improvement (Kircanski & Peris, 2015). Therefore, when treating childhood OCD, it is recommended that cognitive modules are kept brief, focus on cognitive skills that will help children engage successfully in ERP (e.g., externalizing OCD; see *Treatment Elements* below), and quickly proceed to the ERP component of treatment.

Treatment Formats

ERP for childhood OCD can be delivered in several treatment formats (Leonard et al., 2016), including weekly outpatient therapy, web-based therapy, intensive outpatient therapy, and residential programs. Regardless of format, family involvement remains essential. While weekly ERP and more intensive ERP are comparably effective in achieving symptom remission, children receiving intensive treatment show more rapid symptom improvement (Storch et al., 2007). Symptom severity, level of impairment, family preferences, and response to previous treatment (if any) are considered when determining the appropriate treatment format for a child.

Weekly Outpatient Therapy

The traditional format of ERP for child OCD is weekly outpatient therapy, which typically consists of 12 to 14 weekly therapy sessions of 60–90 minutes each. Flexibility can be exercised with regard to the number of sessions; some youth respond in as few as seven sessions (Torp et al., 2019); some treatment manuals include 20 sessions (March & Mulle, 1998); and in clinical practice some youth may need more sessions to achieve symptom remission. Therapy sessions involve psychoeducation, in-session exposures, and homework review (see *Treatment Elements* below). Children complete assigned exposures repeatedly in between sessions, which is essential as ERP is more effective when exposures are conducted close in time (Sperling, Boger, & Potter, 2020). Parents are heavily involved in treatment and are encouraged to attend therapy sessions in part or in full. Frequency of outpatient sessions can be increased to two or three times a week, depending on symptom severity.

Web-Based Therapy

Web-based delivery of ERP for childhood OCD has increased in recent years, which may help increase dissemination of evidence-based treatment for youth, especially during challenging times (e.g., a global pandemic). Although OCD providers perceive low feasibility of delivering ERP to children (Wiese et al., 2022), preliminary studies suggest that therapist-guided ERP (i.e., via a two-way, live video call) is feasible and efficacious. A preliminary trial of 7–16-year-old youth with OCD found that ERP delivered via web camera resulted in greater improvements in OCD-related outcome measures than a waitlist control group (Storch et al., 2011). In a study of 4–8 year-olds with OCD, both video-conference-delivered family-based CBT and clinic-delivered family-based CBT showed similar improvements in OCD symptom outcomes (Comer et al., 2017). Thus, in circumstances in which face-to-face outpatient therapy is not feasible, therapist-guided ERP delivered via the web is a promising alternative. However, the relative efficacy of *self-guided*, web-based ERP (e.g., computer programs or smartphone apps) has not yet been tested in youth OCD (Herbst et al., 2012). See Chapter 10 for a more detailed discussion of technology-mediated treatment for childhood OCD.

Intensive Outpatient Treatment

More intensive treatment options are recommended for children with severe OCD symptoms and functional impairment that cannot be adequately addressed with weekly visits. Due to their condensed, time-limited nature, more intensive treatment formats may also be useful for children who need to travel long distances to receive evidence-based treatment. Intensive outpatient programs (IOP) for childhood OCD typically involve 1.5–3 hours of family-based therapy on 4–5 days a week for 3–6 weeks (Sperling, Boger, & Potter, 2020; Storch et al., 2007), although some work has demonstrated benefits of a one-week intensive protocol (Whiteside et al., 2014). IOP also often includes a group treatment component, which provides opportunities for children to model ERP to one another, as well as receive support from other children experiencing similar difficulties (Boger et al., 2016). Partial hospitalization programs (PHP) are a more intensive outpatient treatment format, in which patients attend therapy for a larger portion of the day (typically 3–4 hours) and engage in more frequent ERP sessions than at the IOP level. PHP often serves as a step-down from residential levels of care, which allows children to gradually transition to managing symptoms at home.

Residential Treatment

Children with severe OCD symptoms who have been unsuccessful at lower levels of care may require more intensive intervention at the residential level. Residential treatment may also be appropriate for children whose OCD interferes with critical domains of functioning (e.g., school attendance, social engagement, completion of daily activities of living, safety concerns) or whose OCD is maintained by circumstances at home such as family accommodation or family discord. Residential treatment provides considerably more hours of coached ERP, increased monitoring to facilitate ritual prevention, increased support for homework completion, and medication management (Leonard et al., 2016). In addition to coached exposures, children complete self-directed exposures seven days a week (Leonard et al., 2016). Residential treatment options also allow for more time and support to address comorbid conditions that may be interfering with OCD treatment (e.g., depression, panic).

Treatment Elements

The following section describes the core treatment elements of ERP for childhood and adolescent OCD. For detailed session-by-session descriptions, readers are referred to manuals such as that by Piacentini, Langley, & Roblek (2007).

Psychoeducation

Following a thorough assessment of a child's specific OCD symptoms (see Chapter 2 on assessment), children and parents are provided psychoeducation about OCD and ERP. OCD can be described as a faulty "fire alarm" that sends fear signals to the child's brain in the absence of threat; describing OCD as a problem in the brain helps to normalize the child's experience, to reduce any feelings of shame, and to reduce any blaming of the child. The therapist describes the OCD cycle, wherein compulsions offer short-term relief from anxiety caused by obsessions, but do not prevent obsessions for long, and maintain the cycle in the long-term. The therapist explains that children have the power to break this cycle by "fighting back against OCD," i.e., by not engaging in the compulsion.

The nature and rationale of ERP is described to the child and parent. Ensuring both the child and parent understand the rationale of ERP is especially important to increase buy-in and compliance, which predicts more successful treatment outcomes (Kircanski & Peris, 2015). Therapists underscore the importance of completing homework or "practice' in between sessions. Therapists may draw on analogies to how becoming skilled at a sport or at playing a musical instrument requires practice in between lessons; similarly, children must practice exposures in between sessions to become better at fighting back against OCD. The therapist describes their role as a "coach" who will guide the child through facing their fears in a systematic way. The therapist emphasizes that while the child will never be forced to do any specific exposure task, and that OCD will be fought at the child's pace, it is important to continue to move forward, no matter how small a "step" is taken.

Parents are actively involved in treatment from the outset. Therapists emphasize that parents are among the child's strongest allies in fighting back against OCD. In addition to receiving psychoeducation about their role in treatment as a "cheerleader" and "co-therapist," parents are provided psychoeducation about family accommodation. Family accommodation refers to behaviors that family members do (or avoid) for the purpose of alleviating their child's OCD-related distress. Common forms of family accommodation include providing reassurance, modifying family schedules or routines, facilitating avoidance behaviors, or participating in OCD rituals (e.g., washing dishes multiple times before a child with contamination fears eats his dinner). Family accommodation promotes avoidant coping among OCD youth and counteracts learning that takes place during ERP (Turner et al., 2018). The therapist normalizes that family accommodation is common among families of a child with OCD, but clearly explains how accommodation reinforces OCD in the long run. The therapist coaches family members in identifying and reducing accommodations throughout treatment. For best treatment outcomes, parents should be actively involved in treatment, unless contraindicated.

Monitoring

In the early stages of treatment before exposure exercises take place, the child and parent are instructed to monitor specific situations that trigger the child's OCD and the related obsession, compulsion, and outcome. This exercise increases the child's and parent's awareness of how the child's OCD manifests, impacts their daily life, and provides information about triggers later used to develop the child's exposure hierarchy. See Table 3.1 for an example of a completed OCD monitoring log.

Table 3.1 Sample OCD monitoring log for a 12-year-old male with OCD symptoms related to contamination, harm, and exactness/symmetry

Situation/trigger	Obsession	Fear thermometer rating (0–10)	Compulsion
Friday afternoon Touched a door handle to enter the waiting room at the doctor's office.	"I'm going to get the other patients' germs and get sick and die."	6	Cleaned my hands using mom's hand sanitizer.
Friday evening Mom served the family steak for dinner.	"I might act on an impulse and stab my brother with my steak knife."	8	Asked brother repeatedly if he was okay. Asked mom to cut my steak for me.
Saturday morning Saw dad cutting up fruit and then touch the plates while preparing breakfast.	"There could be pesticide on those plates that would make us all sick."	5	Re-washed all the plates that dad touched. Insisted that dad washes his hands for 1 minute.
Saturday evening My siblings borrowed my toys and placed them back on my shelf in the "wrong" spots.	"I can't rest easy until my toys are in the exact right spots."	4	Spent 30 minutes rearranging the toys so they were in the exact right spots.

Note: The "fear thermometer rating" column may be added once the child learns how to use the fear thermometer tool.

Cognitive Training

A brief module on cognitive training early in treatment can help prepare children for upcoming ERP exercises. Children are taught to externalize OCD. For younger children, it may help to describe OCD as a "bully" who "bosses around" the child, making them carry out compulsions. Children are then taught to "talk back" at OCD using phrases that do not necessarily argue with the content of the obsessions, but rather highlight the child's ability to resist compulsions (e.g., "I don't have to listen to you, OCD"). Children are also taught helpful self-talk to enhance coping during ERP exercises (e.g., "I can cope with OCD").

It is recommended that cognitive therapy modules are kept to a minimum in treating childhood OCD, and that more emphasis is placed on ERP. This is because if done incorrectly, cognitive restructuring as it is typically applied in anxiety or depressive disorders can serve the function of a self-reassuring mental compulsion (e.g., "Nothing bad will happen because my OCD is wrong"). This behavior can interfere with the learning process during ERP by distracting the child from fully engaging in the exposure exercise. Rather, cognitive approaches that emphasize the learning that occurs with exposures are indicated. For example, the therapist and child can discuss the expectancy the child has about what will happen if they do not engage in the ritual, followed by reinforcing what *actually* happened post-ERP task (i.e., the feared outcome did not occur).

Exposure and Response Prevention

Developing the Exposure Hierarchy

The exposure hierarchy (also referred to as a "symptom hierarchy" or "fear hierarchy") is a list of a child's obsession-triggering situations ordered from most distressing to least distressing. Within these situations, therapists and families also consider how to reduce, delay, or eventually eliminate compulsions within these exercises. Therapists may describe the exposure hierarchy as a ladder, to convey the idea that they will start with easier exposures and work their way up to more difficult exposures. Before hierarchy development, children are taught how to use the fear thermometer to describe how much distress a specific obsession would trigger. Therapists use a visual aid to explain the fear thermometer. While adults use a subjective units of distress scale of 0–100, children often use a simpler scale of 0 (no distress) to 10 (most intense distress experienced). For even younger children, the therapist may use drawings/emojis of facial expressions to represent distress levels. Children practice using the fear thermometer to describe their distress levels in various situations. It can be especially motivating if the therapist is able to bring "fun" into some of these exposure exercises, or to develop exposures that help a child reach their goals. For example, a child who has been avoiding playing baseball with their friends because of fears of contamination when on the fields may be especially motivated to do exposures that involve playing catch outside.

The child, parent (as appropriate) and therapist collaboratively map the child's OCD symptoms onto the exposure hierarchy. Imaginal exposures involve vividly imagining a feared scenario that triggers obsessions – through activities such as writing a story, reading a story, or drawing a picture – without engaging in compulsions. In vivo exposures involve encountering the feared situation without engaging in compulsions. Imaginal exposures are useful when the analogous in vivo exposure would be too distressing for the child to attempt at that point, or would be logistically or ethically impossible. Imaginal and in vivo exposures can also be combined (e.g., writing and reading a story about family members getting killed in a car accident – while sitting in a car). While it is important that the child contributes to the exposure hierarchy, the therapist ensures that a range of fear thermometer ratings are represented in the exposure hierarchy, and that the exposures are targeting the child's core OCD fear.

The exposure hierarchy is a "living document" that can be (and likely will be) adjusted throughout the course of treatment. For example, an exposure task that would have triggered a fear thermometer rating of 8 at the beginning of treatment may only trigger a 5 later in treatment, because the child's learning from other exposures has generalized across situations. Therapists should frequently revisit the exposure hierarchy with the child and parent and revise as appropriate (i.e., adjust ratings, remove tasks that no longer provoke distress, add additional tasks). By the end of treatment, one goal is for children and parents to be able to independently develop exposure exercises with relatively less therapist support. A fear hierarchy looks different for each individual child depending on their OCD presentation. See Tables 3.2 and 3.3 for sample hierarchies for ERP exercises for several presentations of OCD.

Table 3.2 Sample exposure hierarchy for a 14-year-old male with OCD symptoms related to symmetry and scrupulosity

Fear thermometer rating	Exposure task
10	Say, "Hail Satan" underneath my breath in a church, without reciting prayers or drawing a cross afterwards.
10	Say a curse word against God underneath my breath in a church, without reciting prayers or drawing a cross afterwards.
9	Say, "Hail Satan" in a church parking lot, without reciting prayers or drawing a cross afterwards.
9	Spit in a church parking lot, without reciting prayers or drawing a cross afterwards.
8	Write and read out loud a script about Satan and Satan worship, without reciting prayers or drawing a cross afterwards.
8	Watch the *South Park* movie depicting Satan and Saddam Hussain, without reciting prayers or drawing a cross during the movie.
8	Draw a pentagram without reciting prayers or drawing a cross afterwards.
7	Write down "666" without reciting prayers or drawing a cross afterwards.

(Continued)

Table 3.2 (Continued)

Fear thermometer rating	Exposure task
7	Go to bed without reading any passage from the Bible.
6	Read only one passage from the Bible before going to bed.
6	Look at a painting depicting hell without reciting any prayers.
5	Look at a painting depicting hell and recite only one prayer.
5	Sit on the left-side bench during Sunday services, instead of the central bench.
5	Re-order Bible and other biblical books on bedroom bookshelf in the incorrect order before going to church, *and* leave the house without fixing them.
4	Reorder non-biblical books on bedroom bookshelf in non-alphabetical order before going to school, *and* leave the house without fixing them.
4	Read only two passages from the Bible before going to bed.
4	Read a news article about a tragic death, without drawing a cross at all.
3	Read a news article about a tragic death, and draw a cross only once.
3	Wear uneven socks to Sunday morning services, without fixing them.

Table 3.3 Sample exposure hierarchy for a 7-year-old female with OCD symptoms related to contamination

Fear thermometer rating	Exposure task
10	Touch a toilet seat in a public restroom without washing hands afterwards.
10	Rub a cracker on a bathroom floor for five seconds and eat it, without rinsing mouth or washing hands afterwards.
9	Rub a cracker on the floor at therapist's office for five seconds and eat it, without rinsing mouth or washing hands afterwards.
9	Touch the floor in a public restroom without washing hands afterwards.
8	Stand next to the community garbage dump without washing hands or showering afterwards.
8	Rub a cracker on the living room floor for five seconds and eat it, without rinsing mouth or washing hands afterwards
7	Sit in a big hospital's waiting room without washing hands or showering afterwards.
7	Touch the toilet seat at home without washing hands afterwards.

(*Continued*)

Table 3.3 (Continued)

Fear thermometer rating	Exposure task
6	Rub a cracker on an uncleaned tabletop for five seconds and eat it without rinsing mouth or washing hands afterwards.
6	Sit in a small doctor's waiting room without washing hands or showering afterwards.
6	Touch the floor in the therapist's office without washing hands afterwards.
5	Touch the floor in the therapist's office and wash hands for only 10 seconds.
5	Watch a cartoon show clip about a girl who gets sick, without washing hands or showering afterwards.
5	Touch the living room floor without washing hands afterwards.
4	Touch the living room floor and wash hands for only 20 seconds.
4	Toss an uncleaned ball back and forth with siblings without washing hands afterwards
3	Toss an uncleaned ball back and forth with mom without washing hands afterwards

Preparing for the First In-Session Exposure Task

Before starting the first exposure exercise, the therapist lays the groundwork to set the child up for success. This includes reviewing the cognitive skills learned so far, such as externalizing OCD, talking back at OCD, and using encouraging self-talk. The therapist explains to the child and parent each step of the exposure exercise. Whilst the child is given reasonable autonomy in choosing an exposure task, the therapist should make sure the first task is one that the therapist is reasonably confident the child can handle, because this mastery experience will build confidence for future exposures. The therapist also discusses with the child what the child expects will happen, as a "scientist" would generate a hypothesis before an experiment. This prediction will be revisited after the exposure when the child and therapist process what the child has learned.

Facilitating the Exposure Task

In coaching the child through the exposure task, the therapist also models for the parent how to facilitate between-session exposures at home. In addition to asking for the recording of the child's fear thermometer ratings every 1–2 minutes, the therapist may also ask the child to identify OCD thoughts and guide them in talking back at OCD. The therapist must pay close attention to the child to ensure they are not engaging in overt *or* covert compulsions. A child may engage in covert compulsions such as mentally reassuring themselves (e.g., "Nothing bad is going to happen"), distracting themselves (e.g., thinking about something else), or carrying out other mental compulsions (e.g., prayer, repeated phrases). If such covert compulsions are suspected, the therapist asks the child and encourages the child to replace this with other thoughts that are more consistent with ERP learning (e.g., "I may or may not get sick," "I choose to not listen to my OCD," "I can cope with OCD.") In a habituation-based framework, a "rule-of-thumb" is for the therapist to end the exposure task when the child's fear thermometer ratings have decreased by at least 50 percent. In an inhibitory learning framework, the therapist may end the exposure task once the child's expectancy has been violated or simply when the goal for the exposure has been met (e.g., leaving five different picture frames crooked).

Debriefing After the Exposure Task

After the exposure task, the therapist debriefs with the child and parent. The therapist asks the child to report on what happened, in terms of the observable outcome of the task and the progression of the fear thermometer ratings. The therapist shows the child a graph of their fear thermometer ratings recorded during the exposure. This processing is important to ensure the child learns that the feared outcome did not occur, *and* that the child is capable of coping with the distress, which eventually declined. It is also important for the child to not engage in compulsions after leaving the session; parents are instructed to monitor for this. This is another reason within-session habituation can be valuable to the success of exposure (i.e., once a child habituates, they are less likely to "undo" the exposure by engaging in compulsions).

Assigning Out-of-Session Exposure Homework

The therapist assigns out-of-session exposure tasks as homework or "practice." Ideally, the child completes this exposure at least once in-session before it is assigned as homework (Abramowitz, Deacon, & Whiteside, 2019). Out-of-session exposure homework should be completed at least once daily. Therapists must emphasize the importance of homework compliance, and parents are given instructions on their role in facilitating exposures. In their co-therapist role, they will guide the child through the exposure by ensuring compliance, asking for fear thermometer ratings, asking what OCD is saying, coaching the child in talking back at OCD, continuing this until fear thermometer ratings decrease by at least 50 percent, and rewarding the child for completing the task.

Implementing Reward Systems

While parental praise is among the most powerful of rewards for children, systematic reward systems are also developed to maximize child compliance and engagement. Children earn a number of points per exposure task completed, and these points can be "cashed out" for certain rewards. For younger children, points can be gathered in the form of tangible objects, such as "tokens" or "bravery bucks." For older children, keeping a written record of points collected is usually sufficient. For adolescents, monetary compensation may be more motivating. Regardless of what system is chosen, the number of points or compensation earned can be scaled based on the difficulty level of the exposure task. Small rewards that can be earned in the short term are generally recommended over long-term rewards. Parents should immediately and consistently award points (or compensation) after an exposure task is complete. See Table 3.4 for a sample reward system.

Table 3.4 Sample reward system for a 7-year-old female with OCD symptoms related to contamination

Exposure-to-points conversion table	
Exposure task	*Points awarded*
Sit in a big hospital's waiting room for 10 minutes without changing clothes afterwards	8 bravery bucks
Place a cracker on the table for five seconds and eat it without rinsing mouth afterwards.	5 bravery bucks
Read a passage from a book about a girl who gets sick without washing hands afterwards.	2 bravery bucks

Points-to-reward conversion table	
Cost	*Reward*
15 bravery bucks	Family movie night
10 bravery bucks	A trip to the nearby ice cream store
3 bravery bucks	One small toy from a prize box

Note: Examples may be part of a larger hierarchy and rewards list.

For older adolescents, external reward systems may be unnecessary. In such cases, internal motivation is emphasized over external motivation. This includes discussing the adolescent's values and how completing exposure tasks is helping them come closer to the life they want. For example, for an adolescent with harm-related OCD whose fear of hurting others has interfered with their social life and extracurricular activities, knowing that doing exposures will help them overcome OCD and resume these pursuits may be motivation enough.

Progression of Exposures Throughout Treatment

After the first exposure session, each session thereafter follows a similar structure: checking in, reviewing homework, adjusting the exposure hierarchy if needed, choosing and conducting a new in-session exposure, selecting at-home exposure homework, and wrapping up. Unless contraindicated, parents are encouraged to be present at every session. Reviewing homework completion at the beginning of every session highlights the importance of homework compliance. This also provides the opportunity for the therapist to identify challenges with between-session exposure completion, such as non-compliance or engagement in compulsions. If non-compliance is an issue, the therapist takes steps to ensure that both child and parent understand the rationale of ERP, assess motivation, collaboratively problem-solve logistical barriers, and assess if the reward system in place is sufficient. If the child struggles to resist compulsions during at-home ERP tasks, the therapist may review skills learned in therapy to help resist compulsions or adjust the exposure task.

As with the first exposure task, the child is encouraged to choose which exposure tasks to tackle next. While it is common in the habituation-based framework to systematically move up the exposure hierarchy in a graduated manner, doing so it not required. In fact, the inhibitory model of learning proposes that flexibly moving between exposures of varying difficulty levels may accelerate generalization and learning (Craske et al., 2014), assuming the child is willing to do so. For children who are reluctant to attempt more difficult exposures, progressing from easier to more difficult exposures may be more palatable and ensure continued engagement.

Maintenance, Relapse Prevention, and Termination

Termination is considered when children are able to use ERP skills consistently to face OCD triggers on their own in daily life across diverse contexts. To maintain gains obtained during treatment, children are encouraged to live a "bring-it-on lifestyle," wherein day-to-day challenges are treated as opportunities to approach important pursuits without being "bossed around" by OCD. Relapse prevention is discussed. The therapist pre-emptively normalizes the experience of relapse and discusses with the child and parent how they would use ERP skills to handle such a relapse. Booster sessions may also be scheduled at increasingly long intervals.

Treatment Adaptations

ERP has been adapted for several specific populations and delivery formats. ERP for very young children aged 8 and under differs from ERP for older children in that family involvement is essential (with caregivers being the primary driver of treatment), cognitive components are further reduced, and parent behavioral training is incorporated to address common comorbidities in this age group (e.g., tic disorders, learning disabilities) (Flessner, Garcia, & Freeman, 2013). ERP has also been adapted to parent-only formats. Parent-only CBT for childhood OCD typically focuses on providing psychoeducation about OCD and family accommodation, and also coaching the parent in reducing family accommodation (Lebowitz et al., 2020), as well as teaching the parent to help their child externalize OCD, facilitate ERP exercises, and implement contingency management plans (Rosa-Alcázar et al., 2017). A preliminary study comparing parent-only CBT and family-based CBT for 4–8 year-olds with OCD found that both treatment programs showed clinically significant improvements (Rosa-Alcázar et al., 2017). Parent-only ERP may be useful in cases where a child is too young or unwilling to engage in therapy.

Barriers to Successful Treatment Outcomes

Although ERP is efficacious in treating childhood OCD, several clinician and client factors can inhibit successful treatment outcomes. Below, several of the most significant barriers to successful implementation of ERP for childhood OCD are discussed.

Clinician Factors

One factor that prevents therapists from using ERP is that of misconceptions about ERP generally and exposures specifically. A survey of clinicians who treat children with anxiety disorders (including OCD) revealed that many of them held unsubstantiated negative beliefs about the safety, tolerability, and ethicality of ERP (Whiteside et al., 2016). Such misconceptions about ERP may also lead therapists to encourage the use of ineffective strategies, such as relaxation strategies, thought stopping, or distraction. Not only are such techniques ineffective in treating OCD, but they are also detrimental to successful OCD treatment outcomes because they prevent habituation and promote avoidance (Keleher, Jassi, & Krebs, 2020).

Clinician misconceptions regarding logistical aspects of ERP also prevent clinicians from using ERP. For instance, many clinicians believe that exposure sessions need to be 90–120 minutes, although exposures can be effective in sessions of 50–60 minutes (Reid et al., 2017). Lack of adequate training in ERP remains a substantial barrier to clinicians successfully providing ERP treatment for children with OCD. However, didactic training can correct clinicians' misconceptions about ERP (Farrell et al., 2016). Finally, clinicians' own level of comfort with discussing and treating certain "taboo" topics may contribute to hesitancy in conducting ERP for child OCD obsessions related to aggression, sexuality, or religion (Keleher, Jassi, & Krebs, 2020).

Patient factors

Several patient-related factors can also impact treatment outcomes. First, continued family accommodation can limit the success of treatment. If families continue to accommodate children's OCD rituals, ritual prevention is not occurring in all areas of the child's life, which leads to less robust effects of ERP. Reducing family accommodation is associated with more successful clinical outcomes for children with OCD (Merlo et al., 2009). See Chapters 6 and 7 for more information on parent- and family-enhanced versions of treatment.

Greater OCD symptom severity and related impairment are also associated with poorer response to treatment (Turner et al., 2018). Increased severity in OCD symptoms requires more treatment and doses of exposure to result in successful outcomes. Sustaining motivation, treatment adherence, and exposure completion required for symptom improvement can be difficult in severe presentations. More intensive treatment options, such as residential treatment or the addition of medication, may be needed for treatment success. See Chapters 8 and 11 for more information about intensive treatment and pharmacotherapy, respectively.

Children's level of insight into their OCD symptoms can impact treatment response. If insight decreases as treatment progresses, responses to treatment can be negatively impacted (Selles et al., 2020). Additionally, lower levels of insight make it difficult to assess symptoms and identify areas to target (Keleher, Jassi, & Krebs, 2020). Children with lower insight may have difficulty identifying and communicating obsessions and compulsions, which adds an additional barrier to successful treatment (Keleher, Jassi, & Krebs, 2020). Mental compulsions or other covert compulsions may be particularly difficult for therapists to detect during exposures without the child's insight and cooperation. Limited recognition of impairment caused by OCD is also associated with poorer treatment response (Selles et al., 2020), which may explained by lower motivation to engage in ERP.

The presence of a greater number of comorbid mental health disorders is associated with poorer treatment outcomes (Storch et al., 2008). Children with OCD frequently have comorbid attention deficit/hyperactivity disorder (ADHD), disruptive behavior disorders, or major depressive disorder (MDD), all of which are associated with poorer treatment response (Storch et al., 2008). Specifically, comorbid ADHD interferes with ERP effectiveness by reducing attention to the ERP trigger, which prevents successful habituation. Children with disruptive behavior disorders may resist engaging in treatment or resist the therapist's requests. Session time may be spent responding to disruptive behaviors, which detracts from time completing exposures, and results in decreased treatment efficacy. Finally, children with comorbid MDD may experience hopelessness about getting better, which translates to lower motivation to engage in treatment, and greater discouragement in response to relatively normal treatment setbacks.

Individual patient factors also serve as predictors and moderators for successful treatment outcomes. A family history of OCD moderates the effectiveness of CBT interventions, wherein children with a family history of OCD may show poorer treatment outcomes (Turner et al., 2018). Older age also predicts less successful response to treatment (Selles et al., 2020; Turner et al., 2018). Patient decisions related to therapy involvement – e.g., less time spent in therapy, early discontinuation of therapy – also lower effectiveness of treatment (McGuire et al., 2015).

Empirical Support

Research consistently finds that ERP is the most efficacious and effective treatment for childhood OCD (Abramowitz et al., 2018; McGuire et al., 2015). Research studies report that ERP is more effective than other psychological interventions alone or medication alone, and that ERP combined with serotonin re-uptake inhibitors (SRIs) is more effective than either option alone (Abramowitz et al., 2018). For mild to severe cases of childhood OCD, treatments combining ERP and SSRIs are efficacious. Additionally, reductions in symptoms and other treatment benefits are maintained for up to seven years following ERP (McGuire et al., 2015). Importantly, ERP receives the strongest empirical support as the key active ingredient that explains improvements in OCD outcomes, compared to other components of CBT (Abramowitz et al., 2018).

Research supports the uniquely important role that parents play in childhood OCD presentation and treatment (Lebowitz et al., 2020; McGrath &

Abbott, 2019). Parental behaviors, such as accommodation and excessive reassurance, maintain OCD symptoms in children. Meta-analyses indicate that accommodation is the most common family behavior identified and targeted in treatment because it pervades the family system and is antithetical to the principles of ERP (McGrath & Abbott, 2019). Addressing family factors, including accommodation, are a potential mechanism for change in treatment of childhood OCD (McGrath & Abbott, 2019). In line with this finding, parent training interventions and parental involvement in ERP significantly reduce family accommodation and child OCD symptom severity (Dekel et al., 2021).

Parent training is a promising alternative to traditional ERP for children with OCD (Dekel et al., 2021). Supportive Parenting for Anxious Childhood Emotions (SPACE) (Lebowitz et al., 2020) is an example of a parent-based treatment. SPACE is non-inferior to ERP in terms of treatment outcomes, and thus may be an alternative treatment option for childhood OCD and other anxiety disorders (Lebowitz et al., 2020). SPACE has also been adapted to a group parent format (Dekel et al., 2021). At post-treatment, parents who completed SPACE reported significant decreases in parental accommodation behaviors, child OCD symptom severity, and other child anxiety symptoms (Dekel et al., 2021; McGrath & Abbott, 2019). Moreover, meta-analyses indicate that reductions in parental accommodation and child OCD symptoms are maintained several years after completing SPACE (McGrath & Abbott, 2019).

While extensive research has been conducted on the efficacy of ERP for childhood OCD, several areas need to be examined in future research. First, the majority of clinical trials testing the efficacy of ERP for childhood OCD have been conducted in relatively controlled settings (e.g., university-based research clinics), which may limit generalizability to other settings. Additional research on the effectiveness of ERP in community-based settings, and specific barriers to successful outcomes in such settings, is needed. Second, although a majority of youth with OCD respond to ERP, approximately 30–43 percent continue to struggle with OCD after a full course a ERP (McGuire et al., 2015) due to factors such as family dynamics, comorbidity, symptom presentation, or developmental barriers (Storch et al., 2010). Further research is needed to understand how to improve treatment for non-responders, such as supplementing ERP with additional psychological interventions or interdisciplinary services. Third, there is a continued need for effective, widespread dissemination of evidence-based ERP interventions for childhood OCD, in light of limited access to care among many children with OCD and their families. Additional research testing the efficacy of low-cost, scalable adaptations of ERP for childhood OCD (e.g., internet-delivered, self-guided programs) is needed.

Summary

ERP is the gold-standard psychosocial intervention for childhood OCD, and is recommended as first-line intervention for mild to moderate OCD (Geller et al., 2012). ERP is derived from theoretical foundations of cognitive and behavioral models of OCD. Depending on a child's OCD symptom severity and level of functional impairment, ERP can be delivered in one of several treatment formats, including weekly outpatient therapy, web-based therapy, intensive outpatient treatment, and residential treatment. At its core, the central treatment component of ERP is exposure, though this approach also includes psychoeducation, cognitive training, and relapse prevention, with a heavy emphasis on parental involvement throughout treatment. While common barriers to treatment success have been identified, future work is needed to better understand outcomes of ERP in community settings, as well as testing adaptations of ERP to increase effectiveness and dissemination.

References

Abramowitz, J.S., Blakey, S.M., Reuman, L., & Buchholz, J.L. (2018). New directions in the cognitive-behavioral treatment of OCD: Theory, research, and practice. *Behavior Therapy*, 49(3), 311–322.

Abramowitz, J.S., Deacon, B.J., & Whiteside, S.P. (2019). *Exposure therapy for anxiety: Principles and practice*. Guilford Publications.

Barrett, P.M., & Healy, L.J. (2003). An examination of the cognitive processes involved in childhood obsessive-compulsive disorder. *Behaviour Research and Therapy*, 41(3), 285–299.

Boger, K., Sperling, J., Potter, M., & Gallo, K.P. (2016). Treatment overview of an intensive group outpatient cognitive-behavioral therapy for youth anxiety disorders and obsessive-compulsive disorder. *Evidence-Based Practice in Child and Adolescent Mental Health*, 1(2–3), 116–125.

Coles, M.E., Wolters, L.H., Sochting, I., De Haan, E., Pietrefesa, A.S., & Whiteside, S.P. (2010). Development and initial validation of the Obsessive Belief Questionnaire – Child Version (OBQ-CV). *Depression and Anxiety*, 27(10), 982–991.

Comer, J.S., Furr, J.M., Kerns, C.E., Miguel, E., Coxe, S., Elkins, R.M., Carpenter, A.L., Cornacchio, D., Cooper-Vince, C.E., DeSerisy, M., & others. (2017). Internet-delivered, family-based treatment for early-onset OCD: A pilot randomized trial. *Journal of Consulting and Clinical Psychology*, 85(2), 178.

Craske, M.G., Treanor, M., Conway, C.C., Zbozinek, T., & Vervliet, B. (2014). Maximizing exposure therapy: An inhibitory learning approach. *Behaviour Research and Therapy*, 58, 10–23.

Dekel, I., Dorman-Ilan, S., Lang, C., Bar-David, E., Zilka, H., Shilton, T., Lebowitz, E.R., & Gothelf, D. (2021). The feasibility of a parent group treatment for youth with anxiety disorders and obsessive compulsive disorder. *Child Psychiatry & Human Development*, 52, 1044–1049.

Farrell, N.R., Kemp, J.J., Blakey, S.M., Meyer, J.M., & Deacon, B.J. (2016). Targeting clinician concerns about exposure therapy: A pilot study comparing standard vs enhanced training. *Behaviour Research and Therapy*, 85, 53–59.

Flessner, C.A., Garcia, A., & Freeman, J. B. (2013). Treating obsessive-compulsive disorder in the very young child. In E.A. Storch & D. McKay (Eds.), *Handbook of Treating Variants and Complications in Anxiety Disorders* (pp. 125–134). Springer.

Freeman, J., Benito, K., Herren, J., Kemp, J., Sung, J., Georgiadis, C., Arora, A., Walther, M., & Garcia, A. (2018). Evidence base update of psychosocial treatments for pediatric obsessive-compulsive disorder: Evaluating, improving, and transporting what works. *Journal of Clinical Child & Adolescent Psychology*, 47(5), 669–698.

Geller, D.A., March, J., & others. (2012). Practice parameter for the assessment and treatment of children and adolescents with obsessive-compulsive disorder. *Journal of the American Academy of Child & Adolescent Psychiatry*, 51(1), 98–113.

Guzick, A.G., Reid, A.M., Balkhi, A.M., Geffken, G.R., & McNamara, J.P. (2020). That was easy! Expectancy violations during exposure and response prevention for childhood obsessive-compulsive disorder. *Behavior Modification*, 44(3), 319–342.

Herbst, N., Voderholzer, U., Stelzer, N., Knaevelsrud, C., Hertenstein, E., Schlegl, S., Nissen, C., & Külz, A.K. (2012). The potential of telemental health applications for obsessive-compulsive disorder. *Clinical Psychology Review*, 32(6), 454–466.

Keleher, J., Jassi, A., & Krebs, G. (2020). Clinician-reported barriers to using exposure with response prevention in the treatment of paediatric obsessive-compulsive disorder. *Journal of Obsessive-Compulsive and Related Disorders*, 24, 100498.

Kircanski, K., & Peris, T.S. (2015). Exposure and response prevention process predicts treatment outcome in youth with OCD. *Journal of Abnormal Child Psychology*, 43, 543–552.

Kircanski, K., Peris, T.S., & Piacentini, J.C. (2011). Cognitive-behavioral therapy for obsessive-compulsive disorder in children and adolescents. *Child and Adolescent Psychiatric Clinics*, 20(2), 239–254.

Lebowitz, E.R., Marin, C., Martino, A., Shimshoni, Y., & Silverman, W.K. (2020). Parent-based treatment as efficacious as cognitive-behavioral therapy for childhood anxiety: A randomized noninferiority study of supportive parenting for anxious childhood emotions. *Journal of the American Academy of Child & Adolescent Psychiatry*, 59(3), 362–372.

Leonard, R.C., Franklin, M.E., Wetterneck, C.T., Riemann, B.C., Simpson, H.B., Kinnear, K., Cahill, S.P., & Lake, P.M. (2016). Residential treatment outcomes for adolescents with obsessive-compulsive disorder. *Psychotherapy Research*, 26(6), 727–736.

March, J.S., & Mulle, K. (1998). *OCD in children and adolescents: A cognitive-behavioral treatment manual.* Guilford Press.

McGrath, C.A., & Abbott, M.J. (2019). Family-based psychological treatment for obsessive compulsive disorder in children and adolescents: A meta-analysis and systematic review. *Clinical Child and Family Psychology Review*, 22, 478–501.

McGuire, J.F., Piacentini, J., Lewin, A.B., Brennan, E.A., Murphy, T.K., & Storch, E.A. (2015). A meta-analysis of cognitive behavior therapy and medication for child obsessive-compulsive disorder: Moderators of treatment efficacy, response, and remission. *Depression and Anxiety*, 32(8), 580–593. https://doi.org/10.1002/da.22389.

McGuire, J.F., & Storch, E.A. (2019). An inhibitory learning approach to cognitive-behavioral therapy for children and adolescents. *Cognitive and Behavioral Practice, 26*(1), 214–224.

Merlo, L.J., Lehmkuhl, H.D., Geffken, G.R., & Storch, E.A. (2009). Decreased family accommodation associated with improved therapy outcome in pediatric obsessive-compulsive disorder. *Journal of Consulting and Clinical Psychology, 77*(2), 355.

Mowrer, O. (1960). *Learning theory and behavior.* John Wiley & Sons.

Obsessive Compulsive Cognitions Working Group. (2005). Psychometric validation of the obsessive belief questionnaire and interpretation of intrusions inventory – Part 2: Factor analyses and testing of a brief version. *Behaviour Research and Therapy, 43*(11), 1527–1542.

Piacentini, J., Langley, A., & Roblek, T. (2007). *Cognitive behavioral treatment of childhood OCD: It's only a false alarm therapist guide.* Oxford University Press.

Rachman, S. (1998). A cognitive theory of obsessions. In *Behavior and cognitive therapy today* (pp. 209–222). Elsevier.

Reid, A.M., Bolshakova, M.I., Guzick, A.G., Fernandez, A.G., Striley, C.W., Geffken, G.R., & McNamara, J.P. (2017). Common barriers to the dissemination of exposure therapy for youth with anxiety disorders. *Community Mental Health Journal, 53,* 432–437.

Rosa-Alcázar, A.I., Iniesta-Sepúlveda, M., Storch, E.A., Rosa-Alcázar, Á., Parada-Navas, J.L., & Rodríguez, J.O. (2017). A preliminary study of cognitive-behavioral family-based treatment versus parent training for young children with obsessive-compulsive disorder. *Journal of Affective Disorders, 208,* 265–271.

Schuyler, M., & Geller, D.A. (2023). Childhood obsessive-compulsive disorder. *Psychiatric Clinics, 46*(1), 89–106.

Selles, R.R., Højgaard, D.R., Ivarsson, T., Thomsen, P.H., McBride, N.M., Storch, E.A., Geller, D., Wilhelm, S., Farrell, L.J., Waters, A.M., & others. (2020). Avoidance, insight, impairment recognition concordance, and cognitive-behavioral therapy outcomes in pediatric obsessive-compulsive disorder. *Journal of the American Academy of Child & Adolescent Psychiatry, 59*(5), 650–659.

Sperling, J., Boger, K., & Potter, M. (2020). The impact of intensive treatment for pediatric anxiety and obsessive-compulsive disorder on daily functioning. *Clinical Child Psychology and Psychiatry, 25*(1), 133–140.

Storch, E.A., Björgvinsson, T., Riemann, B., Lewin, A.B., Morales, M.J., & Murphy, T.K. (2010). Factors associated with poor response in cognitive-behavioral therapy for pediatric obsessive-compulsive disorder. *Bulletin of the Menninger Clinic, 74*(2), 167–185.

Storch, E.A., Caporino, N.E., Morgan, J.R., Lewin, A.B., Rojas, A., Brauer, L., Larson, M.J., & Murphy, T.K. (2011). Preliminary investigation of web-camera delivered cognitive-behavioral therapy for youth with obsessive-compulsive disorder. *Psychiatry Research, 189*(3), 407–412.

Storch, E.A., Geffken, G.R., Merlo, L.J., Mann, G., Duke, D., Munson, M., Adkins, J., Grabill, K.M., Murphy, T.K., & Goodman, W.K. (2007). Family-based cognitive-behavioral therapy for pediatric obsessive-compulsive disorder: Comparison of intensive and weekly approaches. *Journal of the American Academy of Child & Adolescent Psychiatry, 46*(4), 469–478.

Storch, E.A., Merlo, L.J., Larson, M.J., Geffken, G.R., Lehmkuhl, H.D., Jacob, M.L., Murphy, T.K., & Goodman, W.K. (2008). Impact of comorbidity on cognitive-behavioral therapy response in pediatric obsessive-compulsive disorder. *Journal of the American Academy of Child & Adolescent Psychiatry, 47*(5), 583–592.

Torp, N.C., Weidle, B., Thomsen, P.H., Skarphedinsson, G., Aalberg, M., Nissen, J.B., Melin, K.H., Dahl, K., Valderhaug, R., & Ivarsson, T. (2019). Is it time to rethink standard dosage of exposure-based cognitive behavioral therapy for pediatric obsessive-compulsive disorder? *Psychiatry Research, 281*, 112600.

Turner, C., O'Gorman, B., Nair, A., & O'Kearney, R. (2018). Moderators and predictors of response to cognitive behaviour therapy for pediatric obsessive-compulsive disorder: A systematic review. *Psychiatry Research, 261*, 50–60.

Whiteside, S.P., Deacon, B.J., Benito, K., & Stewart, E. (2016). Factors associated with practitioners' use of exposure therapy for childhood anxiety disorders. *Journal of Anxiety Disorders, 40*, 29–36.

Whiteside, S.P., McKay, D., De Nadai, A.S., Tiede, M.S., Ale, C.M., & Storch, E.A. (2014). A baseline controlled examination of a 5-day intensive treatment for pediatric obsessive-compulsive disorder. *Psychiatry Research, 220*(1–2), 441–446.

Wiese, A.D., Drummond, K.N., Fuselier, M.N., Sheu, J.C., Liu, G., Guzick, A.G., Goodman, W.K., & Storch, E.A. (2022). Provider perceptions of telehealth and in-person exposure and response prevention for obsessive–compulsive disorder. *Psychiatry Research, 313*, 114610.

Wolters, L., Prins, P.J., Garst, G., Hogendoorn, S.M., Boer, F., Vervoort, L., & de Haan, E. (2019). Mediating mechanisms in cognitive behavioral therapy for childhood OCD: The role of dysfunctional beliefs. *Child Psychiatry & Human Development, 50*, 173–185.

Ye, H.J., Rice, K.G., & Storch, E.A. (2008). Perfectionism and peer relations among children with obsessive-compulsive disorder. *Child Psychiatry and Human Development, 39*, 415–426.

4 Cognitive Behavioral Therapy for Adolescent Body Dysmorphic Disorder

*Fanny Alexandra Dietel[1] and
Berta Jane Summers[2]*

[1] *Department of Clinical Psychology and Psychotherapy,
University of Osnabrüeck, Osnabrück, Germany*

[2] *Department of Psychiatry, Massachusetts General Hospital/
Harvard Medical School, Boston, MA*

Introduction

Body dysmorphic disorder (BDD) is a severe mental disorder that most often onsets before the age of 18 years (Bjornsson et al., 2013), yet often remains underrecognized and untreated in this age period. Whilst much of the research examining the efficacy of cognitive behavioral therapy (CBT) for BDD has been conducted in adults, the core principles have been successfully adapted for use in adolescence (Greenberg, Mothi, & Wilhelm, 2016; Krebs et al., 2017; Mataix-Cols et al., 2015). In this chapter, we provide an empirical overview of CBT for adolescent BDD. Further, developmental considerations, caregiver involvement, barriers to treatment, and emerging treatment strategies, such as digital programs, are discussed.

Core components of Cognitive Behavioral Therapy for adolescent Body Dysmorphic Disorder

At its core, CBT for adolescent BDD aims to modify maintaining processes that are specified in the cognitive behavioral model of BDD (Wilhelm, Phillips, & Steketee, 2013; Fang & Wilhelm, 2015). As per this model, ordinary appearance-related thoughts (e.g. "I have blemishes on my forehead.") are exacerbated through various cognitive biases (e.g., perceptual and attentional, like overfocus on unattractive features; or interpretational, like self-defeating cognitions), leading to negative emotions (e.g., anxiety, disgust, shame) that individuals seek to reduce through time-consuming maladaptive behaviors, i.e., safety, ritualized or avoidance behaviors (e.g., extensive mirror checking, grooming, social withdrawal). While these behaviors may lower negative affect in the short term, they maintain the

DOI: 10.4324/9781003386278-4

disorder in the long term as they prevent disconfirmation of underlying core beliefs (e.g., related to perfectionism or low self-esteem) that, in turn, fuel cognitive biases.

This vicious cycle is further embedded within a set of predisposing factors, i.e., overarching sociocultural, developmental, biological, and personality factors. In this respect, some developmentally sensitive topics for adolescent BDD may emerge as recurring foci during treatment. During adolescence, parental and peer influence, such as perceived pressures about and the importance of appearance (e.g., Densham et al., 2017), are typically pronounced. Relatedly, certain family dynamics, including family accommodation of symptoms (van Noppen & Sassano-Higgins, 2017) might further contribute to disorder maintenance, highlighting the need to involve caregivers in treatment, particularly with younger adolescents. Lastly, the pervasive nature of smartphone use among adolescents brings to light the detrimental impact of social media on internalization of body ideals, social comparisons, and body image (Rodgers, 2016). High exposure to these risk factors provides fertile ground for the emergence of BDD symptoms in this vulnerable population.

The Initial Phase of Treatment

Diagnostic and Symptom Assessment

Adolescence is a developmental stage characterized by numerous hormonal, physiological, social, and identity changes (Pfeifer & Berkman, 2018). As such, adolescents who express preoccupations with their appearance should be assessed for BDD by a trained therapist who is able to consider this population's unique characteristics. While there are no diagnostic procedures exclusively designed for adolescents, self-report measures, clinical interviews, and therapist-administered assessments can be utilized to evaluate BDD symptoms.

Shame about their appearance concerns can make adolescents reluctant to disclose the extent of their symptoms (Weingarden & Renshaw, 2015). Thus, cross-informant assessment can be useful for gathering details about the adolescent's engagement in BDD rituals, avoidance of school or social activities, and family accommodation of symptoms. Teachers or guidance counselors can also offer insights into school-related interference and social disengagement associated with BDD. Screening and self-report tools can be used to assess domains of BDD, including appearance preoccupations, distress, and functional impairment. Examples include the Body Dysmorphic Disorder Questionnaire–Adolescent Version (BDDQ-A) (Phillips, 1996) and the Dysmorphic Concerns Questionnaire (DCQ) (Oosthuizen, Lambert, & Castle, 1998).

Diagnostic precision requires the ability to differentiate BDD from other psychiatric disorders that share phenomenological similarities with BDD, such as obsessive-compulsive disorder, social anxiety disorder, and eating disorders. Thus, when assessing an adolescent for BDD, therapists should take care to understand the predominant preoccupations, fears, and behavioral symptom expressions to rule out other possible diagnoses. Structured diagnostic interviews, such as the BDD module of the Structured Clinical Interview for DSM-5 (*Diagnostic and Statistical Manual of Mental Disorders*, 5th edition) (SCID-5) (First & Williams, 2015) or the Body Dysmorphic Disorder Examination (BDDE) (Rosen & Reiter, 1996), can be used to establish a DSM-5 diagnosis; though it is noted that these interviews have largely been validated in adult samples. More comprehensive evaluations of BDD symptoms, severity, and insight can be achieved through the following measures, respectively: the BDD – Symptom Scale (BDD-SS) (Wilhelm et al., 2016), the Yale-Brown Obsessive Compulsive Scale Modified for BDD – Adolescent Version (BDD-YBOCS-A) (Phillips et al., 1997), and the Brown Assessment of Beliefs Scale – Adolescent Version (BABS) (Eisen et al., 1998). Each of these measures is sensitive to change and thus can be used to monitor improvement in treatment.

Once a BDD diagnosis has been established, initial sessions with an adolescent patient should aim to build rapport and set the stage for an effective course of CBT. Importantly, adolescents with BDD often do not present for treatment voluntarily but are instead brought to treatment following a teacher's or caregiver's concern about an observed shift in their mood or withdrawal from their social or school activities. Although their family might be eager for support, youth with BDD often do not believe psychotherapy will help them, as they tend to view their appearance concern as a physical issue, rather than a psychological disorder. Thus, therapists should seek to make treatment feel engaging and meaningful for adolescents in order to enhance the benefits. Early sessions are dedicated to rapport building, educating the adolescent and their support system about BDD and the goals of CBT, and exploring the youth's personal motivation for participating in treatment.

Motivational Enhancement

Motivational interviewing (MI) (Miller & Rollnick, 2002) techniques can be used to explore ambivalence about CBT collaboratively. Central to MI is the cultivation of a non-judgmental therapeutic environment, wherein the therapist skillfully guides the patient in exploring their willingness and readiness to embrace change. Importantly, it is more beneficial to concentrate on the impact that appearance concerns have on the individual's life, rather than debating the legitimacy of the young person's perception. The therapist can use Socratic questioning to guide the patient to consider the potential benefits of committing to the treatment while also recognizing challenges that may arise in the process. For instance, a therapist can invite the patient to explore their motivations for seeking treatment by discussing what matters most to them (e.g., *"What are some things you really care about or wish you could do more?"*). They might also examine ways in which the patient's symptoms negatively affect their daily lives or choices (e.g., *"How do your appearance concerns impact the way you spend your time?"*; *"How do appearance worries get in the way of doing things you love?"*). Further, the therapist can elicit the adolescent's perspective about what therapy could offer them (e.g., *"If your concerns were less overwhelming and didn't take up so much time and energy, what other things would you be able to focus on or enjoy in your life?"*; *"How might that impact your mood and well-being?"*).

Acknowledging ambivalence about treatment and empathizing with the distress caused by BDD helps to build trust and create a safe space for the adolescent to express their concerns. This conversation helps to elicit "change talk" (i.e., the patient's personal reasons for wanting their circumstances to change) and helps cultivate a positive therapeutic alliance, which is associated with better treatment adherence, engagement, and symptom improvement (Wilhelm, Phillips, & Steketee, 2013). It is often necessary to revisit MI strategies throughout treatment.

Psychoeducation

The psychoeducation phase of treatment is an opportunity for the therapist to provide clear information about BDD, normalize the adolescent's symptom experience, address stigma or any misconceptions, demonstrate confidence in CBT, and promote hope and active participation in the treatment process. Information about the prevalence of BDD in adolescence (1–2 percent) (Enander et al., 2018) can help to mitigate feelings of isolation and shame. It is also important to explain that the perception of appearance in BDD is not an accurate reflection of objective reality but rather a manifestation of the disorder itself – in which perceived flaws are amplified while positive aspects are diminished (Veale, 2004). Indeed, individuals with BDD process their appearance differently than those without BDD, such that they do not typically view their body holistically and instead hyperfixate on minute features (Deckersbach et al., 2000; Feusner et al., 2007; 2010). A therapist may introduce this topic by saying, *"Sometimes overly focusing on one thing can make it hard for us to see things accurately. Imagine you're looking at a beautiful painting, but your brain zooms in on one tiny imperfection and then can't focus on anything else. This is something that happens with BDD, it makes it difficult to see the whole picture."*

A therapist can teach the patient about BDD while simultaneously onboarding them to the rationale for CBT by using the cognitive behavioral model of BDD to guide discussions about biopsychosocial factors that likely contributed to the development and maintenance of the patient's personal experience of BDD (Veale, 2004; Wilhelm, Phillips, & Steketee, 2013). Acknowledgment of contributing factors that are outside of the adolescent's control (e.g., genetics, early life experiences, societal messages about beauty ideals, etc.) can help to mitigate shame and self-blame. Conversely, the adolescent's *agency* over BDD can be highlighted through the collaborative identification of current cognitive behavioral treatment targets. For instance, discussion of common unhelpful self-talk patterns they might engage in (e.g., self-criticism, catastrophizing, referential thinking, negative interpretive biases, or beliefs about the importance of appearance) (Buhlmann et al., 2009). Further, the therapist can explain how certain ways of coping with appearance worry (e.g., beauty rituals or avoidance behaviors) can prevent the development of healthier beliefs (Summers & Cougle, 2018). While discussing this information with the adolescent in session, the therapist can elicit the patient's personal examples and visually represent them within the model of BDD, to illustrate the different factors that contribute to their current symptom experience. This personalized approach helps foster deeper insight into the factors driving BDD and identifies targets for treatment.

Caregiver Involvement and Education

Including caregivers (and occasionally teachers) in the education phase of treatment complements the therapeutic process, as successful recovery from BDD is more likely when the adolescent has an encouraging support system and home environment (van Noppen & Sassano-Higgins, 2017). The extent of family involvement should be considered in light of the patient's developmental stage, severity, capacity for autonomy, and individual preferences, when appropriate. Caregivers' involvement in assessment and treatment is particularly important with younger patients, as they can provide structure at home, help the adolescent prioritize between-session therapeutic homework completion, and help fade out compulsive and avoidance behaviors (Greenberg, Mothi, & Wilhelm, 2016). Across ages, it is important for the therapist to set realistic expectations about the challenges and timeline of treatment while teaching caregivers how to recognize and respond patiently and effectively to the adolescent's struggles.

Importantly, it is common for caregivers to inadvertently engage in behaviors that reinforce BDD symptoms. For instance, to quell the adolescent's distress, a family member might repeatedly tell them that they look fine or perfect. While such reassurance may temporarily ease the adolescent's distress in the moment, over time their perceived need for feedback about their looks will continually grow without relief, and participation in this cycle serves to perpetuate their excessive focus on appearance (Jassi et al., 2020). In a similar vein, enabling avoidance behaviors, such as permitting the adolescent to skip school or rearranging schedules to avoid triggering situations, reinforces the adolescent's belief that the avoided activity, person, or environment is intolerable and hinders progress (van Noppen & Sassano-Higgins, 2017). Additionally, frequent or overemphasized comments about appearance at home have been linked to rejection sensitivity and the emergence of symptoms (Densham et al., 2017).

Thus, families should be encouraged to be mindful of appearance-related messaging as such topics could reinforce BDD-related beliefs (e.g., "Appearance is central to a person's self-worth") and behaviors (e.g., mirror-checking, appearance comparisons). Learning about the insidious ways in which daily conversation topics or well-meaning accommodations might be worsening the adolescent's symptoms, caregivers can be intentional about breaking the cycle of BDD and support their child's recovery by reinforcing effective coping and rewarding the adolescent's participation in the therapeutic process.

Promoting Cognitive Change

Cognitive strategies aim to teach individuals with BDD to change their response to negative self-talk and assumptions that activate rituals and avoidance behaviors (Greenberg, Sullivan, & Wilhelm, 2017). Initial sessions seek to promote awareness of internal experiences by having patients monitor automatic thoughts and emotional responses to trigger situations as their homework between sessions. The most commonly used cognitive techniques to change thought processes in BDD include cognitive restructuring and core belief work. However, given that adolescents' developmental capacity for complex reasoning and metacognition varies by age (Weil et al., 2013), younger clients can benefit from a reduced emphasis on traditional thought tracking and challenging in favor of more experiential strategies (Greenberg, Sullivan, & Wilhelm, 2017).

Acceptance-Based Strategies

Mindfulness and cognitive defusion techniques can be used to teach non-judgmental awareness of and ways of "unhooking" from unhelpful thoughts, rather than wrestling with their content (Greenberg, Sullivan, & Wilhelm, 2017; Halliburton & Cooper, 2015; Petersen et al., 2022). Example strategies for externalizing thoughts include making the words silly (e.g., singing to the tune of "Happy Birthday," repeating in slow motion), or artistic (e.g., writing in big, colorful, bubble letters). Metaphors can also be useful for demonstrating ways of responding to intrusive internal experiences. For instance, when introducing the concept of "unhooking" from upsetting feelings (i.e., practicing active defusion of the self and the emotion) about their appearance, a therapist could play "tug of war" in-session and observe how the struggle changes when the patient lets go of the rope. For younger clients, writing coping statements on an index card can serve as a reminder to move through triggers or momentary distress (e.g., *"I won't let this thought get in my way!"*) (Greenberg, Mothi, & Wilhelm, 2016).

Cognitive Restructuring

In early CBT sessions, the therapist orients the adolescent to common unhelpful thought patterns in BDD that often distort the perception of everyday events (e.g., labeling, personalizing, black-and-white thinking, mind-reading, catastrophizing, emotional reasoning) (Wilhelm, Phillips, & Steketee, 2013). Between-session thought logs allow patients to practice gaining awareness of how their thoughts (e.g., *"Everyone at school is disgusted by my acne"*, cognitive distortion, mind-reading) influence feelings (e.g., anxiety, depression, shame), avoidance urges (e.g., refusing to go to school), and appearance rituals (excessive washing, make-up application, researching ways to "fix," mirror-checking). In turn, engagement in BDD behaviors further perpetuates beliefs about the significance of appearance in their lives (*"I won't fit in until my skin looks 'normal.'"*).

Once patients have a better understanding of this pattern, they are taught ways of "challenging" unhelpful thoughts by examining the accuracy of the thought (e.g., *"What is the evidence that people are judging me this way?"*) and its usefulness (e.g., *"Is assuming judgment from others helping me make friends?"*), and by generating alternative perspectives (e.g., *"What would I tell a friend who was feeling this way?"*). The goal of cognitive restructuring is to practice self-awareness of the adolescent's negative self-talk and encourage a shift toward more adaptive, flexible, and balanced thinking (e.g., *"I'm not 100 percent sure people are judging me. I'm more likely to make friends if I go to school than if I skip."*) (Wilhelm, Phillips, & Steketee, 2013). Such a shift reduces emotional distress and enhances the patient's willingness to engage in behavioral work (i.e., exposure and ritual prevention), where experiential learning can take place.

Advanced Cognitive Strategies

Older adolescents may benefit from core belief work, to address low self-esteem (Kuck et al., 2022), more entrenched interpretive biases (Dietel et al., 2021; Schulte et al., 2021), or core beliefs about their value that can reveal themselves during treatment (e.g., *"I'm unlovable."*). Such beliefs are typically addressed toward the end of treatment, once the adolescent has developed greater skills and insight.

To identify core beliefs, therapists may use the "downward arrow" technique (e.g., *"If your skin was imperfect, what would happen?"*; *"If that were true, what would that mean about you?"*). Socratic questioning can then be used to explore the conditions under which the belief was acquired (e.g., peer bullying). To challenge core beliefs, therapists may employ cognitive restructuring techniques, such as disputation (e.g., *"If bullying taught you to believe this, do you want to keep believing your bullies?"*), and targeted behavioral experiments to test and reframe the adolescent's point of view. Relatedly, imagery rescripting methods have shown promise in reducing reactivity to memories of past aversive experiences in BDD and in youth with other mental disorders (e.g., Ghaderi et al., 2022; Willson, Veale, & Freeston, 2016).

To enhance and differentiate self-esteem, the "self-esteem pie" (Wilhelm, Phillips, & Steketee, 2013) can be used to identify the varying influences (e.g., life domains, personal qualities, achievements) on the patient's self-esteem. Typically, this acts as a means of visually illustrating the disproportionate impact of appearance on self-esteem. Drawing from acceptance and commitment therapy for adolescents (Petersen et al., 2022), therapists can explore intrinsic and extrinsic contributors to self-esteem via a value card sort task or metaphors (e.g., *"Imagine you've lived a long life and you are looking back your experiences, what do you want to be remembered for?"*). The therapist and patient can collaboratively create a committed action plan to help the adolescent grow the impact of non-appearance personal qualities on their self-esteem (e.g., personal strengths, achievements, skills), and direct their resources more intentionally toward value-driven activities (e.g., spend more time with friends, build mastery in a hobby, volunteer or take part in community events).

Promoting Behavioral Change

Exposure hierarchies serve as a road map for pacing and achieving meaningful behavioral goals. The hierarchy takes into consideration the adolescent's specific appearance anxiety triggers (e.g., school, social activities, pictures, being seen without make-up) and organizes steps based on their anticipated level of anxiety or discomfort in each situation (i.e., "subjective unit of distress" (SUD), on a 0–100 scale). Youth with BDD engage in behavioral avoidance and compulsive rituals aimed at checking, "fixing," or hiding their perceived appearance flaw. As noted, in the short term, mirror-checking, compulsive grooming, skin-picking, comparing oneself to others, camouflaging perceived flaws, reassurance-seeking, surgery-seeking, parental accommodation, and substance use can provide relief, but they also perpetuate the illness. Thus, in addition to approaching feared situations (exposures), the therapist works with patients and/or caregivers to fade, and eventually eliminate, engagement in these rituals over the course of treatment (i.e., ritual prevention) (Wilhelm et al., 2013). Strategies for fading rituals might include delaying engagement (e.g., waiting until lunch to check mirror), setting time limits (e.g., 30 minutes to get ready in the morning, instead of one hour), or reducing degree (e.g., applying less make-up).

Exposure and response prevention (ERP) exercises can be designed in the form of "behavioral experiments" in-session to "test" out the adolescent's fear. For instance, an adolescent who is self-conscious about their "frizzy hair," might benefit from a behavioral experiment in which they plan to go swimming with friends (exposure) and allow their hair to get wet without hiding, styling, or avoiding their friends seeing it dry naturally (ritual prevention). Prior to the behavioral experiment, the adolescent identifies and challenges unhelpful thoughts (e.g., *"My friends will be embarrassed to be around me with my frizzy hair."*), and operationalize their feared outcome (e.g., *"They will ignore me after my hair gets wet"*). Afterward, the adolescent and therapist reflect discrepancies between the feared and the actual outcome and identify take-away lessons (e.g., *"My friends treated me the same, even when my hair got frizzy."*). Exposures should be repeated frequently and in different contexts to ingrain lessons.

Caregivers can support the adolescent's progress by helping to identify situations and behaviors the adolescent struggles within the context of BDD, and encouraging them to move through between-session exposure practices. It can be useful to consider the utility of a developmentally appropriate reward system for achieving specific goals in ritual reduction or consistency with between-session homework assignments (Greenberg, Sullivan, & Wilhelm, 2017). Younger adolescents may respond best to snacks or enjoyable activities whilst older adolescents may respond best to greater privileges and autonomy (e.g., the ability to use the car). In the event of low homework compliance, the therapist can revisit motivational enhancement strategies to explore and problem-solve barriers with the patient (e.g., situational circumstances, low motivation, challenges with exposure pacing) (Greenberg, Mothi, & Wilhelm, 2016, Wilhelm, Phillips, & Steketee, 2013).

Promoting Perceptual and Body Image Change

As noted, individuals with BDD exhibit biases when processing bodily features. Specifically, BDD has been associated with local processing of faces (e.g., Feusner et al., 2007), selective attention to self-rated unattractive over attractive facial features (e.g., Greenberg et al., 2014; Kollei et al., 2017), and attractiveness-based judgment biases (e.g., Dondzilo et al., 2021, Dietel et al., 2023). Further, individuals with BDD symptoms have been shown to experience aversive reactions to their reflection, including negative thoughts and emotions (e.g., anxiety, shame, disgust) (e.g., Schoenenberg & Martin, 2022; Windheim, Veale, & Anson, 2011). Mirror exposures serve to modify these mechanisms by (1) fostering holistic, non-judgmental processing of the body, (2) reducing aversive reactions, and (3) promoting adaptive mirror use.

Overall, in the preparatory phase, therapists should work with the adolescent to devise a mirror hierarchy that includes a range of reflective surfaces (e.g., mirrors, windows, smartphone cameras) and contextual influences (e.g., lighting, distance from mirror, clothing worn, presence of others). Hierarchy steps should be organized by discomfort (SUDS) and avoidance; exposures typically start at a SUDS of approximately 40–50 and increase in intensity.

The therapist can illustrate the effects of mirror-gazing by having the patient look at one of the therapist's facial features (e.g., the nose of the therapist) in the mirror for one minute. The therapist can ask the patient to describe their observations (e.g., perceptual changes). Most patients will report an overfocus on the facial feature, which offers the therapist an opportunity to discuss the effects of localized processing on body image.

In the exposure phase, we recommend using a full-length, distortion-free mirror if possible. Features of the exposure (e.g., lighting, distance) should be determined as per the mirror hierarchy. The therapist should remain next to the patient without obstructing their view. During the exposure, the patient is asked to describe their appearance in a non-judgmental fashion (that is, without using negative statements), devoting equal time per body part, covering all body parts systematically (e.g., from top to bottom) (see Wilhelm, Phillips, & Steketee, 2013). Some helpful metaphors for this procedure could be: *"Describe yourself as you would to a painter that has to paint you, but does not see you!"*; *"Describe yourself as you would to a blind person that would love to get to know you!"*). Therapists may also provide examples for non-judgmental statements throughout the first exposure.

During the exposure, the therapist should regularly check for discomfort ratings and reactions, gently limit maladaptive behaviors, and verbally reward steps of the exposure. With adolescents, therapists may introduce some alterations, such as ending the exposure with a fun pose (e.g., a "Superman" pose). Exposures should last for at least one full-body description; repetition often allows for some reduction in discomfort and/or cognitive change within the session. Mirror exposures should be conducted in different settings and circumstances to enhance the generalizability of this exercise. When ready, patients may practice on their own, preferably multiple times a week. Caregivers can be coached to facilitate these exercises.

Apart from mirror exposures, other interventions may be implemented to foster a positive relationship with one's body. For example, therapists might focus on body neutrality interventions (e.g., based on functionality appreciation, see Perry et al., 2019) or build self-care habits that do not focus on improving appearance (e.g., getting massages, taking baths). However, therapists should carefully assess the evolution of these habits over time to prevent them from becoming ritualistic behaviors.

Relapse Prevention

Progressing toward the end of treatment might be a challenging moment for both the adolescent and their caregivers. In this phase, it is critical to highlight the progress that has been made and foster the autonomy of patients, as well as provide support where needed.

To take inventory of progress, therapists should evaluate symptom improvement via objective measures (e.g., BDD-YBOCS, BABS) and collaboratively review and consolidate the helpful lessons, strategies, and encouraging mantras/reframes collected over the different phases of treatment (e.g., using a narrative storyline with memory signals and/or assemble a "toolbox" of lessons and skill reminders for the patient to have handy).

To prevent relapse, it is important to prepare patients and their support system for periodic worsening of symptoms (e.g., during times of stress, loss, or transitions), while explaining that this is not a sign of unsuccessful treatment, but rather inherent in BDD (Phillips et al., 2006). Thus, a safety plan with relevant contact persons should be maintained.

To promote awareness of symptoms and continued practice of treatment strategies, adolescents should engage in regular "self-check-ins" (e.g., via journaling), to reflect on their mood, recent self-talk, and engagement in appearance-related rituals or avoidance. Weekly check-ins can also be facilitated by the adolescent's caregiver using a traffic light system (i.e., rating the symptom severity on a red-yellow-green scale). In general, for younger adolescents, it is important to involve their support system more extensively in the final phase of treatment to establish beneficial systemic support for relapse prevention. As treatment nears completion, therapy sessions can be gradually spaced out to occur bi-weekly or monthly. Booster sessions can be scheduled as necessary to provide additional support if needed.

Challenges in Treatment

During the treatment of adolescent BDD, challenging situations may emerge that require individualized intervention to accommodate the needs and safety of the patient. In the following, we present three common challenges and how to target them in treatment.

Fixation on Cosmetic Interventions

Desire for cosmetic solutions, including plastic surgery, is common among individuals with BDD, as 64–71 percent of adult patients report having sought or received cosmetic procedures (Crerand et al., 2005). The prevalence of BDD in cosmetic settings is high (13.2 percent; see Veale et al., 2016), despite BDD remaining a contraindication for plastic surgery (ISAPS, 2017). Notably, plastic surgery patients with, versus without, BDD tend to be younger, have lower self-esteem, and greater psychopathology (e.g., Dey et al., 2015; Mulkens et al., 2012). Individuals with BDD may typically engage in research about cosmetic treatments or consult multiple doctors for their appearance concerns ("doctor shopping"). If symptoms are severe, adolescents may repeatedly request that caregivers facilitate cosmetic procedures. Critically, if interventions are denied or unaffordable, individuals with severe BDD may turn to harmful and potentially fatal "do-it-yourself" interventions (e.g., self-mutilation to alter a perceived flaw) (see O'Sullivan et al., 1999; Veale, 2000).

For therapists, it is essential to include information on the link between BDD and cosmetic information from the start of treatment. Importantly, the adolescent should be made aware of the undesired effects of cosmetic interventions in the context of a BDD diagnosis, namely symptom continuation or worsening after the procedure. That is, most individuals with BDD are unsatisfied with the results of cosmetic procedures, which induces new concerns about the operated region; alternatively, concerns can also shift to a new body part (e.g., Phillips, 1996; Picavet et al., 2013). Therapists may collaboratively explore short- and long-term consequences of cosmetic treatments and highlight the known pattern of detrimental effects. Ideally, an agreement of abstinence from cosmetic interventions for the duration of treatment should be made early in CBT. Therapists should regularly monitor urges to seek cosmetic procedures and discuss them in a non-judgmental manner (e.g., via MI).

Poor Insight

Insight refers to the degree of conviction in appearance beliefs and the ability to recognize that one's own beliefs may or may not be true (First & Williams, 2015). Overall, insight has been found to be poor or absent in a majority of individuals with BDD. Strikingly, compared to adults, youth with BDD have even poorer insight, with up to 79 percent reporting delusional beliefs or ideas of reference (e.g., believing that others take special notice of their perceived flaws) (Albertini & Phillips, 1999; Phillips et al., 2006). Patients may hold rigid beliefs about being hideous, worthless, or unlovable because of their appearance, even when presented with disconfirmatory evidence (e.g., positive feedback from others). Low insight is associated with increased symptom severity and suicidality (Eisen et al., 1998; Mancuso, Knoesen, & Castle, 2010; Phillips et al., 2014), more therapeutic ambivalence, preference of cosmetic over psychological treatment and, in some studies, poorer treatment response in CBT (e.g., Greenberg et al., 2019; Neziroglu et al., 2001). Importantly, recent research shows that insight is dynamic, with negative affect and lower self-esteem predicting subsequent insight reductions (Schulte et al., 2021). Thus, therapists may use emotion regulation training and advanced work on self-esteem and core beliefs to build stable insight over time. Insight can be assessed and monitored throughout treatment via established measures (e.g., the BABS).

Suicidality

With lifetime rates of 67–81 percent and 44 percent, respectively, suicidal ideation and attempts appear exacerbated in adolescent BDD, compared to rates in adult BDD (Albertini & Phillips, 1999; Phillips et al., 2006). Suicidality may be fostered by various risk factors, including normatively higher body dissatisfaction in adolescence, poor insight, low self-esteem, comorbid depression, and greater risk for impulsive and aggressive behaviors in adolescence (e.g., Albertini & Phillips, 1999; Crow et al., 2008; Phillips et al., 2006).

Given this risk, therapists should prioritize patient safety and initiate the appropriate level of care throughout treatment. Regular assessment of self-harm behaviors and suicidality is important, particularly in the context of certain risk factors (e.g., depression, poor insight). Therapists should remain cognizant of other factors suggestive of imminent risk (e.g., agitation, insomnia) and, if depression or other comorbidities become primary, they should be addressed first. During crises, potentially destabilizing interventions (e.g., exposures) should be discontinued. Adjunctive psychiatric treatment (e.g., medication management) can be considered to facilitate stabilization. Safety plans should be created early in treatment, with the involvement of the caregiver and members of the adolescent's support system.

Effectiveness of Cognitive Behavioral Therapy for Adolescent Body Dysmorphic Disorder

Thus far, five studies have investigated the effectiveness of CBT in treating adolescent BDD. Overall, these studies have examined effects of CBT as a standalone and combined approach within different settings, thus providing valuable insights into outcomes for symptoms and associated features (e.g., insight) achieved with specific CBT rationales.

In a first case study ($N = 6$), Krebs et al. (2012) assessed the efficacy of age-appropriate CBT for BDD that was based on extant adult approaches (e.g., Veale & Neziroglu, 2010; Wilhelm, Phillips, & Steketee, 2013). The program was adapted for this developmental stage (e.g., easy language, age-appropriate worksheets, parental involvement), consisting of psychoeducation, ritual and response prevention, and relapse prevention. The concurrent case series indicated a score improvement on the BDD-YBOCS of 44 percent at post-treatment, and 57 percent at follow-up, providing initial evidence for the effectiveness of CBT for adolescent BDD.

Greenberg, Mothi, and Wilhelm (2016) extended this effort in a pilot open trial with $N = 13$ adolescents aged 13 to 17 years, evaluating the feasibility, acceptability, and outcome of CBT for adolescent BDD. This 12- to 22-session program incorporated psychoeducation, cognitive strategies, exposure and ritual prevention, mindfulness and perceptual retraining, and relapse prevention. Post-treatment assessments revealed significant improvements in BDD symptoms (50–68 percent, for intention-to-treat versus completers) and associated features (e.g., insight, mood) with effects maintained at 6-month follow-up. Overall, 75 percent of adolescents starting treatment and 100 percent of completers were classified as responders, with large effect sizes.

Krebs et al. (2017) examined long-term outcomes of CBT for adolescent BDD in a trial with $N = 26$ participants with a mean age of 16.2 years. Following this integrated program, BDD symptoms significantly decreased from pre- to post-treatment and remained stable over the 12-month follow-up period. At this point, 50 percent of participants were classified as responders, indicating a sustained positive treatment response, while 23 percent were identified as remitters. Further, participants demonstrated significant improvements in all secondary outcome measures.

In a randomized controlled trial, Mataix-Cols et al. (2015) compared the outcomes of CBT with a psychoeducation control condition in a trial with $N = 30$ adolescents with BDD and their families. This age-adapted CBT protocol included psychoeducation, ritual and response prevention, and relapse prevention, with additional modules implemented as needed (e.g., mirror-retraining). Findings indicated that adolescents in the CBT, versus those in psychoeducation only, exhibited significantly greater improvement both at post-treatment and at the 2-month follow-up, with insight, depression, and quality of life concurrently improving. Importantly, 40 percent of individuals in the CBT, versus 6.7 percent in the control condition, were classified as responders, thus indicating differential benefits of CBT.

In a recent study, Rautio et al. (2022) investigated the effectiveness of multimodal treatment for adolescent BDD in two outpatient specialist clinics located in Sweden ($N = 96$) and the UK ($N = 44$). In this naturalistic setting, treatment consisted of CBT and, in 72 percent of cases, adjunct pharmacotherapy, primarily serotonin re-uptake inhibitors. At the conclusion of treatment, 79 percent of the participants were classified as responders, indicating a significant improvement in BDD symptoms, while 59 percent were categorized as full or partial remitters.

The findings indicate that CBT is effective in treating adolescent BDD within different settings, approaches, and multimodal programs. Treatment effects extend to associated features and psychosocial functioning, and are maintained for 12 months, thus demonstrating sustained benefit. Nonetheless, the underlying mechanisms and predictors of treatment response remain unclear and research into prevention strategies is very much needed.

Treatment Barriers to Cognitive Behavioral Therapy

As noted, efficacious CBT protocols for adolescent BDD exist. However, across studies, only about a third of individuals with diagnosable BDD had received a diagnosis and mental health treatment for BDD (Buhlmann et al., 2011; Marques et al., 2011; Schulte et al., 2020). Apart from other factors (e.g., misdiagnosis among health care providers), this stark contrast between the need for and provision of treatment may be explained by treatment barriers that those affected experience during help-seeking. Overall, such treatment barriers may be categorized as: (1) financial and logistic barriers (e.g., high costs for sessions); (2) perceived stigma, shame, and discrimination to disclose appearance concerns; and (3) treatment perception and satisfaction, such as the impression that previous treatment had not worked (Marques et al., 2011). Thus far, four studies have been conducted to assess self-reported treatment barriers for adult BDD in different health care systems, including the US, Australia, and Germany (Buhlmann et al., 2011, Marques et al., 2011; Schulte et al., 2020; McCausland et al., 2021). Across these studies, shame- and stigma-related barriers emerged as the most commonly reported barriers to treatment, including discomfort about discussing appearance concerns with a professional and convictions that providers would not understand these concerns. Results from these studies further indicated strong preference of wanting to address appearance concerns independently or through cosmetic interventions (Marques et al., 2011; McCausland et al., 2021). While financial and logistic barriers appeared somewhat secondary and varied more per health system under study, high session costs for CBT were among the most commonly reported barriers in a study from Australia, a country with universal health care

(McCausland et al., 2021). Despite the current lack of treatment barrier studies in adolescent BDD, we might assume that they mirror or exceed the extent for adults, given that main personal treatment barriers, like shame, are highly prevalent in adolescence (e.g., Möllmann et al., 2017). Further, as adolescents are less independent than adults in seeking mental health care, parental or caregiver influences (e.g., financial restrictions, dismissal of BDD symptoms as "normal") may further play a role in delaying necessary treatment.

Taken together, these findings demonstrate the important need to improve the early detection of adolescent BDD in mental health care, primary care and cosmetic intervention settings, e.g., via routine screenings (Schneider & Storch, 2017). Further, the accessibility of prevention and intervention programs for adolescent BDD should be enhanced, e.g., through stepped care or digitalized approaches (see, e.g., Kuck et al., 2022), as well as through broad educative campaigns covering BDD. Using specialized techniques outlined in this chapter (e.g., targeting low insight, shame), therapists are advised to monitor emerging barriers during treatment and offer individual approaches to address them (e.g., provide digital programs).

Digital Cognitive Behavioral Therapy Interventions

Digital interventions administered through (video) calls, web-based platforms, smartphones, or wearable devices have gained attention both in research and clinical practice (see Hirandandi et al., 2023, for a review). Most digital programs are based on CBT, delivering modules in an age-appropriate fashion while employing gamification principles (e.g., quizzes, level structures, rewards) (see Fleming, Poppelaars, & Thabrew, 2023) that may appeal to digitally proficient youth (see Granic, Lobel, & Engels, 2014). Thus, digital interventions constitute low-threshold, scalable, cost-efficient, flexible, available tools that could lower extant treatment barriers.

Thus far, two digital CBT programs for adolescent BDD have been developed. "ImaginYouth" (Hartmann et al., 2021) is a therapist-guided, web-based intervention for clinical BDD in youth aged 15 to 21 years. It comprises six modules of CBT (i.e., psychoeducation, cognitive restructuring, work on self-esteem, exposure and response prevention, mirror retraining, and relapse prevention). "AINA" (Kuck et al., 2022) is an unguided self-help program for the prevention and early intervention of adolescent BDD (adolescents aged 14–21 years) featuring seven modules drawn from psychoeducation, cognitive strategies, and self-esteem work. Notably, AINA was deemed acceptable to the target population (Kuck et al., 2022), indicating its potential as a prevention and early intervention tool.

Overall, following pending evaluation, therapists may consider using these digital programs as an adjunct to CBT. However, future research is needed to determine effectiveness in naturalistic settings and indicated decision rules for their use in practice.

Summary

In this chapter, we describe CBT strategies for adolescent BDD, and the unique challenges and vulnerabilities faced by patients during this critical developmental stage. Caregiver involvement in treating adolescent BDD is crucial for creating a supportive home environment, assisting with therapy homework, and reducing compulsive behaviors. They can also offer valuable insights, reinforce therapeutic techniques, and help the adolescent apply skills learned in therapy to daily life. Caregivers should be mindful of inadvertently reinforcing BDD symptoms through excessive appearance-related comments or enabling avoidance behaviors. Therapists should work to establish a strong therapeutic alliance, include motivational enhancement and value-identification strategies to inspire genuine treatment investment from the adolescent, and pay attention to clinical risk factors including fixation on cosmetic interventions, poor insight, and suicidality. The efficacy of CBT for adolescent BDD has been demonstrated in several studies, showing significant improvements in BDD symptoms, associated features, and psychosocial functioning. Continued efforts are needed to address treatment barriers (e.g., low treatment accessibility, shame and stigma-related beliefs, preference for cosmetic interventions) and improve early detection of BDD in adolescents.

References

Albertini, R.S., & Phillips, K.A. (1999). Thirty-three cases of body dysmorphic disorder in children and adolescents. *Journal of the American Academy of Child & Adolescent Psychiatry, 38*(4), 453–459. https://doi.org/10.1097/00004583-199904000-00019.

Bjornsson, A.S., Didie, E.R., Grant, J.E., Menard, W., Stalker, E., & Phillips, K.A. (2013). Age at onset and clinical correlates in body dysmorphic disorder. *Comprehensive Psychiatry, 54*(7), 893–903. http://www.ncbi.nlm.nih.gov/pmc/articles/PMC3779493/.

Buhlmann, U. (2011). Treatment barriers for individuals with body dysmorphic disorder: An internet survey. *The Journal of Nervous and Mental Disease, 199*(4), 268–271. https://doi.org/10.1097/NMD.0b013e31821245ce.

Buhlmann, U., Teachman, B.A., Naumann, E., Fehlinger, T., & Rief, W. (2009). The meaning of beauty: Implicit and explicit self-esteem and attractiveness beliefs in body dysmorphic disorder. *Journal of Anxiety Disorders, 23*(5), 694–702. https://doi.org/10.1016/j.janxdis.2009.02.008.

Crerand, C.E., Phillips, K.A., Menard, W., & Fay, C. (2005). Nonpsychiatric medical treatment of body dysmorphic disorder. *Psychosomatics, 46*(6), 549–555. https://doi.org/10.1176/appi.psy.46.6.549.

Crow, S., Eisenberg, M.E., Story, M., & Neumark-Sztainer, D. (2008). Suicidal behavior in adolescents: Relationship to weight status, weight control behaviors, and body dissatisfaction. *International Journal of Eating Disorders, 41*(1), 82–87. https://doi.org/10.1002/eat.20466.

Deckersbach, T., Savage, C.R., Phillips, K.A., Wilhelm, S., Buhlmann, U., & Rauch, S.L. (2000). Characteristics of memory dysfunction in body dysmorphic disorder. *Journal of the International Neuropsychology Society, 6*(6), 673–681. https://doi.org/10.1017/s1355617700666055.

Densham, K., Webb, H.J., Zimmer-Gembeck, M.J., Nesdale, D., & Downey, G. (2017). Early adolescents' body dysmorphic symptoms as compensatory responses to parental appearance messages and appearance-based rejection sensitivity. *Body Image, 23*, 162–170. https://doi.org/10.1016/j.bodyim.2017.09.005.

Dey, J.K., Ishii, M., Phillis, M., Byrne, P.J., Boahene, K.D.O., & Ishii, L.E. (2015). Body dysmorphic disorder in a facial plastic and reconstructive surgery clinic: Measuring prevalence, assessing comorbidities, and validating a feasible screening instrument. *JAMA Facial Plastic Surgery, 17*(2), 137–143. https://doi.org/10.1001/jamafacial.2014.1492.

Dietel, F.A., Jacobs, L., Onken, R., Buhlmann, U., MacLeod, C., & Dondzilo, L. (2023). Association between judgment biases during facial processing and body dysmorphic symptomatology. *Cognitive Therapy and Research*. https://doi.org/10.1007/s10608-023-10399-0.

Dietel, F.A., Möllmann, A., Bürkner, P.-C., Wilhelm, S., & Buhlmann, U. (2021). Interpretation bias across body dysmorphic, social anxiety and generalized anxiety disorder – A multilevel, diffusion model account. *Cognitive Therapy and Research, 45*(4), 715–729. https://doi.org/10.1007/s10608-020-10180-7.

Dondzilo, L., Dietel, F.A., Buhlmann, U., & MacLeod, C. (2021). The role of biases in the judgement processing of (un)attractive faces in body dysmorphic symptomatology. *Behaviour Research and Therapy, 144*, 103919. https://doi.org/10.1016/j.brat.2021.103919

Eisen, J.L., Phillips, K.A., Baer, L., Beer, D.A., Atala, K.D., & Rasmussen, S.A. (1998). The Brown Assessment of Beliefs Scale: Reliability and validity. *American Journal of Psychiatry, 155*(1), 102–108. https://doi.org/10.1176/ajp.155.1.102.

Enander, J., Ivanov, V.Z., Mataix-Cols, D., Kuja-Halkola, R., Ljótsson, B., Lundström, S., Pérez-Vigil, A., Monzani, B., Lichtenstein, P., & Rück, C. (2018). Prevalence and heritability of body dysmorphic symptoms in adolescents and young adults: A population-based nationwide twin study. *Psychological Medicine, 48*(16), 2740–2747. https://doi.org/10.1017/S0033291718000375.

Fang, A., & Wilhelm, S. (2015). Clinical features, cognitive biases, and treatment of body dysmorphic disorder. *Annual Review of Clinical Psychology, 11*, 187–212. https://doi.org/10.1146/annurev-clinpsy-032814-112849.

Feusner, J.D., Bystritsky, A., Hellemann, G., & Bookheimer, S. (2010). Impaired identity recognition of faces with emotional expressions in body dysmorphic disorder. *Psychiatry Research, 179*(3), 318–323. https://doi.org/10.1016/j.psychres.2009.01.016.

Feusner, J.D., Townsend, J., Bystritsky, A., & Bookheimer, S. (2007). Visual information processing of faces in body dysmorphic disorder. *Archives of General Psychiatry, 64*(12), 1417–1425. https://doi.org/10.1001/archpsyc.64.12.1417.

First, M.B., & Williams, J.B.W. (2015). *Structured clinical interview for DSM-5 disorders*. American Psychiatric Publishing.

Fleming, T., Poppelaars, M., & Thabrew, H. (2023). The role of gamification in digital mental health. *World Psychiatry*, 22(1), Article 1. https://doi.org/10.1002/wps.21041.

Ghaderi, A., Welch, E., Zha, C., & Holmes, E.A. (2022). Imagery rescripting for reducing body image dissatisfaction: A randomized controlled trial. *Cognitive Therapy and Research*, 46(4), 721–734. https://doi.org/10.1007/s10608-022-10295-z.

Granic, I., Lobel, A., & Engels, R.C.M.E. (2014). The benefits of playing video games. *American Psychologist*, 69(1), Article 1. https://doi.org/10.1037/a003485.

Greenberg, J.L., Sullivan, A., & Wilhelm, S. (2017). Treating children and adolescents with body dysmorphic disorder. In K.A. Phillips (Ed.), *Body dysmorphic disorder: Advances in research and clinical practice* (pp. 397–409). Oxford University Press.

Greenberg, J.L., Mothi, S.S., & Wilhelm, S. (2016). Cognitive-behavioral therapy for adolescent body dysmorphic disorder: A pilot study. *Behavior Therapy*, 47(2), 213–224. https://doi.org/10.1016/j.beth.2015.10.009.

Greenberg, J.L., Phillips, K.A., Steketee, G., Hoeppner, S.S., & Wilhelm, S. (2019). Predictors of response to cognitive-behavioral therapy for body dysmorphic disorder. *Behavior Therapy*, 50(4), 839–849. https://doi.org/10.1016/j.beth.2018.12.008.

Greenberg, J.L., Reuman, L., Hartmann, A.S., Kasarskis, I., & Wilhelm, S. (2014). Visual hot spots: An eye tracking study of attention bias in body dysmorphic disorder. *Journal of Psychiatric Research*, 57, 125–132. https://doi.org/10.1016/j.jpsychires.2014.06.015.

Halliburton, A.E., & Cooper, L.D. (2015). Applications and adaptations of acceptance and commitment therapy (ACT) for adolescents. *Journal of Contextual Behavioral Science*, 4(1), 1–11. https://doi.org/10.1016/j.jcbs.2015.01.002.

Hartmann, A.S., Schmidt, M., Staufenbiel, T., Ebert, D.D., Martin, A., & Schoenenberg, K. (2021). Imaginyouth – A therapist-guided internet-based cognitive-behavioral program for adolescents and young adults with body dysmorphic disorder: Study protocol for a two-arm randomized controlled trial. *Frontiers in Psychiatry*, 12. https://www.frontiersin.org/articles/10.3389/fpsyt.2021.682965.

Hiranandani, S., Ipek, S.I., Wilhelm, S., & Greenberg, J.L. (2023). Digital mental health interventions for obsessive compulsive and related disorders: A brief review of evidence-based interventions and future directions. *Journal of Obsessive-Compulsive and Related Disorders*, 36, 100765. https://doi.org/10.1016/j.jocrd.2022.100765.

ISAPS (International Society of Aesthetic Plastic Surgery). (2017). *Patient safety recommendations on body dysmorphic disorder – Practical points*. https://www.isaps.org/media/n0zpigfg/body-dysmorphic-disorder.pdf.

Jassi, A.D., Baloch, A., Thomas-Smith, K., & Lewis, A. (2020). Family accommodation in pediatric body dysmorphic disorder: A qualitative study. *Bulletin of the Menninger Clinic*, 84(4), 319–336. https://doi.org/10.1521/bumc.2020.84.4.319.

Kollei, I., Horndasch, S., Erim, Y., & Martin, A. (2017). Visual selective attention in body dysmorphic disorder, bulimia nervosa and healthy controls. *Journal of Psychosomatic Research*, 92, 26–33. https://doi.org/10.1016/j.jpsychores.2016.11.008.

Krebs, G., Fernández de la Cruz, L., Monzani, B., Bowyer, L., Anson, M., Cadman, J., Heyman, I., Turner, C., Veale, D., & Mataix-Cols, D. (2017). Long-term outcomes of cognitive-behavioral therapy for adolescent body dysmorphic disorder. *Behavior Therapy*, 48(4), 462–473. https://doi.org/10.1016/j.beth.2017.01.001.

Krebs, G., Turner, C., Heyman, I., & Mataix-Cols, D. (2012). Cognitive behaviour therapy for adolescents with body dysmorphic disorder: A case series. *Behavioural and Cognitive Psychotherapy*, 40(4), 452–461. https://doi.org/10.1017/S1352465812000100.

Kuck, N., Dietel, F.A., Nohr, L., Vahrenhold, J., & Buhlmann, U. (2022). A smartphone app for the prevention and early intervention of body dysmorphic disorder: Development and evaluation of the content, usability, and aesthetics. *Internet Interventions*, 28, 100521. https://doi.org/10.1016/j.invent.2022.100521.

Mancuso, S.G., Knoesen, N.P., & Castle, D.J. (2010). Delusional versus nondelusional body dysmorphic disorder. *Comprehensive Psychiatry*, 51(2), 177–182. https://doi.org/10.1016/j.comppsych.2009.05.001.

Marques, L., Weingarden, H.M., LeBlanc, N.J., & Wilhelm, S. (2011). Treatment utilization and barriers to treatment engagement among people with body dysmorphic symptoms. *Journal of Psychosomatic Research*, 70(3), 286–293. https://doi.org/10.1016/j.jpsychores.2010.10.002.

Mataix-Cols, D., Fernández de la Cruz, L., Isomura, K., Anson, M., Turner, C., Monzani, B., Cadman, J., Bowyer, L., Heyman, I., Veale, D., & Krebs, G. (2015). A pilot randomized controlled trial of cognitive-behavioral therapy for adolescents with body dysmorphic disorder. *Journal of the American Academy of Child & Adolescent Psychiatry*, 54(11), 895–904. https://doi.org/10.1016/j.jaac.2015.08.011.

McCausland, J., Paparo, J., & Wootton, B.M. (2021). Treatment barriers, preferences and histories of individuals with symptoms of body dysmorphic disorder. *Behavioural and Cognitive Psychotherapy*, 49(5), 582–595.

Miller, W.R. & Rollnick, S. (2002). *Motivational interviewing: Preparing people for change* (2nd ed.). Guilford Press.

Möllmann, A., Dietel, F.A., Hunger, A., & Buhlmann, U. (2017). Prevalence of body dysmorphic disorder and associated features in German adolescents: A self-report survey. *Psychiatry Research*, 254, 263–267. https://doi.org/10.1016/j.psychres.2017.04.063.

Mulkens, S., Bos, A.E.R., Uleman, R., Muris, P., Mayer, B., & Velthuis, P. (2012). Psychopathology symptoms in a sample of female cosmetic surgery patients. *Journal of Plastic, Reconstructive & Aesthetic Surgery*, 65(3), 321–327. https://doi.org/10.1016/j.bjps.2011.09.038.

Neziroglu, F., Stevens, K.P., McKay, D., & Yaryura-Tobias, J.A. (2001). Predictive validity of the overvalued ideas scale: Outcome in obsessive-compulsive and body dysmorphic disorders. *Behaviour Research and Therapy*, 39(6), 745–756. https://doi.org/10.1016/S0005-7967(00)00053-X.

Oosthuizen, P., Lambert, T., & Castle, D. (1998). Dysmorphic concern: Prevalence and associations with clinical variables. *Australian and New Zealand Journal of Psychiatry*, 32, 129–132. https://doi.org/10.3109/00048679809062719.

O'Sullivan, R.L., Phillips, K.A., Keuthen, N.J., & Wilhelm, S. (1999). Near-fatal skin picking from delusional body dysmorphic disorder responsive to fluvoxamine. *Psychosomatics*, 40(1), 79–81. https://doi.org/10.1016/S0033-3182(99)71276-4.

Perry, M., Watson, L., Hayden, L., & Inwards-Breland, D. (2019). Using body neutrality to inform eating disorder management in a gender diverse world. *The*

Lancet Child & Adolescent Health, 3(9), Article 9. https://doi.org/10.1016/S2352-4642(19)30237-8.

Petersen, J., Hayes, L., Gillard, D., & Ciarrochi, J. (2022). ACT for children and adolescents. In M.P. Twoig, M.E. Levin, & J.M. Petersen (Eds.), *The Oxford Handbook of Acceptance and Commitment Therapy*. Oxford University Press.

Pfeifer, J.H., & Berkman, E.T. (2018). The development of self and identity in adolescence: Neural evidence and implications for a value-based choice perspective on motivated behavior. *Child Development Perspectives*, *12*(3), 158–164. https://doi.org/10.1111/cdep.12279.

Phillips, K.A. (1996). *The broken mirror: Understanding and treating body dysmorphic disorder*. Oxford University Press.

Phillips, K.A., Didie, E.R., Menard, W., Pagano, M.E., Fay, C., & Weisberg, R.B. (2006). Clinical features of body dysmorphic disorder in adolescents and adults. *Psychiatry Research*, *141*(3), 305–314. https://doi.org/10.1016/j.psychres.2005.09.014.

Phillips, K.A., Hart, A.S., Simpson, H.B., & Stein, D.J. (2014). Delusional versus nondelusional body dysmorphic disorder: Recommendations for DSM-5. *CNS Spectrums*, *19*(1), 10–20. https://doi.org/10.1017/S1092852913000266.

Phillips, K.A., Hollander, E., Rasmussen, S.A., Aronowitz, B.R., Decaria, C., & Goodman, W.K. (1997). A severity rating scale for body dysmorphic disorder: Development, reliability, and validity of a modified version of the Yale-Brown Obsessive Compulsive Scale. *Psychopharmacology Bulletin*, *33*, 17.

Picavet, V.A., Gabriëls, L., Grietens, J., Jorissen, M., Prokopakis, E.P., & Hellings, P.W. (2013). Preoperative symptoms of body dysmorphic disorder determine postoperative satisfaction and quality of life in aesthetic rhinoplasty. *Plastic and Reconstructive Surgery*, *131*(4), 861. https://doi.org/10.1097/PRS.0b013e3182818f02.

Rautio, D., Gumpert, M., Jassi, A., Krebs, G., Flygare, O., Andrén, P., Monzani, B., Peile, L., Jansson-Fröjmark, M., Lundgren, T., Hillborg, M., Silverberg-Mörse, M., Clark, B., Fernández de la Cruz, L., & Mataix-Cols, D. (2022). Effectiveness of multimodal treatment for young people with body dysmorphic disorder in two specialist clinics. *Behavior Therapy*, *53*(5), 1037–1049. https://doi.org/10.1016/j.beth.2022.04.010.

Rodgers, R.F. (2016). the relationship between body image concerns, eating disorders and internet use, Part II: An integrated theoretical model. *Adolescent Research Review*, *1*(2), 121–137. https://doi.org/10.1007/s40894-015-0017-5.

Rosen, J.C., & Reiter, J. (1996). Development of the body dysmorphic disorder examination. *Behaviour Research and Therapy*, *34*(9), 755–766. https://doi.org/10.1016/0005-7967(96)00024-1.

Schneider, S.C., & Storch, E.A. (2017). improving the detection of body dysmorphic disorder in clinical practice. *Journal of Cognitive Psychotherapy*, *31*(4), Article 4. https://doi.org/10.1891/0889-8391.31.4.230.

Schoenenberg, K., & Martin, A. (2022). Cognitive-affective reactions to a non-judgmental and judgmental mirror gazing task in individuals with body dysmorphic concerns. *Journal of Behavior Therapy and Experimental Psychiatry*, *77*, 101779. https://doi.org/10.1016/j.jbtep.2022.101779.

Schulte, J., Dietel, F.A., Wilhelm, S., Nestler, S., & Buhlmann, U. (2021). Temporal dynamics of insight in body dysmorphic disorder: An ecological momentary assessment study. *Journal of Abnormal Psychology*, *130*(4), 365–376. https://doi.org/10.1037/abn0000673.

Schulte, J., Schulz, C., Wilhelm, S., & Buhlmann, U. (2020). Treatment utilization and treatment barriers in individuals with body dysmorphic disorder. *BMC Psychiatry*, *20*(1), 69. https://doi.org/10.1186/s12888-020-02489-0.

Summers, B.J., & Cougle, J.R. (2018). An experimental test of the role of appearance-related safety behaviors in body dysmorphic disorder, social anxiety, and body dissatisfaction. *Journal of Abnormal Psychology*, *127*(8), 770–780. https://doi.org/10.1037/abn0000387.

van Noppen, B., & Sassano-Higgins, S. (2017). The family and body dysmorphic disorder: Impact, responses, and a suggested family-based treatment approach. In K.A. Phillips (Ed.), *Body dysmorphic disorder: Advances in research and clinical practice* (pp. 411–427). Oxford University Press.

Veale, D. (2000). Outcome of cosmetic surgery and "DIY" surgery in patients with body dysmorphic disorder. *Psychiatric Bulletin*, *24*(6), 218–221. https://doi.org/10.1192/pb.24.6.218.

Veale D. (2004). Advances in a cognitive behavioural model of body dysmorphic disorder. *Body Image*, *1*(1), 113–125. https://doi.org/10.1016/S1740-1445(03)00009-3.

Veale, D., Gledhill, L.J., Christodoulou, P., & Hodsoll, J. (2016). Body dysmorphic disorder in different settings: A systematic review and estimated weighted prevalence. *Body Image*, *18*, 168–186. https://doi.org/10.1016/j.bodyim.2016.07.003.

Veale, D., & Neziroglu, F. (2010). *Body dysmorphic disorder: A treatment manual.* John Wiley & Sons.

Weil, L.G., Fleming, S.M., Dumontheil, I., Kilford, E.J., Weil, R.S., Rees, G., Dolan, R.J., & Blakemore, S.J. (2013). The development of metacognitive ability in adolescence. *Consciousness and Cognition*, *22*(1), 264–271. https://doi.org/10.1016/j.concog.2013.01.004.

Weingarden, H., & Renshaw, K.D. (2015). Shame in the obsessive compulsive related disorders: A conceptual review. *Journal of Affective Disorders, 171*, 74–84.

Wilhelm, S., Phillips, K.A., & Steketee, G. (2013). *Cognitive-behavioral therapy for body dysmorphic disorder: A treatment manual.* Guilford Press.

Wilhelm, S., Greenberg, J.L., Rosenfield, E., Kasarskis, I., & Blashill, A.J. (2016). The Body Dysmorphic Disorder Symptom Scale: Development and preliminary validation of a self-report scale of symptom specific dysfunction. *Body Image*, *17*, 82–87.

Willson, R., Veale, D., & Freeston, M. (2016). Imagery rescripting for body dysmorphic disorder: A multiple-baseline single-case experimental design. *Behavior Therapy*, *47*(2), 248–261. https://doi.org/10.1016/j.beth.2015.08.006.

Windheim, K., Veale, D., & Anson, M. (2011). Mirror gazing in body dysmorphic disorder and healthy controls: Effects of duration of gazing. *Behaviour Research and Therapy*, *49*(9), 555–564. https://doi.org/10.1016/j.brat.2011.05.003.

5 Behavioral Therapy for Tic Disorders and Body-Focused Repetitive Behavior Disorders

Kesley A. Ramsey,[1] *Ainsley K. Patrick,*[1] *and Joseph F. McGuire*[1]

[1] *Division of Child and Adolescent Psychiatry, Johns Hopkins University School of Medicine, Baltimore, MD*

Tourette's and other chronic tic disorders (collectively, TS) and body-focused repetitive behaviors (BFRBs), such as hair-pulling, predominantly onset in childhood and are associated with significant functional impairment and affect quality of life.[1-4] Fortunately, several evidence-based treatments exist, including pharmacotherapy[5,6] and behavioral therapies such as habit reversal training (HRT) and the Comprehensive Behavioral Intervention for Tics (CBIT).[7,8]

In this chapter we present information on behavior therapy for TS and associated obsessive-compulsive and related disorders (OCRDs), conditions characterized by BFRBs such as trichotillomania (TTM) and skin-picking disorder (SPD). The chapter first provides details on the theoretical background and intervention components of behavioral therapy for these conditions. Next, evidence for the efficacy of these behavioral interventions is summarized succinctly. Finally, the chapter concludes with a discussion on future directions for behavior therapy for TS and BFRBs.

History of Behavioral Therapy for Tic Disorders and Body-Focused Repetitive Behavior Disorders

First described by Azrin and Nunn,[9] HRT is a behavioral intervention originally designed to eliminate nervous habits and tics. HRT is a multi-component intervention that can consist of several therapeutic strategies, including awareness training, competing response training, generalization training, self-monitoring, relaxation training, behavioral rewards, and social support.[9,10] Although it can consist of multiple components, initial research suggests that awareness training, competing response training, and social support are the core components of HRT that drive symptom change.[11-13] Over the past 20 years, HRT has been applied as a behavioral intervention for youth with a variety of conditions and has emerged as the

DOI: 10.4324/9781003386278-5

first-line treatment for TS[14] and associated OCRDs that are characterized by the presence of BFRBs, such as hair-pulling[6,15,16] and skin-picking.[17]

Theoretical Foundations of Behavioral Therapy for Tic Disorders and Body-Focused Repetitive Behavior Disorders

Behavioral interventions for TS and BFRBs are initially grounded within a tension-reduction model.[9] The tension-reduction model posits that tics and/or BFRB symptoms (e.g., hair-pulling, skin-picking) are maintained over time through a cycle of negative reinforcement. For instance in TS, tic expression is influenced by a variety of factors, including premonitory urge sensations.[18] Premonitory urges are uncomfortable, aversive somatic phenomena, which commonly precede tics and can be temporarily alleviated by tic occurrence.[19–21] Once a tic is expressed, individuals with TS generally experience short-term relief from the uncomfortable urge sensation; however, this can make it more likely for the tic behavior to be maintained over time. Similarly for related BFRBs, individuals with TTM experience a comparable physical, sensation-based tension that precedes the hair-pulling behavior, and engagement in hair-pulling brings about a sense of relief afterwards. In the absence of intervention, this pattern of tension-relief can reinforce TS and related BFRB symptoms over time.

More recent conceptualizations have recognized that TS and BFRB symptoms become associated with a variety of internal and external factors through associative learning processes (e.g., classical conditioning, operant learning processes).[22,23] Internal factors may include physiological urge sensations and emotional states (e.g., stress, anxiety), while external factors may include environmental contexts (e.g., home, school).[18,24] While often having clear associations at the outset, tics and BFRB symptoms can even be expressed without awareness (e.g., engagement in tics without recognition, engagement in automatic hair-pulling).[25,26] Behavioral therapies such as HRT aim to disrupt the negative reinforcement cycle and related processes that maintain tics,[27] TTM,[28] and SPD.[29]

Behavioral Therapy for Tic Disorders

In youth, HRT for TS generally centers on four main components: psychoeducation about TS, awareness training, competing response training, and social (parental) support.[12,30] In psychoeducation, clinicians provide youth and their caregivers essential information that includes the etiology of TS, symptom phenomenology, developmental trajectory, and when to implement evidence-based interventions based on symptom severity.[31] Awareness training refers to building awareness for a tic targeted in treatment. This may include activities such as noticing the behavior itself, as well as early detection of the behavior (e.g., awareness for premonitory urges that may precede the tic, earliest tic movements or sounds). Competing response training involves teaching patients physically incompatible behaviors designed to be implemented upon the detection of the targeted tic or its antecedents. After consistently detecting the targeted tic or its earliest antecedent (i.e., the premonitory urge for the tic), a competing response can be implemented that is intended to inhibit expression of the targeted tic. Finally, social support in HRT entails having a support person – such as a parent or caregiver – reinforce the implementation of awareness training and competing response training outside of therapy sessions. Greater adherence to these core therapeutic skills results in greater reductions in symptom severity.[32] Additional components of HRT, such as self-monitoring and behavioral rewards, can also be implemented as part of the treatment course. Self-monitoring allows youth to practice building awareness of tics and related antecedents (i.e., premonitory urges), which can be helpful later to build mastery over implementing competing responses contingent upon such awareness. Meanwhile, behavioral rewards can be utilized to reinforce the consistent implementation of HRT skills outside of session and increase motivation to participate in treatment.

Building upon the initial foundation of HRT, the CBIT serves as a natural extension of the original HRT principles.[13] While CBIT contains the core therapeutic elements of HRT (i.e., psychoeducation about TS, awareness training, competing response training, and social support), it also incorporates additional therapeutic skills such relaxation training and functional assessment/intervention to address internal and external factors that influence tic expression.[13] In relaxation training, patients learn specific skills (e.g., diaphragmatic breathing, progressive muscle relaxation) to manage stress – a factor that commonly increases tic expression. The functional assessment evaluates situations and environments (e.g., antecedents) that exacerbate tic severity, and defines the outcomes of those situations when tic expression is worse (e.g., consequences). Building on this assessment, the functional intervention strives to apply functional strategies to decrease antecedents that exacerbate tic expression and reduce consequences that may unintentionally maintain and/or worsen tic expression. Both HRT and CBIT are behavioral interventions that are designed to disrupt the negative reinforcement cycle that maintains tic expression over time. Whilst HRT primarily focuses on targeting internal factors (e.g., premonitory urges), CBIT targets both internal (e.g., premonitory urges, anxiety) and external (e.g., situational, contextual) factors that maintain tic expression over time.[27]

Behavioral Therapy for Body-Focused Repetitive Behavior Disorders

After providing general psychoeducation about the specific BFRB, its general phenomenology, and treatment recommendations, HRT for

BFRB symptoms such as TTM or SPD typically includes the following core behavioral therapeutic components: awareness training, stimulus control, and competing response training.[33,34] In awareness training, strategies are provided and practiced to increase awareness of the BFRB itself (e.g., hair-pulling, skin-picking), as well as any antecedent sensations (e.g., urges) that precede the symptom. Common strategies include assigning self-monitoring exercises to track the occurrence of BFRBs outside of session. Once self-monitoring exercises are completed and specific factors identified (e.g., "I pull my hair in the bathroom using tweezers", "I pick my skin when I'm stressed"), stimulus control strategies can be utilized. Stimulus control strategies refer to a variety of methods that serve as "speed bumps" designed to reduce the probability of engaging in the target behavior (e.g., hair-pulling, skin-picking). For instance, stimulus control strategies for hair-pulling behaviors based on the self-monitoring example might be limiting access to the tweezers and/ or not keeping them in the bathroom. Meanwhile, stimulus control strategies for skin-picking behaviors based on the self-monitoring example might entail covering one's fingertips with finger cots when experiencing anxiety. Finally, as greater awareness of symptom occurrence is achieved via self-monitoring, competing responses can be utilized to engage in a behavior that is physically incompatible to the target behavior for a short period of time – contingent upon detecting the earliest sign of target behavior (e.g., crossing arms when experiencing urge to pull hair and/ or pick skin). While many contemporary behavioral interventions for BFRBs draw on the original elements of HRT as described by Azrin and Nunn,[9,28] some treatment protocols (primarily in adult samples, but also in some adolescent samples) have been expanded to incorporate additional components such as cognitive strategies, relaxation training, and acceptance-based strategies.[33,35,36]

Evidence-Base for Behavioral Therapy for Tic Disorders and Body-Focused Repetitive Behavior Disorders

Behavioral Therapy for Youth with Tic Disorders

Following the administration of the Yale Global Tic Severity Scale (YGTSS),[37,38] treatment recommendations for youth with TS are based on tic symptom severity (see McGuire et al.[39] for empirical guidance on benchmarks of tic severity). For individuals with mild symptom severity, psychoeducation about TS and watchful waiting to monitor symptom progression are recommended. For individuals with moderate symptom severity or greater, behavioral interventions – such as HRT and CBIT – are universally recommended as a first-line treatment, due to their efficacy and low side-effect profiles.[40,41] Behavioral interventions for TS have been the subject of extensive clinical investigation,[8] with research reports on youth as young as 5 years of age[42] and as old as 75.[43]

Across randomized controlled trials, behavioral interventions have demonstrated efficacy for treating youth[44] and adults[45] with TS. Behavior therapy has consistently shown moderate-to-large effects across randomized controlled trials relative to comparison conditions (effect size = 0.67–0.94).[14] Moreover, evidence suggests that different tic symptom clusters respond equally well to behavioral interventions for TS,[46] and that specific bothersome tics can remit from behavioral interventions.[47] For individuals who exhibit a treatment response to behavior therapy for TS, therapeutic gains are found to be sustained for up to six months.[48,49] Perhaps most notably, youth who respond to behavior therapy for TS in childhood have been found to continue to benefit from this treatment in adulthood – demonstrating the potential of this intervention to alter the developmental trajectory of TS.[50] A number of clinical characteristics have been identified as factors that influence treatment responder status in behavioral therapy, including medication status,[51] comorbid attention deficit hyperactivity disorder,[14] and behavior therapy homework adherence.[32]

Behavioral Therapy for Youth with Body-Focused Repetitive Behavior Disorders

Behavioral therapies – such as HRT – have the strongest evidence base for BFRB symptoms such as hair-pulling and skin-picking.[7,33,52,53] Despite its strong empirical support, there is a paucity of randomized controlled clinical trials examining the benefit of behavioral therapies for youth with TTM and SPD.[16,17,52]

Across the available randomized controlled trials, behavioral interventions have demonstrated efficacy for treating youth with TTM and SPD.[6,15–17] In these trials, behavior therapy has shown medium-to-large effects relative to comparison conditions for hair-pulling (effect size = 0.56–2.74)[15,16] and skin-picking behaviors (effect size = 0.50–1.42).[17,52] For youth who experience a treatment response to behavior therapy for BFRBs, evidence suggests that therapeutic gains are maintained for at least 6 months.[28,54] Indeed, long-term naturalistic follow-up studies suggest that youth with hair-pulling do not experience clinically meaningful improvement in hair-pulling symptoms in the absence of evidence-based treatments like behavior therapy.[55] However, further investigation is needed to determine the influence of patient-specific factors on behavioral treatment outcomes. For instance, given the importance of self-monitoring in behavior therapy for BFRBs like hair-pulling, initial evidence suggests that automatic hair-pulling behaviors (i.e., those that occur outside a patient's awareness) are less responsive to HRT in comparison to more focused hair-pulling behaviors (i.e., those that occur within a patient's awareness).[56]

Future Directions

Despite the promise of behavior therapy and its benefits, some youth do not respond to this intervention. Therefore, further research is necessary to advance our understanding of TS and BFRBs in youth, facilitating implementation of interventions that can effect meaningful clinical change.

One clear future direction for this line of research is that the evidence base for BFRBs needs to catch up with that of TS. There is a paucity of large, well-designed randomized clinical trials investigating the effects of behavioral interventions for youth with BFRBs.[57] Given the importance of early intervention for these childhood-onset disorders, there is a critical need for research investigations conducted by independent sites to establish the efficacy of behavioral interventions for this clinical population.

Understanding the mechanisms that underlie the etiology and treatment of TS and BFRBs can ultimately improve clinical outcomes for youth.[8,22,58,59] Promising mechanisms include associative learning,[22] cognitive control,[60] emotional regulation,[61,62] psychological flexibility,[63] and urge intolerance.[64,65] By understanding the underlying mechanisms of the etiology and treatment of TS and BFRBs, we can inform precise strategies to enhance treatments and/or develop new interventions to help youth achieve wellness.

Pinpointing the mechanisms that underlie behavioral interventions for TS and BFRBs would also afford opportunities to optimize treatment.[8,22,58,59] A number of strategies have been proposed to enhance behavioral treatment outcomes for TS, one of which includes the optimization of critical learning processes involved in behavioral interventions (e.g., reinforcement/reward learning, inhibiting tic expression).[8,22] Cognitive enhancers, such as d-cycloserine (DCS), administered in conjunction with behavioral interventions, may enhance therapeutic learning and ultimately improve TS treatment outcomes.[27,66] Even trials with null findings[67] can provide critical information to inform pathways toward treatment optimization.

While behavioral interventions have been shown to be efficacious for TS and BFRBs, many patients remain symptomatic after treatment.[8,17,54] Future research can explore whether augmented behavioral interventions or novel psychosocial treatment approaches can benefit youth within these clinical populations. For instance – while relaxation treatment has been integrated into behavioral treatment of TS, evidence suggests that this therapeutic element alone may prove insufficient for reducing tic severity.[67] Novel intervention protocols that incorporate third-wave cognitive behavioral therapy elements such as mindfulness may prove beneficial for affect modulation and urge tolerance among individuals with TS.[61,64,65,68] Early clinical trials of a mindfulness-based stress reduction (MBSR) intervention for tics found that adolescents and adults with TS experienced reductions in self-reported functional impairment.[69,70] McGuire and colleagues[76] found that a modularized behavioral intervention that incorporated mindfulness strategies significantly reduced tic-related impairment among youth with TS. For BFRBs, clinical investigations have focused on the merits of enhancing HRT with acceptance commitment therapy (ACT)[36,71,72] and dialectical behavior therapy (DBT)[73,74] for TTM. Flessner and colleagues[75] found that acceptance-enhanced behavior therapy was beneficial for reducing BFRB symptoms among five individuals diagnosed with either TTM or SPD. One trial found that ACT alone reduced symptom severity among adolescents and adults with hair-pulling, yielding similar clinical outcomes relative to trials of HRT combined with ACT.[76]

Across all the TS and related BFRBs covered in this chapter, clinical researchers universally agree there is a strong need for well-powered, thoughtfully designed randomized controlled trials to validate the efficacy of behavioral therapies.[6,17,52,59] Furthermore, the majority of clinical investigations of behavior therapy for TS and BFRBs recruit adults; more research is needed to establish best treatment practices among youth with these conditions, particularly for youth with BFRBs. It is important to consider the notable developmental differences between children and adults (e.g., differences in premonitory urge awareness in TS in youth versus adults).[77] Mechanistic processes likely differ across youth and adults. Consequently, clinical outcomes from adult literature cannot be widely applied to youth with TS and BFRBs. Furthermore, the delivery of clinical interventions needs to be adapted to ensure that youth are able to engage and learn clinical skills at a developmentally appropriate level. Finally, in optimizing the design of clinical trials for behavior therapies in youth, it is critical that valid assessment instruments are implemented in these investigations to document clinically significant symptom change. Therefore, future researchers should strive to validate TS and BFRB-symptom instruments among pediatric populations[78,75] and establish meaningful severity benchmarks for these conditions.[39] Taken together, further research is needed on TS and BFRBs among youth to advance our understanding of these conditions and achieve optimal clinical outcomes.

Summary

This chapter reviewed behavioral interventions for youth with TS and BFRBs such as hair-pulling and skin-picking in youth. This chapter provided a brief overview on the conceptual models that underlie the etiology and behavioral treatment for these conditions. Next, the practical components of each type of behavioral therapy were discussed, with an emphasis placed on awareness training and competing response training strategies. Afterward, the empirical support for behavior therapy for TS and BFRBs was presented, which demonstrated that behavior therapy has considerable therapeutic benefit and, in some cases, can alter the course of the illness trajectory. Despite these achievements and growing evidence base, further research on behavior therapy is essential to determine underlying mechanisms that can optimize clinical outcomes. As some patients remain non-responsive to behavior therapy, more work is needed to consider optimization approaches and/or new psychosocial treatments to assist youth with TS and/or BFRBs in achieving wellness.

References

1 Conelea, C.A. et al. Exploring the impact of chronic tic disorders on youth: Results from the Tourette Syndrome Impact Survey. *Child Psychiatry Hum. Dev.* **42**, 219–242 (2011).

2 Franklin, M.E. et al. The child and adolescent trichotillomania impact project: Descriptive psychopathology, comorbidity, functional impairment, and treatment utilization. *J. Dev. Behav. Pediatr. JDBP* **29**, 493–500 (2008).

3 Ricketts, E.J. et al. Academic, interpersonal, recreational, and family impairment in children with Tourette syndrome and attention-deficit/hyperactivity disorder. *Child Psychiatry Hum. Dev.* **53**, 3–15 (2022).

4 Tucker, B.T.P., Woods, D.W., Flessner, C.A., Franklin, S.A., & Franklin, M.E. The Skin Picking Impact Project: phenomenology, interference, and treatment utilization of pathological skin picking in a population-based sample. *J. Anxiety Disord.* **25**, 88–95 (2011).

5 Cavanna, A.E. Current and emerging pharmacotherapeutic strategies for Tourette syndrome. *Expert Opin. Pharmacother.* **23**, 1523–1533 (2022).

6 Farhat, L.C. et al. Pharmacological and behavioral treatment for trichotillomania: An updated systematic review with meta-analysis. *Depress. Anxiety* **37**, 715–727 (2020).

7 Jones, G., Keuthen, N., & Greenberg, E. Assessment and treatment of trichotillomania (hair pulling disorder) and excoriation (skin picking) disorder. *Clin. Dermatol.* **36**, 728–736 (2018).

8 McGuire, J.F. et al. Behavior therapy for tic disorders: An evidenced-based review and new directions for treatment research. *Curr. Dev. Disord. Rep.* **2**, 309–317 (2015).

9 Azrin, N.H. & Nunn, R.G. Habit-reversal: A method of eliminating nervous habits and tics. *Behav. Res. Ther.* **11**, 619–628 (1973).

10 Azrin, N.H. & Peterson, A.L. Treatment of tourette syndrome by habit reversal: A waiting-list control group comparison. *Behav. Ther.* **21**, 305–318 (1990).

11 Himle, M.B., Woods, D.W., Piacentini, J.C., & Walkup, J.T. Brief review of habit reversal training for Tourette syndrome. *J. Child Neurol.* **21**, 719–725 (2006).

12 Woods, D.W., Miltenberger, R.G., & Lumley, V.A. Sequential application of major habit-reversal components to treat motor tics in children. *J. Appl. Behav. Anal.* **29**, 483–493 (1996).

13 Woods, D.W. et al. *Managing Tourette syndrome: A behavioral intervention for children and adults (Therapist guide).* Oxford University Press (2008).

14 McGuire, J.F. et al. A meta-analysis of behavior therapy for Tourette syndrome. *J. Psychiatr. Res.* **50**, 106–112 (2014).

15 Bloch, M.H. et al. Systematic review: Pharmacological and behavioral treatment for trichotillomania. *Biol. Psychiatry* **62**, 839–846 (2007).

16 McGuire, J.F. et al. Treating trichotillomania: A meta-analysis of treatment effects and moderators for behavior therapy and serotonin reuptake inhibitors. *J. Psychiatr. Res.* **58**, 76–83 (2014).

17 Selles, R.R., McGuire, J.F., Small, B.J., & Storch, E.A. A systematic review and meta-analysis of psychiatric treatments for excoriation (skin-picking) disorder. *Gen. Hosp. Psychiatry* **41**, 29–37 (2016).

18 Silva, R.R., Munoz, D.M., Barickman, J., & Friedhoff, A.J. Environmental factors and related fluctuation of symptoms in children and adolescents with Tourette's disorder. *J. Child Psychol. Psychiatry* **36**, 305–312 (1995).

19 Leckman, J.F., Walker, D E., & Cohen, D.J. Premonitory urges in Tourette's syndrome. *Am. J. Psychiatry* **150**, 98–102 (1993).

20 McGuire, J.F. et al. The premonitory urge revisited: An individualized premonitory urge for tics scale. *J. Psychiatr. Res.* **83**, 176–183 (2016).

21 Woods, D.W., Piacentini, J., Himle, M.B., & Chang, S. Premonitory Urge for Tics Scale (PUTS): Initial psychometric results and examination of the premonitory urge phenomenon in youths with tic disorders. *J. Dev. Behav. Pediatr.* **26**, 397–403 (2005).

22 Essoe, J.K.-Y., Ramsey, K.A., Singer, H.S., Grados, M., & McGuire, J.F. Mechanisms underlying behavior therapy for Tourette's disorder. *Curr. Dev. Disord. Rep.* (2021) doi:10.1007/s40474-021-00225-1.

23 Friman, P.C., Finney, J.W., & Christophersen, E.R. Behavioral treatment of trichotillomania: An evaluative review. *Behav. Ther.* **15**, 249–265 (1984).

24 Himle, M.B. et al. Variables associated with tic exacerbation in children with chronic tic disorders. *Behav. Modif.* **38**, 163–183 (2014).

25 Azrin, N.H. & Nunn, G. *Habit control in a day.* Pocket Books (1978).

26 Flessner, C.A. et al. The Milwaukee Inventory for Styles of Trichotillomania – Child Version (MIST-C): Initial development and psychometric properties. *Behav. Modif.* **31**, 896–918 (2007).

27 Essoe, J.K.-Y., Grados, M.A., Singer, H.S., Myers, N.S., & McGuire, J.F. Evidence-based treatment of Tourette's disorder and chronic tic disorders. *Expert Rev. Neurother.* **19**, 1103–1115 (2019).

28 Rahman, O., McGuire, J., Storch, E.A., & Lewin, A.B. Preliminary randomized controlled trial of habit reversal training for treatment of hair pulling in youth. *J. Child Adolesc. Psychopharmacol.* **27**, 132–139 (2017).

29 Capriotti, M.R., Ely, L.J., Snorrason, I., & Woods, D.W. Acceptance-enhanced behavior therapy for excoriation (skin-picking) disorder in adults: A clinical case series. *Cogn. Behav. Pract.* **22**, 230–239 (2015).

30 Ricketts, E.J. & Bauer, C.C. Habit reversal training for tics. In *The clinician's guide to treatment and management of youth with Tourette syndrome and tic disorders*, 43–70. Academic Press (2018).

31 Wu, M.S. & McGuire, J.F. Psychoeducation about tic disorders and treatment. in *The clinician's guide to treatment and management of youth with Tourette syndrome and tic disorders*, 21–42. Academic Press (2018).

32 Essoe, J.K.-Y. et al. Homework adherence predicts therapeutic improvement from behavior therapy in Tourette's disorder. *Behav. Res. Ther.* 140, 103844 (2021).

33 Franklin, M.E., Zagrabbe, K., & Benavides, K.L. Trichotillomania and its treatment: A review and recommendations. *Expert Rev. Neurother.* 11, 1165–1174 (2011).

34 Teng, E J., Woods, D.W., & Twohig, M.P. Habit reversal as a treatment for chronic skin picking: A pilot investigation. *Behav. Modif.* 30, 411–422 (2006).

35 Petersen, J., Capel, L., Levin, M., & Twohig, M. Moderators and processes of change in a pilot randomized controlled trial of acceptance-enhanced behavior therapy for trichotillomania in adolescents. *J. Obsessive-Compuls. Relat. Disord.* 35, 1–10 (2022).

36 Twohig, M.P. et al. A pilot randomized controlled trial of online-delivered ACT-enhanced behavior therapy for trichotillomania in adolescents. *Cogn. Behav. Pract.* 28, 653–668 (2021).

37 Leckman, J.F. et al. The Yale Global Tic Severity Scale: Initial testing of a clinician-rated scale of tic severity. *J. Am. Acad. Child Adolesc. Psychiatry* 28, 566–573 (1989).

38 McGuire, J.F. et al. A multicenter examination and strategic revisions of the Yale Global Tic Severity Scale. *Neurology* 90, e1711–e1719 (2018).

39 McGuire, J.F. et al. Defining tic severity and tic impairment in Tourette disorder. *J. Psychiatr. Res.* 133, 93–100 (2021).

40 Murphy, T.K., Lewin, A.B., Storch, E.A., & Stock, S. Practice parameter for the assessment and treatment of children and adolescents with tic disorders. *J. Am. Acad. Child Adolesc. Psychiatry* 52, 1341–1359 (2013).

41 Pringsheim, T. et al. Practice guideline recommendations summary: Treatment of tics in people with Tourette syndrome and chronic tic disorders. *Neurology* 92, 896–906 (2019).

42 Bennett, S. et al. Development and open trial of a psychosocial intervention for young children with chronic tics: The CBIT-JR Study. *Behav. Ther.* 51, 659–669 (2020).

43 McGuire, J.F. & Storch, E.A. Behavior therapy for a 75-year-old woman with chronic motor tic disorder. *Neuropsychiatry* 3, 477–481 (2013).

44 Piacentini, J. et al. Behavior therapy for children with Tourette disorder: A randomized controlled trial. *JAMA* 303, 1929–1937 (2010).

45 Wilhelm, S. et al. Randomized trial of behavior therapy for adults with Tourette's disorder. *Arch. Gen. Psychiatry* 69, 795–803 (2012).

46 McGuire, J.F. et al. A cluster analysis of tic symptoms in children and adults with Tourette syndrome: Clinical correlates and treatment outcome. *Psychiatry Res.* 210, 1198–1204 (2013).

47 McGuire, J.F. et al. Bothersome tics in patients with chronic tic disorders: characteristics and individualized treatment response to behavior therapy. *Behav. Res. Ther.* 70, 56–63 (2015).

48 McGuire, J.F. et al. Effect of behavior therapy for tourette's disorder on psychiatric symptoms and functioning in adults. *Psychol. Med.* 50, 2046–2056 (2020).

49 Woods, D.W. et al. Behavior therapy for tics in children: acute and long-term effects on psychiatric and psychosocial functioning. *J. Child Neurol.* 26, 858–865 (2011).

50 Espil, F.M. et al. Long-term outcomes of behavior therapy for youth with Tourette disorder. *J. Am. Acad. Child Adolesc. Psychiatry* **61**, 764–771 (2022).

51 Sukhodolsky, D.G. et al. Moderators and predictors of response to behavior therapy for tics in Tourette syndrome. *Neurology* **88**, 1029–1036 (2017).

52 Schumer, M.C., Bartley, C.A., & Bloch, M.H. Systematic review of pharmacological and behavioral treatments for skin picking disorder. *J. Clin. Psychopharmacol.* **36**, 147–152 (2016).

53 Skurya, J., Jafferany, M., & Everett, G.J. Habit reversal therapy in the management of body focused repetitive behavior disorders. *Dermatol. Ther.* **33**, e13811 (2020).

54 Franklin, M.E., Edson, A.L., Ledley, D.A., & Cahill, S.P. Behavior therapy for pediatric trichotillomania: A randomized controlled trial. *J. Am. Acad. Child Adolesc. Psychiatry* **50**, 763–771 (2011).

55 Schumer, M.C., Panza, K.E., Mulqueen, J.M., Jakubovski, E., & Bloch, M.H. Long-term outcome in pediatric trichotillomania. *Depress. Anxiety* **32**, 737–743 (2015).

56 McGuire, J.F., Myers, N.S., Lewin, A.B., Storch, E.A., & Rahman, O. The influence of hair pulling styles in the treatment of trichotillomania. *Behav. Ther.* **51**, 895–904 (2020).

57 Woods, D.W. & Houghton, D.C. Evidence-based psychosocial treatments for pediatric body-focused repetitive behavior disorders. *J. Clin. Child Adolesc. Psychol. Off. J. Soc. Clin. Child Adolesc. Psychol. Am. Psychol. Assoc. Div. 53* **45**, 227–240 (2016).

58 Walther, M.R., Ricketts, E.J., Conelea, C.A., & Woods, D.W. Recent advances in the understanding and treatment of trichotillomania. *J. Cogn. Psychother.* **24**, 46–64 (2010).

59 Woods, D.W., Himle, M.B., Stiede, J.T., & Pitts, B.X. Behavioral interventions for children and adults with tic disorder. *Annu. Rev. Clin. Psychol.* **19**, 233–260 (2023).

60 McGuire, J.F. et al. Cognitive control processes in behavior therapy for youth with Tourette's disorder. *J. Child Psychol. Psychiatry* **63**, 296–304 (2022).

61 Ramsey, K.A. et al. The role of affect lability on tic severity and impairment in youth with Tourette's disorder. *J. Obsessive-Compuls. Relat. Disord.* **27**, 100578 (2020).

62 Roberts, S., O'Connor, K., & Bélanger, C. Emotion regulation and other psychological models for body-focused repetitive behaviors. *Clin. Psychol. Rev.* **33**, 745–762 (2013).

63 Houghton, D.C. et al. Measuring the role of psychological inflexibility in trichotillomania. *Psychiatry Res.* **220**, 356–361 (2014).

64 Ramsey, K.A. et al. Urge intolerance predicts tic severity and impairment among adults with Tourette syndrome and chronic tic disorders. *Front. Psychiatry* **13**, (2022).

65 Ramsey, K.A., Essoe, J.K.Y., Storch, E.A., Lewin, A.B., Murphy, T.K., & McGuire, J.F. (2021). Urge intolerance and impairment among youth with Tourette's and chronic tic disorders. *Child Psychiatry & Human Development*, **52**, 761–771.

66 McGuire, J.F. et al. Optimizing behavior therapy for youth with Tourette's disorder. *Neuropsychopharmacology* 1–6 (2020) doi:10.1038/s41386-020-0762-4.

67 Peterson, A.L., Blount, T.H., Villarreal, R., Raj, J.J., & McGuire, J.F. Relaxation training with and without Comprehensive Behavioral Intervention for Tics

for Tourette's disorder: A multiple baseline across participants consecutive case series. *J. Behav. Ther. Exp. Psychiatry* **74**, 101692 (2022).

68 Reese, H. Mindfulness for tics. in *The Clinician's Guide to Treatment and Management of Youth with Tourette Syndrome and Tic Disorders*, 279–299 (2018). doi:10.1016/B978-0-12-811980-8.00013-3.

69 Reese, H.E. et al. Mindfulness-based stress reduction for Tourette syndrome and chronic tic disorder: A pilot study. *J. Psychosom. Res.* **78**, 293–298 (2015).

70 Reese, H.E. et al. Feasibility and acceptability of an online mindfulness-based group intervention for adults with tic disorders. *Pilot Feasibility Stud.* **7**, 82 (2021).

71 Crosby, J., Dehlin, J., Mitchell, P., & Twohig, M. Acceptance and commitment therapy and habit reversal training for the treatment of trichotillomania. *Cogn. Behav. Pract.* **19**, 595–605 (2012).

72 Woods, D.W., Wetterneck, C.T., & Flessner, C.A. A controlled evaluation of acceptance and commitment therapy plus habit reversal for trichotillomania. *Behav. Res. Ther.* **44**, 639–656 (2006).

73 Keuthen, N.J. et al. Pilot trial of dialectical behavior therapy-enhanced habit reversal for trichotillomania. *Depress. Anxiety* **27**, 953–959 (2010).

74 Keuthen, N.J. et al. DBT-enhanced cognitive-behavioral treatment for trichotillomania: A randomized controlled trial. *J. Behav. Addict.* **1**, 106–114 (2012).

75 McGuire, J.F. et al. Evidence-based assessment of compulsive skin picking, chronic tic disorders and trichotillomania in children. *Child Psychiatry Hum. Dev.* **43**, 855–883 (2012).

76 Lee, E.B., Homan, K.J., Morrison, K.L., Ong, C.W., Levin, M.E., & Twohig, M.P. Acceptance and commitment therapy for trichotillomania: A randomized controlled trial of adults and adolescents. *Behavior modification*, **44**, 70–91 (2020).

77 Sambrani, T., Jakubovski, E., & Müller-Vahl, K.R. New insights into clinical characteristics of Gilles de la Tourette syndrome: Findings in 1032 patients from a single German center. *Front. Neurosci.* **10**, 415 (2016).

78 Farhat, L.C. et al. Measuring treatment response in pediatric trichotillomania: A meta-analysis of clinical trials. *J. Child Adolesc. Psychopharmacol.* **30**, 306–315 (2020).

6 Family-based Conceptualization and Treatment of Pediatric Obsessive-Compulsive Disorder

Sisi Guo[1] and Tara S. Peris[1]

[1] *UCLA Semel Institute for Neuroscience and Human Behavior, University of California, Los Angeles, CA*

Obsessive-compulsive disorder (OCD) is a chronic and debilitating disorder with common onset in childhood (Fineberg et al., 2019). Cognitive behavioral therapy (CBT) is considered the gold-standard intervention for pediatric OCD, yet many youths do not respond or exhibit only partial response, even when CBT is used in combination with pharmacotherapy (Freeman et al., 2014; Fineberg et al., 2020). One mechanism for improving treatment response is to address common family dynamics that are known to interfere with CBT treatment response for pediatric OCD (Peris et al., 2012; Murphy & Flessner, 2015). Family-based interventions have garnered attention as an alternative or augmentation to individual CBT to optimize treatment outcomes (Freeman et al., 2018; Peris et al., 2017; Piacentini et al., 2011; Lewin et al., 2014). In this chapter, we (1) identify family factors associated with child and adolescent OCD; (2) review the current evidence base for family interventions for OCD; and (3) provide a case study of pediatric OCD using a family-based conceptualization and treatment. In doing so, we document both advancements and challenges in the development of effective treatments for complex families and highlight important future directions in family-based interventions.

Family Factors in Pediatric Obsessive-Compulsive Disorder

OCD is a distressing condition for most families to navigate. Its symptoms may be difficult to understand, shift over time, or appear to be disruptive or challenging in one setting but non-existent (or well managed) in another. These challenges understandably take a toll. Most families report high levels of stress, and family conflict and blame are common phenomena. Indeed, compared to parents of children without a clinical disorder, parents of children with OCD report higher levels of anxiety

DOI: 10.4324/9781003386278-6

and depression, greater use of maladaptive coping strategies, and poorer adjustment (Derisley et al., 2005). Youth OCD symptom severity and impairment are also linked to parental distress, caregiver strain, social and occupational impairments, and disrupted family routines (Storch et al., 2009; Stewart et al., 2017). The impacts of OCD reverberate throughout the family system and siblings of youth with OCD report higher levels of internalizing problems and poorer sibling relationships relative to peers without mental health problems (Labouliere et al., 2014; Browings et al., 2023). As with all forms of youth psychopathology, these challenges are clearly bidirectional, with OCD symptoms disrupting routine family life, and the home environment simultaneously shaping the development and course of the condition.

By far, the family factor that has received the most attention in the pediatric OCD literature is accommodation (Peris et al., 2008; Storch et al., 2007; Wu et al., 2016). Accommodation is a process by which family members begin to participate in OCD symptoms and rituals, often with a goal of providing relief or avoiding a difficult OCD episode. Accommodation can occur in many forms and can range from participating in a compulsion or providing reassurance to facilitating avoidance or purchasing items needed for a ritual (e.g., soap). It is often insidious in its onset inasmuch as parents make small gestures aimed at helping a child in distress. Although well-intentioned, these gestures are negatively reinforcing and typically grow and expand over time. The result is that the vast majority of youth with OCD receive some form of accommodation from their families, with 99 percent of parents providing at least one form of accommodation, and 77 percent providing accommodations on a daily basis (Storch et al., 2007; Leibowitz et al., 2012). Symptom accommodation is not only linked to OCD symptom severity and functioning (e.g., Garcia et al., 2010; Strauss, Hale, & Stobie, 2015; Wu et al., 2016), but it is also a mechanism of treatment outcome (Merlo et al., 2009). Parental changes in symptom accommodation precede reductions in child symptom severity (Piacentini et al., 2011), and changes in accommodation have been shown to mediate CBT outcome for youth OCD (Peris et al., 2017). Together, these findings suggest that symptom accommodation is an important target of family intervention.

Unfortunately, accommodation can be quite difficult to change. It is closely linked to symptom severity such that more severe cases of OCD tend to have higher levels of family accommodation (Storch et al., 2007; Pinto, Noppen, & Calvocoressi, 2013; Wu et al., 2016). In addition, it is not uncommon for youth to protest, tantrum, or grow aggressive when parents attempt to disengage from accommodation. Indeed, families with higher levels of conflict report more adverse outcomes when they attempt to change patterns of accommodation compared to families with lower levels of discord (Peris et al., 2008). By contrast, families with higher levels of cohesion – a variable that reflects the degree to which families collaborate and support each other when problem solving – report faring better. Conflict, blame, and poor cohesion are relatively common, and they each independently predict poor CBT response, even when controlling for symptom severity at the outset of treatment (Peris et al., 2012). Moreover, they exert additive effects such that treatment response declines as the level of family dysfunction increases. Taken together, this work highlights that it can be difficult for some families to change patterns of accommodation without more structured guidance from the therapist, and, in some cases, addressing broader family dynamics (e.g., conflict, blame).

Another family correlate of pediatric OCD is expressed emotion (EE) – a measure of the affective climate of the home environment. High EE in caregivers – characterized by strong criticism, hostility, and/or emotional over-involvement – is among the most robust predictors of outcome in both the child and adult psychopathology literature (Peris & Miklowitz, 2015). Compared to parents of children without a clinical diagnosis, parents of children with OCD display higher EE (Hibbs et al., 1991; Peris et al., 2012). Within-family differences have also been found; caregivers exhibited more criticism toward their child with OCD than an unaffected sibling (Przeworski et al., 2012). High EE is associated with worse OCD symptom severity at baseline and poorer treatment outcomes (Peris & Miklowitz, 2015). Peris and colleagues (2012) also identified EE as a predictor of treatment outcome for pediatric OCD. Although the mechanism of action is not well understood, one hypothesis is that EE creates an affectively charged home environment whereby stressful dynamics between family members interact with a child's biological vulnerabilities to exacerbate symptoms such as OCD and complicate its recovery (Peris & Miklowitz, 2015).

Observational studies of parent-child interactions have also identified some distinct features in OCD families. Compared to non-clinical families, parents of youth with OCD were more aversive during a problem-solving task, while the children were less warm and more withdrawn (Mantz & Abbott, 2020). Youth with OCD and their parents also displayed lower levels of confidence and positive problem solving compared to parent-child dyads with other anxiety disorders (Barrett, Shortt, & Healy, 2002). Finally, children with OCD showed less warmth and confidence in their ability to solve the problem, and more withdrawal and doubt during their interaction with parents compared to their anxious peers (Mantz & Abbott, 2020). Notably, the negative parent-child interactions that are characteristic of OCD families appear responsive to treatment. Schlup and colleagues (2011) found that after a course of family-involved CBT, mother-child interactions during a problem-solving task improved relative to the waitlist control group.

Family-Based Intervention for Obsessive-Compulsive Disorder

Exposure-based CBT is the treatment of choice for pediatric OCD based on reviews of the literature and expert consensus guidelines (Freeman et al., 2018; Storch et al., 2020). For youth with mild to moderate OCD, CBT is recommended as the first-line treatment, while for youth with severe OCD, CBT plus pharmacotherapy is considered the best starting point (Geller & March, 2012; Avasthi, Sharma, & Grover, 2019; Fineberg et al., 2020). Although CBT has been proven to reduce symptoms and improve functioning, a meaningful number of youths fail or only partially respond to treatment (McGrath & Abbott, 2019). Only 40 percent of youth have an excellent response to CBT in controlled treatment trials, and 50 percent of youth (including treatment responders) remain symptomatic following combined treatment of CBT and sertraline (POTS, 2004; Ivarsson et al., 2015; Storch et al., 2013). Several factors have been shown to limit treatment efficacy for pediatric OCD. These include symptom severity at the outset of treatment, comorbidities such as tic disorder and oppositional defiant disorder, and family functioning (Garcia et al., 2010; Torp et al., 2015; Murphy & Flessner, 2015). Importantly, however, family factors consistently emerge as a potentially modifiable treatment target with clear links to CBT response (Stewart et al., 2017).

Virtually all protocols for pediatric OCD involve some degree of family involvement. However, its timing, intensity, and targets vary. In most standard child-focused protocols, emphasis is on teaching youth with OCD to identify, approach, and tolerate their obsessions (exposures), while refraining from compulsive behaviors that they previously engaged in to manage distress (response prevention). Most CBT sessions are completed with the child alone, while caregivers play a limited role, receiving psychoeducation about OCD, learning about homework, and occasionally assisting in exposure practices (Freeman et al., 2014; March & Mulle, 1998; Piacentini, Langley, & Roblek, 2007). When family specific interventions are used, there is no consensus on how family members should be involved in treatment or which types of techniques should be used. In part, this reflects the methodological differences in how family-based interventions have been designed and tested. To date, most family-based interventions only included attendance by family members and did not explicitly target specific family factors (Freeman et al., 2014; McGrath & Abbott, 2019). These interventions have produced favorable outcomes by significantly reducing OCD symptoms and family accommodation, although the latter construct was not consistently assessed (McGrath & Abbott, 2019). However, it has been difficult to ascertain the additive value of family intervention as they have not been reliably tested against a robust control group (i.e., individual CBT). Moreover, with limited exception (Peris et al., 2017), these treatments have often failed to shift relevant family dynamics or to meaningfully shift putative underlying mechanisms.

When studies have focused on specific family factors in OCD treatment, the most common target has been family accommodation (McGrath & Abbott, 2019). Although accommodation is well recognized as a maladaptive family behavior, treatment approaches to reduce the behavior vary widely across studies. Moreover, most family-based interventions have only targeted accommodation as a family factor, when the behavior likely occurs in a larger suite of other negative family variables such as high EE, conflict, and poor cohesion. The heterogeneous treatment approach and the limited attention to other environmental factors likely contributes to the different outcomes reported in family-based interventions thus far, with effect sizes ranging from small to large (McGrath & Abbott, 2019). To optimize clinical response, treatment must consider and target the range of negative family variables implicated in the development and maintenance of OCD. Indeed, a recent meta-analysis showed that there is a greater reduction in family accommodation when more family factors are addressed in treatment (McGrath & Abbott, 2019).

Positive Family Interaction Therapy (PFIT; Peris & Piacentini, 2016) is an exemplar family-based intervention that takes a mechanism approach by targeting several key family variables (i.e., conflict, cohesion, expressed emotions) to reduce OCD behaviors and family accommodations. PFIT was developed to address broader family dynamics that often make it difficult for families to disengage from accommodation. It focuses on collaborative family problem solving, parental distress tolerance –particularly during exposures, and peaceful disengagement from difficult OCD episodes. To improve the affective environment around the child, parents learn to regulate their emotions through labeling, monitoring, and early intervention (e.g., walking away from difficult and often emotionally-charged OCD episodes to prevent escalation and teaching self-soothing skills to the parent and child). As a way to promote cohesion and reduce conflict, parents also learn to engage in positive and collaborative communication with their children to resolve family problems. In a randomized controlled trial (RCT), PFIT outperformed an alternative family CBT intervention with a more traditional approach (i.e., weekly psychoeducation, session review, and homework discussion). This included superior OCD improvement as measured by remission rate, symptom severity, and functional impairment, and family changes as measured by conflict, accommodation, and cohesion. Of note, the study sample was fairly diverse compared to other OCD treatment trials with one-third of families identifying as a race other than White. Moderation analysis showed that racially minoritized families responded better to PFIT than the control group, highlighting the potential for such intervention to optimize treatment response for diverse families (Peris et al., 2020).

Case Study

In this section, we present the case study of "Sarah" to illustrate a family-based intervention for child OCD that targets individual symptoms and family variables. Sarah was a nine-year-old European-American cisgender girl who came to our intensive outpatient program for treatment of severe OCD. Sarah lived with her mother "Claudia", father "Ralph", and 13-year-old sister "Jessica". She met all developmental milestones and had no significant medical history. Sarah was previously treated for selective mutism when she was in the second grade.

Assessment and Case Conceptualization

At the intake evaluation, the therapist met with Sarah and her mother Claudia to gather information about the presenting problems. According to the family, Sarah first developed symptoms of OCD when she was six years old and the family vacationed on a cruise ship that had a recent rotavirus outbreak. At that time, Sarah began to worry excessively about people spitting in her food and the whole family becoming sick. The obsessions subsided after the trip but reemerged on another family vacation five months ago. Claudia reported that Sarah became fearful of getting sick, refused to go into the ocean to swim, and "did not sleep for a whole week". Over the next five months, Sarah's OCD symptoms evolved and intensified. She participated in weekly supportive therapy but made little improvement.

By the time of the evaluation, Sarah's most bothersome obsession was contamination from dirt, bodily functions (e.g., burping, coughing, and breathing), and "essence" from certain foods (e.g., "wet" fruits, meat and animal products). To avoid these contaminants, Sarah would wash her hands up to 50 times each day, clean various personal and household items, and avoid touching surfaces and individuals she viewed as "dirty". Sarah believed Claudia was the dirtiest person in the family and would closely monitor her movement or question her whereabouts. Interestingly, Claudia was also the family member that provided the most accommodations for Sarah, including helping Sarah use any object that was deemed dirty (e.g., opening door handles, picking up items dropped on the floor) and cleaning items while Sarah watched and critiqued their cleanliness (e.g., laundering clothes that Sarah wore once). The rest of the family also accommodated Sarah's OCD by not sitting on her designated chair, entering her room, eating certain foods around her, or using the same utensils as her. In addition to contamination obsessions, Sarah also had "just right" symptoms that were less bothersome; she had to perform certain tasks such as pushing chairs into tables and arranging gym mats until she achieved a "just right" feeling.

Claudia reported that Sarah would have "outbursts" several times a week when she was asked to resist a compulsion or the family refused to follow through with accommodations. During these episodes, Sarah would scream at family members, throw objects at them, and make threats that she did not want to live or that she would hurt her family. However, the family acknowledged that Sarah had no intention to harm herself and others and she was always scared by her own "outbursts".

During the intake, the therapist used the Children's Yale-Brown Obsessive-Compulsive Scale (CY-BOCS; Scahill et al., 1997) to gather information about Sarah's OCD symptoms, and the Family Accommodation Scale for Obsessive-Compulsive Disorder (FAS; Calvocoressi et al., 1999) to understand the type and degree of accommodations provided by Sarah's family. Throughout the interview, the therapist paid close attention to how OCD affected each person in the family, their insight about their role on OCD, and their motivation to change. Lastly, the therapist used the intake to observe the parent-child dyad interact in a relatively novel and emotionally challenging situation (i.e., discussing the child's presenting problem and its impact on the family). During the interview, Sarah presented as nervous and withdrawn; she clung to Claudia's side, made little eye contact, and rarely spoke even when directly prompted by the therapist. At times, Sarah would mutter under her breath or grunt loudly, which appeared to frustrate Claudia. Claudia requested that Sarah "speak up" if she disagreed with the information she provided and repeatedly apologized to the therapist about Sarah's "bad attitude". Claudia showed a wide range of emotions during the interview – anxiety about Sarah's worsening OCD and outbursts, guilt for the accommodations she provided and her own history of OCD, and anger about Sarah's low motivation to get better.

Taken together, the therapist viewed Sarah as a nine-year-old with severe OCD characterized by obsessions and compulsions related to contamination and "just right" urges (CY-BOCS score = 31). The family provided extensive accommodations that not only maintained Sarah's OCD but also disrupted the entire family's daily routines (FAS score = 36). Accommodation was conceptualized as the parents' effort to alleviate Sarah's distress and their own, as Claudia also reported fears about contamination. Finally, the family demonstrated low cohesion and high conflict; their interactions were characterized by blame and criticism, overinvolvement, and poor affect regulation and communication. Based on this conceptualization, the therapist formulated a treatment plan that combined standard exposure and response prevention (ERP) with active parent participation in treatment. In doing so, the therapist aimed to decrease Sarah's OCD and address family risk factors that were maintaining her symptoms and interfering with family functioning.

Treatment Plan and Execution

The therapist formulated the treatment plan to include (1) child-focused ERP sessions to decrease obsessions and compulsions, (2) parent sessions to reduce family accommodations, affect dysregulation and other negative parent-child interactions, and (3) joint family meetings to generalize adaptive coping skills across family members and settings. Reduction of family accommodation and negative parent-child interactions were theorized as the mechanisms of change.

The first part of treatment focused on psychoeducation about OCD and the goals of treatment. In the child ERP sessions, Sarah learned that (1) obsessions and compulsions feed into each other in a negative cycle, (2) obsessions can go away on their own without compulsions, and (3) treatment will teach her to tolerate the distress from obsessions without doing a compulsion. In the parent sessions, the therapist provided similar psychoeducation about the OCD cycle and the rationale for exposure-based CBT. This traditional psychoeducation was enhanced by further teaching the parents that (1) accommodation is a part of the OCD cycle, and one that serves a similar function as compulsions, providing only temporary relief and maintaining the OCD, (2) a goal of treatment is to refrain from accommodation and support exposure-based approaches, (3) which requires parents to be able to monitor and manage the emotions that come up in treatment, and (4) accordingly, treatment will teach them emotion regulation and problem-solving skills to support disengagement from accommodation. Through psychoeducation, the therapist helped Sarah and her parents externalize OCD as a common problem to solve rather than blame each other. Psychoeducation also taught the family that while compulsions and accommodations were initially performed to help with Sarah's distress, they had become harmful over time and must be changed to improve Sarah's and the family's functioning. In this early stage of treatment, a parent-only session was also conducted to explore and validate the full spectrum of emotions that parents were feeling. The therapist normalized feelings of frustration and blame that the parents were feeling while simultaneously conveying the need to monitor and manage these feelings to respond in effective ways to OCD. The parents were asked to notice their emotions in different situations with Sarah, and separately, to begin to develop a list of the ways in which they accommodated OCD symptoms.

The second part of treatment focused on emotion regulation skills. Sarah and Claudia displayed a range of emotions at the intake, including anxiety, frustration, and anger. The therapist selected this treatment module to provide the family with some adaptive coping skills that would be consistently reinforced throughout the rest of treatment. This proved highly important for Sarah as she struggled to communicate her distress at the outset of treatment. She was unable to separate from Claudia for the first few sessions and refused to talk other than in grunts or moans when the therapist asked her a question or prompted her to do an exposure. During these exchanges, Claudia spoke on behalf of Sarah but was visibly frustrated and frequently blamed Sarah for "not trying hard enough". To address these problems, the therapist introduced the concept of affect labeling to help the family identify their emotions in stressful situations, such as participating in an intensive treatment program and resisting OCD urges. Paralleling the individual child sessions, the parents also learned to use the feelings wheel and feelings thermometer to label and monitor the intensity of their emotions, particularly the feeling of anxiety/anger in the context of OCD treatment (e.g., when resisting a compulsion or refraining from accommodating to the symptoms). Finally, the therapist taught Sarah and her parents self-soothing skills that they could use when they noticed their distress rising on the feeling thermometer. Specific strategies included relaxation (e.g., deep breathing, progressive muscle relaxation) and mindfulness/

grounding techniques (e.g., using all five senses to observe your surroundings). The goal of this treatment module was to provide Sarah and her parents with a common language to communicate their feelings and identify moments when they can engage in adaptive coping in order to reduce distress and respond to difficult situations more effectively. The parents were thus encouraged to recognize and monitor their emotions in a way that paralleled Sarah's distress ratings in the upcoming exposure sessions. They continued to develop their list of accommodations and to gain awareness of patterns that served to continue the OCD cycle.

In the third stage of family treatment, the therapist worked with Sarah and her parents to translate the accommodation list into a hierarchy that could be used to begin to disengage from symptom accommodation. This hierarchy was viewed as distinct from the hierarchy developed in individual sessions because it asked parents to list OCD symptoms, how hard it would be for *them* to disengage from accommodation, and, separately, how hard it would be for Sarah to tolerate. Sarah was asked to do the same exercise. These separate symptom hierarchies became a platform for discussion. Parents were able to note places where they overestimated how difficult certain changes in routine might be, and Sarah was able to communicate what she felt ready to address. With therapist support, they worked together to create a "joint hierarchy" that was their roadmap for disengaging from accommodation.

The goal of the hierarchy development was to teach the family about a gradual stepwise approach to taking on appropriate new challenges that would maximize the chance of successful practice. For the parents, the symptom hierarchy was also a good model for teaching the concept of scaffolding. Specifically, Sarah's parents were taught to use the feelings thermometer to identify situations or modify exposures to be sufficiently challenging so that Sarah had the opportunity to learn without becoming overwhelmed. For Claudia, the ability to label and compare distress ratings was particularly useful, as she saw over time that her expectations of Sarah's reaction did not always match with Sarah's own experience. Moreover, the anticipated distress ratings from both the parents and Sarah often exceeded the actual experience of distress in the moment.

Using the symptom hierarchy as a guide, the therapist and Sarah began to complete exposures in session to target her fears of contamination from dirt (e.g., picking up items from the floor, re-wearing clothes she had worn before, washing herself in the shower), germs and bodily fluids (e.g., using the same utensils that others have used, sitting near people when they breathe and eat, visiting a hospital), and "essence" from specific foods (e.g., eating "wet" fruits such as strawberry and mango, eating vegetarian food that touches meat). Additionally, treatment also targeted Sarah's "just right" symptoms (e.g., moving furniture before a "just right" feeling is achieved, resisting re-writing and re-reading). In the parent sessions, the therapist collaborated with parents to reduce their accommodations at home. Similar to individual exposures, family accommodations were removed gradually and systematically based on the reported difficulty. For example, Claudia first stopped helping Sarah use or clean objects that were perceived to be less dirty (e.g., car doors, items dropped on the floor at home). Once Sarah tolerated these changes, Claudia refrained from helping her with using "dirtier" items (e.g., clinic doors, items from outside, laundry). Likewise, Claudia gradually removed her reassurance about the cleanliness of items and people; she first reduced the frequency of her responses, then stopped responding altogether, and eventually asked Sarah to answer questions on her own if she had the urge to know.

Despite having a hierarchy to withdraw accommodations, the parental changes did not always go according to plan. For example, when Claudia attempted to reduce the number of reassurances she offered to Sarah about the cleanliness of items, Sarah would increase her questioning, follow her around, and escalate to tantrums. This angered Claudia, who would fluctuate between shouting back and attempting to console Sarah with reason. In these situations, the therapist provided additional parent training. Specifically, Claudia learned to validate Sarah's distress (i.e., "I can tell this is really hard for you when I'm not answering you as usual"), help Sarah label the distress as OCD (i.e., "This is your OCD"), suggest a coping skill (i.e., "Is there something you learned from your therapist that you can do to feel better?"), and ultimately walk away. For many parents, the hardest but most important part is walking away when the child is visibly distressed. However, by walking away, the parent is modeling emotion regulation and giving the child an opportunity to self-soothe. Walking away also proved useful when Sarah's contamination fears triggered Claudia's own OCD. For example, Sarah's avoidance of washing "dirty parts" of her body worried Claudia and during Sarah's shower she would often "scrub her down" to ensure she was cleaned properly. When the therapist asked Sarah to wash herself, Claudia struggled to let go of her accommodation.

The therapist provided additional psychoeducation about personal hygiene but ultimately also encouraged Claudia to recognize that if her distress is too high, she should walk away and allow Sarah to manage the exposure on her own. Claudia agreed; she asked Ralph to assist with Sarah's shower exposures, which at times involved minimal cleaning for the purpose of over-correction.

To promote cohesion and reduce conflict, the therapist also taught Sarah and Claudia collaborative problem solving to address OCD and non-OCD issues at home. Despite notable improvements in session, Claudia still reported ongoing "outbursts" at home. The therapist introduced functional analysis to the family. Specifically, Sarah and Claudia were asked to identify problematic behaviors they would like to change, examine the events that led up to the behaviors (antecedent), and how each family member responded after the behaviors (consequences). With the therapist's aid, Sarah and Claudia brainstormed solutions, assessed the costs and benefits of each one, and finally chose one solution to try out at home. For example, Claudia reported an incident where Sarah screamed at her for bringing out strawberries during a playdate. Through the functional analysis, Sarah learned that Claudia saw her take bites of strawberries in session and believed she was ready to do the same at home. Claudia learned that Sarah was expecting her usual snacks and was not prepared to eat the fruit that she still felt "uncomfortable" around. Moreover, she was embarrassed and nervous about what her friend would think. After some brainstorming, the family agreed that it was important to introduce fruits Sarah previously avoided in the home, but the exposure required more planning and practice around family members first before peers. Claudia also agreed that if Sarah continues to struggle with these exposures, she will walk away to give Sarah space to use her coping tools. These problem-solving sessions allowed Claudia and Sarah to hear each other's perspective in a calm and neutral environment, identify shared goals, and think more flexibly about how to solve a problem.

Over the course of treatment, Sarah and her parents made significant improvement in reducing OCD-related compulsions and accommodations. By the end of treatment, Sarah had stopped asking parents to help her avoid potential contaminants and was able to tolerate previously feared places, objects, and foods independently. Although Sarah still experienced obsessions, she was generally able to resist the urge to perform a compulsion or purposefully challenge her OCD with an exposure. Likewise, Sarah's parents – particularly

Claudia – learned to withdraw accommodation by regulating their own emotions in times of distress, collaborating with Sarah to resolve conflict, and increasing positive communication. In supporting Sarah in daily exposures, the parents also sent the positive message to Sarah that she is capable of handling distress; rather than helping her escape from challenging events, they were modeling and reinforcing her courageous behaviors of confronting her fears, labeling her emotions, and using adaptive coping tools to self-soothe. In lieu of accommodating Sarah's OCD behaviors, the family was able to spend more time together doing more positive and non-OCD activities, which the therapist continuously encouraged throughout treatment. Taken together, Sarah had made significant improvement and was ready to transition from our intensive outpatient program to weekly outpatient therapy (CY-BOCS score = 7). The parents also made significant improvement by reducing their accommodations and improving family functioning (FAS score = 2).

Summary and Future Directions

Several family factors are implicated in the development and course of pediatric OCD. These include parental accommodations, high EE such as criticism and hostility, family conflict and poor cohesion, and negative parent-child interactions. Despite the growing evidence that the family ecosystem surrounding a child with OCD is a prime target for treatment, few family-based interventions have been effectively designed and tested to demonstrate their efficacy over individual CBT. The few family-involved interventions for pediatric OCD have limited their focus to reduce accommodations. However, they rarely take into consideration other relevant variables and are not mechanism-based to identify specific models of change. This gap in research and treatment is concerning as many youths with OCD do not respond sufficiently to the current gold-standard care; they remain symptomatic, and their family continue to experience disruptions to their daily living as a result. Below, we outline recommendations for research, treatment, and training to optimize care of childhood OCD.

Future Directions in Research

Family accommodations have been shown in research to be a critical parenting factor that maintains OCD symptoms and negatively impacts outcomes in therapy. In response, treatment studies are increasingly targeting this negative behavior by integrating parents in treatment sessions with and without the child, producing favorable results for both parent and child functioning. We recommend that researchers invest equally in related system-level variables such as expressed emotions and conflict, as they are common in families affected by OCD but rarely directly targeted in treatment. A recent meta-analysis showed that when more family factors are targeted in treatment, there is greater reduction of family accommodations (McGrath & Abbott, 2019).

Future research should also elucidate how to effectively integrate family members in treatment and for whom. There is significant heterogeneity in how caregivers are involved, from psychoeducation only to more skills-training. Dismantling studies that compare different permutations of family involvement is challenging but necessary to identify the active ingredients in family treatment (e.g., problem solving, emotion regulation, communication skills training, psychoeducation). Likewise, more research is needed to determine the optimal dosage of family involvement. To date, the number of hours parents spent in treatment does not appear to influence child outcome, and there is insufficient data to assess its impact on family functioning (McGrath & Abbott, 2019). The degree of family involvement may also depend on who makes up the family. There is some evidence that parent-involved treatment is more beneficial for certain groups, such as younger children and families with higher parental distress (Breinholst et al., 2012). Following this line of research, it is possible that the degree of parental involvement depends on factors such as family structure and cultural background and values.

To date, family-based interventions have not demonstrated additional benefits over individual treatment for pediatric OCD when symptom improvement is the primary measure of outcome; more randomized trials with a robust control group are needed to determine whether family treatment can improve clinical outcomes of the non- and partial responders to individual CBT. When assessing the efficacy of family-based interventions, it is also important to move beyond individual symptomatology; family-based variables such as cohesion, conflict, and parent-child relationships are meaningful outcomes to consider in determining the immediate and long-term success of treatments. Theoretically, the inclusion of caregivers in treatment should help generalize skills and extend gains in the treatment of child problems (Forehand, Jones, & Parent, 2013). Compared to individually focused CBT, family-based interventions may also be more acceptable and sustainable because parents are systematically integrated and engaged in treatment. Relatedly, it is important for treatment research to use accurate and timely assessment of parental and family factors.

Routine monitoring of systems-level variables (e.g., maladaptive parenting behaviors and parent-child conflict) along with traditional indicators of change (e.g., symptom severity) throughout treatment is critical to study moderators and mediators of change.

Future Directions in Treatment and Training

In recent years, competency models have gained popularity to translate EBTs into routine clinical settings. For clinicians who are treating pediatric OCD in the context of a complex family system, we recommend the adoption of a common-factors approach by flexibly using conceptualizations and techniques from multiple empirically-supported protocols (Sburlati et al., 2011).

First, it is important for clinicians to examine the impact that systems-level factors such as family structure, parent-child relationships, and parenting behaviors have on the child's behaviors. This can be achieved by conducting a thorough evaluation and gathering relevant data using evidence-based measures. Another way to enhance treatment outcomes is the building of positive relationships with different family members. Given the important role of family in the maintenance and treatment of child outcomes, it is important to build rapport and trust with the parents as well as the child when establishing care. In the context of CBT treatment, we recommend that clinicians pay close attention to the specific parenting behaviors that contribute to negative child outcomes (e.g., blame, criticism, accommodations) and how negative outcomes are transferred between family members (e.g., modeling, reinforcement, conflict). It is also important that clinicians design, execute, and adapt a CBT formulation and treatment plan. When treating a child with OCD, outcomes are likely to be enhanced if clinicians can tailor the degree of parental involvement in treatment based on the family's functioning, parent-child relationship, and parents' willingness and ability to assist. Again, this may require the clinician to conduct a comprehensive evaluation at the outset of treatment. Finally, in terms of specific CBT techniques, we recommend that clinicians target maladaptive parenting factors that have been linked to negative child outcomes in empirical research (e.g., family accommodations, conflict, blame, and hostility).

For beginning clinicians, several factors are important to keep in mind when working with a complex family system: (a) the reciprocal relationship between parents and children, (b) establishment of a therapeutic alliance with all family members without overly identifying with any particular individual, (c) comprehensive assessment of relevant systems-level factors that could affect treatment, and (d) individualization of treatment based on those family variables. For new clinicians, it is also important to know the dynamics of the relationship between the child's OCD behaviors and the family's functioning. Once again, a thorough assessment of the family environment, establishment of positive rapport, and open communication are crucial to identifying and managing negative family variables such as conflict and emotional dysregulation over the course of treatment.

To provide effective treatment for pediatric OCD, it is also important to take a competency-based approach to training. Specifically, we recommend clinical training programs to educate future clinicians about common factors that inform the change process in family interventions. Students should not only gain exposure to a variety of empirically-supported protocols but also recognize the overarching approach and techniques that are relevant to multiple evidence-based practices (Karam & Sprenkle, 2010). Moreover, students should receive training to analyze findings from empirical studies, select evidence-based measurement tools, and adapt evidence-based protocols for "real-world" settings to translate EBTs into their daily clinical practice (Kaslow et al., 2012).

References

Avasthi, A., Sharma, A., & Grover, S. (2019). Clinical practice guidelines for the management of obsessive-compulsive disorder in children and adolescents. *Indian Journal of Psychiatry, 61*(Suppl 2), 306.

Barrett, P., Shortt, A., & Healy, L. (2002). Do parent and child behaviours differentiate families whose children have obsessive-compulsive disorder from other clinic and non-clinic families? *Journal of Child Psychology and Psychiatry, 43*(5), 597–607.

Breinholst, S., Esbjørn, B.H., Reinholdt-Dunne, M.L., & Stallard, P. (2012). CBT for the treatment of child anxiety disorders: A review of why parental involvement has not enhanced outcomes. *Journal of Anxiety Disorders, 26*(3), 416–424.

Brownings, S., Hale, L., Simonds, L. M., & Jassi, A. (2023). Exploring the experiences and responses of siblings living with a brother or sister with obsessive compulsive disorder. *Psychology and Psychotherapy: Theory, Research and Practice, 96*(2), 464–479.

Calvocoressi, L., Mazure, C.M., Kasl, S.V., Skolnick, J., Fisk, D., Vegso, S. J., . . . & Price, L.H. (1999). Family accommodation of obsessive-compulsive symptoms: Instrument development and assessment of family behavior. *The Journal of Nervous and Mental Disease, 187*(10), 636–642.

Derisley, J., Libby, S., Clark, S., & Reynolds, S. (2005). Mental health, coping and family-functioning in parents of young people with obsessive-compulsive disorder and with anxiety disorders. *British Journal of Clinical Psychology, 44*(3), 439–444.

Fineberg, N.A., Dell'Osso, B., Albert, U., Maina, G., Geller, D., Carmi, L., . . . & Zohar, J. (2019). Early intervention for obsessive compulsive disorder: an expert consensus statement. *European Neuropsychopharmacology, 29*(4), 549–565.

Fineberg, N.A., Hollander, E., Pallanti, S., Walitza, S., Grünblatt, E., Dell'Osso, B.M., . . . & Menchon, J.M. (2020). Clinical advances in obsessive-compulsive disorder: A position statement by the International College of Obsessive-Compulsive Spectrum Disorders. *International Clinical Psychopharmacology, 35*(4), 173.

Forehand, R., Jones, D.J., & Parent, J. (2013). Behavioral parenting interventions for child disruptive behaviors and anxiety: What's different and what's the same. *Clinical Psychology Review, 33*(1), 133–145.

Freeman, J., Benito, K., Herren, J., Kemp, J., Sung, J., Georgiadis, C., . . . & Garcia, A. (2018). Evidence base update of psychosocial treatments for pediatric obsessive-compulsive disorder: Evaluating, improving, and transporting what works. *Journal of Clinical Child & Adolescent Psychology, 47*(5), 669–698.

Freeman, J., Garcia, A., Frank, H., Benito, K., Conelea, C., Walther, M., & Edmunds, J. (2014). Evidence base update for psychosocial treatments for pediatric obsessive-compulsive disorder. *Journal of Clinical Child & Adolescent Psychology, 43*(1), 7–26.

Garcia, A.M., Sapyta, J.J., Moore, P.S., Freeman, J.B., Franklin, M.E., March, J.S., & Foa, E.B. (2010). Predictors and moderators of treatment outcome in the Pediatric Obsessive Compulsive Treatment Study (POTS I). *Journal of the American Academy of Child & Adolescent Psychiatry, 49*(10), 1024–1033.

Geller, D.A., & March, J. (2012). Practice parameter for the assessment and treatment of children and adolescents with obsessive-compulsive disorder. *Journal of the American Academy of Child and Adolescent Psychiatry, 51*(1), 98–113. https://doi.org/10.1016/j.jaac.2011.09.019.

Hibbs, E.D., Hamburger, S.D., Lenane, M., Rapoport, J.L., Kruesi, M.J., Keysor, C.S., & Goldstein, M.J. (1991). Determinants of expressed emotion in families of disturbed and normal children. *Journal of Child Psychology and Psychiatry, 32*(5), 757–770.

Ivarsson, T., Skarphedinsson, G., Kornør, H., Axelsdottir, B., Biedilæ, S., Heyman, I., . . . & March, J. (2015). The place of and evidence for serotonin reuptake inhibitors (SRIs) for obsessive compulsive disorder (OCD) in children and adolescents: Views based on a systematic review and meta-analysis. *Psychiatry Research, 227*(1), 93–103.

Karam, E.A., & Sprenkle, D.H. (2010). The research informed clinician: A guide to training the next generation MFT. *Journal of Marital and Family Therapy, 36*, 307–319.

Kaslow, N.J., Broth, M.R., Smith, C.O., & Collins, M.H. (2012). Family-based interventions for child and adolescent disorders. *Journal of Marital and Family Therapy, 38*(1), 82–100.

Labouliere, C.D., Arnold, E.B., Storch, E.A., & Lewin, A.B. (2014). Family-based cognitive-behavioral treatment for a preschooler with obsessive-compulsive disorder. *Clinical Case Studies, 13*(1), 37–51.

Lebowitz, E.R., Panza, K.E., Su, J., & Bloch, M.H. (2012). Family accommodation in obsessive–compulsive disorder. *Expert Review of Neurotherapeutics, 12*(2), 229–238.

Lewin, A.B., Park, J.M., Jones, A.M., Crawford, E.A., De Nadai, A.S., Menzel, J., . . .& Storch, E.A. (2014). Family-based exposure and response prevention therapy for preschool-aged children with obsessive-compulsive disorder: A pilot randomized controlled trial. *Behaviour Research and Therapy, 56*, 30–38.

Mantz, S.C., & Abbott, M.J. (2020). Parent-child interactions and childhood OCD: Comparing OCD families with other clinical and non-clinical families. *Journal of Obsessive-Compulsive and Related Disorders, 26*, Article 100549.

March, J.S., & Mulle, K. (1998). *OCD in children and adolescents: A cognitive-behavioral treatment manual.* Guilford Press.

Merlo, L.J., Lehmkuhl, H.D., Geffken, G.R., & Storch, E.A. (2009). Decreased family accommodation associated with improved therapy outcome in pediatric obsessive–compulsive disorder. *Journal of Consulting and Clinical Psychology*, 77(2), 355.

McGrath, C.A., & Abbott, M.J. (2019). Family-based psychological treatment for obsessive compulsive disorder in children and adolescents: A meta-analysis and systematic review. *Clinical Child and Family Psychology Review*, 22, 478–501.

Murphy, Y.E., & Flessner, C.A. (2015). Family functioning in paediatric obsessive compulsive and related disorders. *British Journal of Clinical Psychology*, 54(4), 414–434.

Peris, T.S., Bergman, R.L., Langley, A., Chang, S., McCracken, J.T., & Piacentini, J. (2008). Correlates of accommodation of pediatric obsessive-compulsive disorder: Parent, child, and family characteristics. *Journal of the American Academy of Child & Adolescent Psychiatry*, 47(10), 1173–1181.

Peris, T.S., & Miklowitz, D.J. (2015). Parental expressed emotion and youth psychopathology: New directions for an old construct. *Child Psychiatry & Human Development*, 46, 863–873.

Peris, T.S., & Piacentini, J. (2016). *Helping families manage childhood OCD: Decreasing conflict and increasing positive interaction, Therapist guide.* Oxford University Press.

Peris, T.S., Rozenman, M.S., Bai, S., Perez, J., Thamrin, H., & Piacentini, J. (2020). Ethnicity moderates outcome in family focused treatment for pediatric obsessive compulsive disorder. *Journal of Anxiety Disorders*, 73, 102229.

Peris, T.S., Rozenman, M.S., Sugar, C.A., McCracken, J.T., & Piacentini, J. (2017). Targeted family intervention for complex cases of pediatric obsessive-compulsive disorder: a randomized controlled trial. *Journal of the American Academy of Child & Adolescent Psychiatry*, 56(12), 1034–1042.

Peris, T.S., Sugar, C.A., Bergman, R.L., Chang, S., Langley, A., & Piacentini, J. (2012). Family factors predict treatment outcome for pediatric obsessive-compulsive disorder. *Journal of consulting and clinical psychology*, 80(2), 255.

Peris, T.S., Yadegar, M., Asarnow, J.R., & Piacentini, J. (2012). Pediatric obsessive compulsive disorder: Family climate as a predictor of treatment outcome. *Journal of Obsessive-Compulsive and Related Disorders*, 1(4), 267–273.

Piacentini, J., Bergman, R. L., Chang, S., Langley, A., Peris, T., Wood, J.J., & McCracken, J. (2011). Controlled comparison of family cognitive behavioral therapy and psychoeducation/relaxation training for child obsessive-compulsive disorder. *Journal of the American Academy of Child & Adolescent Psychiatry*, 50(11), 1149–1161.

Piacentini, J., Langley, A., & Roblek, T. (2007). *Cognitive behavioral treatment of childhood OCD: It's only a false alarm therapist guide.* Oxford University Press.

Pinto, A., Van Noppen, B., & Calvocoressi, L. (2013). Development and preliminary psychometric evaluation of a self-rated version of the Family Accommodation Scale for Obsessive-Compulsive Disorder. *Journal of Obsessive-Compulsive and Related Disorders*, 2(4), 457–465.

Przeworski, A., Zoellner, L.A., Franklin, M.E., Garcia, A., Freeman, J., March, J.S., & Foa, E.B. (2012). Maternal and child expressed emotion as predictors of treatment response in pediatric obsessive–compulsive disorder. *Child Psychiatry & Human Development*, 43, 337–353.

Shurlati, F.S., Schniering, C.A., Lyneham, H.J., & Rapee, R.M. (2011). A model of therapist competencies for the empirically supported cognitive behavioral treatment of child and adolescent anxiety and depressive disorders. *Clinical Child and Family Psychology Review*, 14, 89–109.

Scahill, L., Riddle, M.A., McSwiggin-Hardin, M., Ort, S.I., King, R.A., Goodman, W.K., . . . & Leckman, J. F. (1997). Children's Yale-Brown obsessive compulsive scale: reliability and validity. *Journal of the American Academy of Child & Adolescent Psychiatry, 36*(6), 844–852.

Schlup, B., Farrell, L., & Barrett, P. (2011). Mother-child interactions and childhood OCD: Effects of CBT on mother and child observed behaviors. *Child & family behavior therapy, 33*(4), 322–336.

Stewart, S.E., Hu, Y.P., Leung, A., Chan, E., Hezel, D.M., Lin, S.Y., . . . & Pauls, D.L. (2017). A multisite study of family functioning impairment in pediatric obsessive-compulsive disorder. *Journal of the American Academy of Child & Adolescent Psychiatry, 56*(3), 241–249.

Storch, E.A., Bussing, R., Small, B.J., Geffken, G.R., McNamara, J.P., Rahman, O., . . . & Murphy, T.K. (2013). Randomized, placebo-controlled trial of cognitive-behavioral therapy alone or combined with sertraline in the treatment of pediatric obsessive–compulsive disorder. *Behaviour research and therapy, 51*(12), 823–829.

Storch, E.A., Geffken, G.R., Merlo, L.J., Jacob, M.L., Murphy, T.K., Goodman, W.K., . . . & Grabill, K. (2007). Family accommodation in pediatric obsessive–compulsive disorder. *Journal of Clinical Child and Adolescent Psychology, 36*(2), 207–216.

Storch, E.A., Lehmkuhl, H., Pence, S.L., Geffken, G.R., Ricketts, E., Storch, J.F., & Murphy, T.K. (2009). Parental experiences of having a child with obsessive-compulsive disorder: Associations with clinical characteristics and caregiver adjustment. *Journal of Child and Family Studies, 18*, 249–258.

Storch, E.A., Peris, T.S., De Nadai, A., Piacentini, J., Bloch, M., Cervin, M., . . . & Goodman, W. K. (2020). Little doubt that CBT works for pediatric OCD. *Journal of the American Academy of Child and Adolescent Psychiatry, 59*(7), 785–787.

Strauss, C., Hale, L., & Stobie, B. (2015). A meta-analytic review of the relationship between family accommodation and OCD symptom severity. *Journal of Anxiety Disorders, 33*, 95–102.

The Pediatric OCD Treatment Study Team (POTS) (2004). Cognitive-behavior therapy, sertraline, and their combination for children and adolescents with obsessive-compulsive disorder: the Pediatric OCD Treatment Study (POTS) randomized controlled trial. *Jama, 292*(16), 1969–1976.

Torp, N.C., Dahl, K., Skarphedinsson, G., Compton, S., Thomsen, P.H., Weidle, B., . . . & Ivarsson, T. (2015). Predictors associated with improved cognitive-behavioral therapy outcome in pediatric obsessive-compulsive disorder. *Journal of the American Academy of Child & Adolescent Psychiatry, 54*(3), 200–207.

Wu, M.S., McGuire, J.F., Martino, C., Phares, V., Selles, R.R., & Storch, E.A. (2016). A meta-analysis of family accommodation and OCD symptom severity. *Clinical Psychology Review, 45*, 34–44.

7 Parental Involvement in Pediatric Obsessive-Compulsive Disorder Treatment

Cynthia Onyeka,[1] *and*
Abigail Candelari, PhD.[1,2]

[1] *Department of Psychiatry and Behavioral Sciences, Baylor College of Medicine, Houston, TX*

[2] *Ben Taub Hospital, Harris Health System, Houston, TX*

Author Note

Correspondence regarding this manuscript should be sent to Ogechi "Cynthia" Onyeka, Ph.D., Department of Psychiatry and Behavioral Sciences, Baylor College of Medicine, 1977 Butler Boulevard, Houston, TX, 77030. Email: Ogechi.onyeka@bcm.edu.

Overview

Pediatric obsessive-compulsive disorder (OCD) is a neuropsychiatric disorder defined by obsessive thoughts (i.e., unwanted, repetitive, intrusive cognitions) and subsequent compulsive behaviors and/or mental acts (Demaria et al., 2021; Storch et al., 2007). Pediatric OCD is diverse in presentation and, when left untreated, follows a chronic course that can present significant functional impairment in a child's life and across their lifespan (Albert et al., 2010; Wu et al., 2018).

Pediatric OCD has been described as a "family-based illness", as the development and maintenance of symptoms are often associated with a variety of parental and/or caregiver factors. For many children, OCD symptoms and behaviors present at home and impact quality of life for both the child and family. Empirical evidence strongly suggests family functioning, parental modeling, and family accommodation (the extent to which caregivers endorse OCD symptoms by participating in the rituals) play a role in symptom severity, resulting in in a feedback loop impacting functional impairment across all parties (Lebowitz et al., 2012; Stewart et al., 2017; Waters & Barrett, 2000). Patterns of family functioning, parent-child interactions, and parental factors all likely impact symptom expression and presentation, suggesting the need for a family-based framework for treatment.

DOI: 10.4324/9781003386278-7

Given the significant role of parents and caregivers, treatment for pediatric OCD (cognitive behavioral therapy [CBT] with exposure and response prevention [ERP]) is the gold-standard intervention) often includes parental involvement in varying forms (POTS, 2004; Geller & March, 2012). The extent to which parents and/or caregivers are involved in treatment does vary depending on the intervention, but typically all exhibit key active ingredients. This chapter will first present a thorough conceptualization of parent-focused pediatric OCD treatment, centering the family context in symptom presentation and orientation of treatment. Next, the differences in treatment delivery will be reviewed, followed by significant parental factors to consider in treatment. A recent empirical example of a parent-based treatment, the Supportive Parenting for Anxious Childhood Emotions (SPACE) program, will then be discussed, concluded by a summary and recommendations for future work.

Conceptualizing the Family as a Vehicle for Treatment

Importance of the Family Context

There is considerable evidence to suggest that family context and related functioning are imperative vehicles for sustainable treatment development and delivery (Freeman et al., 2008, 2014b; Lebowitz et al., 2020). Given the embeddedness of the child within the family system, it is important to consider the reciprocal roles of the parent/caregivers and child on the development and maintenance of symptoms. Regarding pediatric OCD, this begins at the genetic level where there is compelling evidence to suggest that OCD has a strong hereditary component (Monzani et al., 2014; Nesdat et al., 2010). Heritability estimates hover around 48–60 percent for OCD according to family and twin studies, suggesting that an individual's genetic load presents a significant risk factor (Monzani et al., 2014; Waters & Barrett, 2000). However, both genetic and environmental factors (including the family system) play a role in symptom presentation and severity.

Broadly, the family system is a key factor in transdiagnostic mental health symptom severity and related treatment outcomes. Children are first socialized to comprehend, express, and regulate emotions within the family context. Due to their dependence on their caregivers, children are highly vulnerable to family processes and interactions that impact their overall emotional well-being (e.g., children are less likely to adaptively regulate their emotions if their parents are unable to; Blaustein & Kinniburgh, 2010). For example, contextual factors such as parental psychopathology and family dynamics can all impact the severity of child symptoms, functional impairment, and treatment progress (Kazdin & Weisz, 1998; Selles et al., 2020). Pediatric OCD presents a unique lens through which to contextualize the role of family in symptoms and treatment in that parents/caregivers often participate in (i.e., accommodate) their child's symptoms (i.e., rituals and avoidance). This then presents an accommodation cycle where parents unknowingly perpetuate existing symptoms in order to temporarily reduce distress (Lebowitz et al., 2012). Understanding how a parent may become involved in this cycle is an important component of treatment conceptualization. Moreover, incorporating parenting behaviors into individual treatment itself has increasingly been recognized as critical to amplifying intervention outcomes (Peris et al., 2017; see Chapter 6).

Why Parental Involvement in Treatment?

Cognitive and behavioral-oriented family interventions have long been considered as the model of choice when involving parents in treatment of a wide range of childhood psychopathology (e.g., attention-deficit/hyperactivity disorder, oppositional defiant disorder, eating disorders, etc.; Mash & Barkley, 2014). The cognitive-behavioral intervention model consists of addressing the affective and cognitive features of the parent-child relationship and targeting behaviors (Freeman et al., 2008; Sanders, 1996). There is empirical support for paradigms of this nature, where parents serve as an integral vehicle to deliver active ingredients of the treatment such as psychoeducation, coaching, behavior change, and relapse prevention (Everett, Martin, & Zalewski, 2021; Farmer et al., 2002). With respect to pediatric OCD, several studies suggest that parental involvement is necessary in pediatric OCD treatment to support the previously discussed treatment components as well as to design and practice exposures, a key portion of ERP (Freeman et al., 2014a; Freeman et al., 2018; Storch et al., 2010. Given the importance of parents and family context, treatments involving a significant parental component or family-focused interventions are more likely to be more effective and associated with long-term treatment gains than interventions that solely target the child (Waters & Barrett, 2000; Peris et al., 2017). Moreover, parent-focused interventions can empower parents through 'transfer of control' (Ginsburg & Schlossberg, 2002) via skill transfer and task-shifting from the therapist to the family, and from the family to the child. This is important given the functional and relational impairment OCD can present in a family (Peris et al., 2017). More recently, an entirely parent-based treatment in which therapists only work with parents, without meeting with children, has also been proposed and shows promise in the treatment of youth with OCD (Lebowitz & Shimshoni, 2018).

Parental Factors

When discussing the importance of parental involvement in OCD treatment, it is important to consider the parent-level processes and within-family interactions that contextualize childhood OCD.

Family Accommodation

Children often rely on their caregivers to cope with the anxiety associated with intrusive, obsessive thoughts and facilitate the compulsions that provide temporary relief. In response, many caregivers will search for ways to reduce distress or prevent behavioral outbursts. Although well-intentioned, some may unwittingly reinforce avoidance by engaging in family accommodation. Family accommodation is broadly defined as any behavior on the part of family members (usually parents or caregivers) that helps a loved one cope with their mental health condition or alleviates symptomatic distress (Shimshoni et al., 2019). It is negatively reinforced by reduced distress in the short term, but ultimately perpetuates symptomology.

Family accommodation is very common in OCD. Studies suggest that it is related to poor role definition, intrusiveness, and limited boundaries (Calvocoressi et al., 1995). Moreover, accommodation does not permit for corrective learning of obsessive fears. Examples of accommodation include participating in the child's compulsions by altering routines and helping the child avoid fearful stimuli (Marien et al., 2009; Shimshoni et al., 2019). By continuing to engage in the accommodating behavior, parents may concurrently experience negative reinforcement. Engaging in accommodating behaviors can help provide personal respite for parents by comforting children, allowing them to move on to additional plans for the day, or simply preventing disruptive behaviors from occurring (Marien et al., 2009). Family accommodation is associated with greater symptom severity, caregiver burden, and functional impairment (Shimshoni et al., 2019; Van Noppen et al., 2021). As such, addressing family accommodation is an integral component of pediatric OCD treatment. Similar to response prevention for compulsions or avoidance behavior, families are taught to reduce accommodating behaviors in treatment.

Expressed Emotion and Parental Conflict

Negative family processes can also impact intervention outcomes, given the involvement of the family system during treatment. Factors such as expressed emotion (EE) and parental conflict may provoke OCD symptoms by sustaining and exacerbating their presentation (Waters & Barrett, 2000). EE refers to critical comments, emotional overinvolvement, and hostility within the family environment (Waters & Barrett, 2000). A family is considered to have high EE when at least one family member exhibits one or more of the above characteristics. Stemming from early schizophrenia literature, EE has been associated with increased symptom severity and high relapse rates (Brown et al., 1962; Miklowitz et al., 1988). Similar trends are demonstrated in adolescents with depression, aggression, and delinquency (Hale et al., 2011) and adults with OCD (Koujalgi et al., 2014). While the literature is limited regarding EE and pediatric OCD, there is some data to suggest that high EE is associated with symptom severity. Przeworski and colleagues (2012) demonstrated that high child and maternal EE were associated with increased pre-treatment symptom severity, but not post-treatment symptom severity (Przeworski et al., 2012). Peris & Miklowitz (2015) also discuss the importance of considering the family-based environmental determinants of high EE (e.g., toxic family stress) in symptom presentation and intervention.

Similarly, family conflict refers to active opposition, criticism, and hostility among family members within the family system (Lin, Schleider, & Eaton, 2021). Highly conflictual family environments are hypothesized to impact a child's emotion expression and regulation through social learning. Conversely, families characterized with lower levels of parental blame, lower levels of parental conflict, and higher family cohesion were more likely to respond to family-focused CBT for OCD (Peris et al., 2012).

Chambless and Steketee (1999) demonstrated that different characteristics of EE may impact OCD severity differently among adults. The authors demonstrated that family hostility increased a patient's chance of dropping out of treatment six times over. Perceived criticism from family members was also identified as a strong predictor of reduced treatment outcomes for OCD (Chambless & Steketee, 1999). The authors determined that family-based treatments to reduce EE may help support treatment gains as OCD is embedded in a family context (also see Chapter 6).

Evidence-Base for Pediatric Obsessive-Compulsive Disorder Treatment

Presently, first-line treatment for mild to moderate pediatric OCD is CBT and the combination of CBT and medication is selected for moderate to severe OCD (de Haan et al., 1998; Geller & March, 2012; Freeman et al., 2018). Specifically, ERP is the main component of CBT for pediatric OCD, where its efficacy is demonstrated whether applied alone or in combination with other techniques (Freeman et al., 2018; Lewin et al., 2014; Rosa-Alcazar et al., 2015). ERP builds upon Mowrer's Two-Factor Theory of Learning, where a performed response is reinforced by fear reduction (Krypotos et al., 2015; Mowrer, 1951). In other words, maladaptive avoidance is developed when a conditioned fear response evokes compulsions or avoidance, which is endorsed by temporary fear reduction. ERP aims to disrupt the negative reinforcement cycle by exposing children to feared thoughts and situations (conditioned stimuli) while preventing rituals and/or avoidance (Barret et al., 2008; Freeman et al., 2014a).

The evidence base for ERP is strong – according to the *Journal of Clinical Child and Adolescent Psychology*'s evidence-based treatment (EBT) evaluation criteria (Southam-Gerow & Prinstein, 2014, family-focused individual CBT is defined as a Level 1: Well-Established treatment for pediatric OCD. This indicates family-focused CBT demonstrated the statistically significant superiority of family-focused CBT to pill or psychological placebo or to another treatment or equivalent to already well-established treatments in multiple, independent studies (e.g., Barrett et al., 2008; Freeman et al., 2014b; Grunes et al., 2001; Piacentini et al., 2011; POTS, 2004). CBT produces clinically significant improvement for the majority of children. In a meta-analysis, Öst and colleagues (2016), identified five randomized controlled trials demonstrating the superiority of CBT to placebo ($g = .93$) and seven demonstrating its superiority to waitlist control ($g = 1.53$). An additional meta-analysis conducted around the same time found similar results, where large effect sizes for CBT (particularly when involving multiple components such as parental involvement and relapse prevention) were demonstrated in reducing OCD symptoms for children and adolescents (Rosa-Alcázar et al., 2015). Moreover, in the first meta-analysis assessing treatment efficacy, treatment response, and remission rates for pediatric OCD, McGuire and colleagues (2015) determined that CBT demonstrated large treatment effects.

Parent-Focused Interventions

Given the role of family accommodation in symptom presentation and maintenance, parent-only interventions for pediatric OCD have also been developed. Randomized controlled trials (RCTs) evaluating parental involvement in treatment for child anxiety disorders to date may have found such mixed results because these treatments have historically not involved parents effectively (Brienholst et al., 2012; Cobham et al., 2010). Since humans are born unequipped, both physically and psychologically, to deal with danger, parents play an important role in scaffolding these skills throughout development. Children's innate anxiety responses in the context of actual danger are adaptive (i.e., avoidance, escape, or safety-seeking behaviors); however, anxiety responses become maladaptive when they repeatedly occur in the context of harmless stimuli. Parents and other caregiver figures are needed for protection, helping children learn to evaluate risk in the environment, and helping children self-regulate negative affect (Iniesta-Sepúlveda et al., 2017).

Further, the attachment literature postulates that parental responses to anxiety could be characterized as repeated "triggering" of the attachment system, leading parents to protect their children, provide reassurance, and aid in their children's development of self-regulation of negative emotions (Siqueland, Rynn, & Diamond, 2005; van Leeuwen et al., 2020). Parents are required to intervene when anxiety reaches clinical levels; for example, parents of children with anxiety disorders are frequently asked for reassurance, and asked to change other behaviors/routines (i.e., parental accommodation). Parental accommodation perpetuates the cycle of anxiety because it allows the child to avoid facing feared situations, thereby reinforcing beliefs that the child is unable to cope with their own negative emotions, and that actually harmless situations should be feared.

Parent-Focused Pediatric Obsessive-Compulsive Disorder Treatment– the SPACE Program

SPACE (Lebowitz et al., 2014a) is a manualized treatment approach where parents of anxious youth participate in the treatment without their children present. The primary goal is to increase parental support and reduce parental accommodation, thereby reducing child anxiety symptom severity over the course of treatment. By focusing on changing parent responses to child anxiety as the **primary mechanism of change**, SPACE incorporates our theoretical understanding of the etiology and maintenance of childhood anxiety disorders, and offers an efficacious treatment for child anxiety. While SPACE was developed based on the vast literature on accommodation in childhood OCD and was developed with this population in mind, only preliminary support exists for OCD (Lebowitz, 2013; Lebowitz & Shimshoni, 2018).

Efficacy of SPACE

In a randomized, non-inferiority trial comparing SPACE to traditional CBT with parent involvement (N = 124, ages 7–14), SPACE was non-inferior to CBT (Lebowitz et al., 2020). Compared to CBT, SPACE resulted in higher reductions of family accommodation. SPACE was rated favorably by families in terms of treatment credibility and treatment satisfaction. Although youth with OCD were not included in the original SPACE trial, accommodation of avoidance and safety behaviors are similarly frequent in these populations and are conceptualized transdiagnostically in SPACE; thus, it is expected that SPACE would be similarly effective for youth with OCD, though this remains an empirical question. That said, several case studies and series have suggested that SPACE is likely an effective option for at least some youth with OCD.

Lebowitz and Shimshoni (2018) illustrate a case example where barriers including lack of motivation and resistance to treatment prevented a pediatric OCD patient from benefiting from ERP, and instead benefited from the SPACE treatment protocol which systematically reduces family accommodation of rituals. In a sample of 24 parent-child dyads (eight of whom had OCD) who participated in SPACE, Dekel et al. (2021) found significant decreases in the severity of child anxiety/OCD symptoms; however, this data did not examine an OCD-only group due to sample size. Despite a lack of strong empirical evidence, SPACE has become very popular among child OCD specialists, as it appears clinically intuitive and has a very strong theoretical foundation. Further randomized controlled trials are needed to evaluate whether SPACE is an appropriate supplement to traditional CBT for pediatric OCD or to determine whether SPACE versus CBT personalization based on family characteristics is advantageous.

Overview of SPACE

The first phase of SPACE involves psychoeducation. Parents are introduced to the systematic conceptualization of childhood anxiety, and to the rationale for treating children with anxiety disorders via parents. Parents are engaged in a discussion of prior attempts to directly change their child's behavior/decrease their child's anxiety, and the results. The therapist then identifies reasons that past approaches have not been successful with the parent. Importantly, the first phase of treatment involves ensuring that parents to not internalize any feelings of self-blame or beliefs that they have been "parenting wrong."

The second phase of treatment involves the parents and therapist collaboratively reviewing the family's daily routine and habits, with a focus on identification of accommodating behaviors. The family is asked to record these types of behaviors over the course of the week. Next, the therapist helps the family identify target problems to address. The therapist and parents collaboratively create a plan to inform the child about the upcoming changes they will begin to experience in their daily routine.

In the next phase of treatment, the therapist and parents plan specific behavioral changes which the parents will implement. An example of a plan for a child struggling with separation anxiety is outlined below.
    Plan:

- Parents will not respond to more than one phone call per day.
- Parents will kiss the child goodnight/complete the bedtime routine one time per night.
- The patient (child) will be rewarded for every day they meet their goal of not calling more than one time and not requesting more than one goodnight ritual.
- The child will be informed of this in advance.

For children with OCD, similar behavioral changes are implemented, either focusing on parental participation in the child's compulsive behaviors and/or modifying routines to accommodate compulsions. An example of a plan for a child presenting with contamination OCD symptoms is presented below.

Plan:

- Parents will not provide "special" handwashing soap for child.
- Parents will not supervise the child washing their hands before dinner.
- The child will be informed of this in advance.

Importantly, the success of the plan only relies on the parent's ability to change their behavior. Success is not determined by the child's reactions to the plan or willingness to cooperate with the plan.

The remainder of treatment involves discussion of additional target problems, and creating additional plans to target these problems. Difficulties in accomplishing the planned changes are carefully monitored by the therapist, and changes are made accordingly at each session if required. At the end of treatment, the family's progress towards the goals of treatment is reviewed and the therapist assists the parents with relapse prevention/planning for any similar problems which may arise in the future.

SPACE offers an alternative for families who may not benefit from traditional treatment approaches. For example, SPACE may be the best treatment option for certain groups of children including those who are resistant to attending treatment, who have motivated parents who engage in substantial accommodation, and whose OCD is so severe that they refuse to engage with a provider in traditional one-on-one therapy. Future work should investigate whether matching families to CBT or SPACE based on these or other characteristics would offer a more personalized approach.

Conclusion

Pediatric OCD has been described as a "family-based illness," and the delivery and application of treatment should follow a similar approach. Family-based CBT with robust parent involvement has developed the strongest scientific evidence base, with the consensus now emphasizing a considerable degree of parent involvement to help support ERP at home and reduce family accommodation. Recently, the field has also seen the emergence of an entirely parent-led approach, the SPACE program, that may provide an effective alternative for some youth with OCD, though this remains untested. Regardless, SPACE has become very popular among childhood OCD specialists, and thus an empirical test of its efficacy and/or its non-inferiority to ERP is a high priority for the field.

Regarding parental involvement in pediatric OCD intervention, a targeted treatment approach may be the most appropriate clinically. Wei & Kendall (2014) discussed the importance of assessing parent/family factors prior to anxiety treatment to ensure that parental involvement can be the most effective. For example, family-based interventions might be the most beneficial when a high-level of parent-child conflict, expressed emotion, or family accommodation is present, though questions of treatment moderation in CBT vs. SPACE remain untested.

After establishing a stronger evidence base for SPACE for childhood OCD, future research should investigate how to systematically and effectively screen for parent/family factors at pretreatment to ensure treatment fit and also identify which treatment components should be included (CBT with ERP augmented with parental involvement, family-based CBT, or parent training/SPACE). Similar to utilizing modular treatment designs, a targeted treatment approach is beneficial as clinicians can select and arrange treatment components to match the needs of patients (Wei & Kendall, 2014). Doing so can help individualize treatment to the patient and increase the likelihood of treatment adherence.

References

Albert, U., Bogetto, F., Maina, G., Saracco, P., Brunatto, C., & Mataix-Cols, D. (2010). Family accommodation in obsessive–compulsive disorder: Relation to symptom dimensions, clinical and family characteristics. *Psychiatry Research*, 179(2), 204–211. https://doi.org/10.1016/j.psychres.2009.06.008.

Bariola, E., Gullone, E., & Hughes, E.K. (2011). Child and Adolescent Emotion Regulation: The Role of Parental Emotion Regulation and Expression. *Clinical Child and Family Psychology Review*, 14(2), 198–212. https://doi.org/10.1007/s10567-011-0092-5.

Barrett, P.M., Farrell, L., Pina, A.A., Peris, T.S., & Piacentini, J. (2008). Evidence-based psychosocial treatments for child and adolescent obsessive–compulsive disorder. *Journal of Clinical Child & Adolescent Psychology*, 37(1), 131–155. https://doi.org/10.1080/15374410701817956.

Blaustein, M.E., & Kinniburgh, K.M. (2010). *Treating traumatic stress in children and adolescents: How to foster resilience through attachment, self-regulation, and competency* (pp. xii, 372). Guilford Press.

Brown, G.W., Monck, E.M., Carstairs, G.M., & Wing, J.K. (1962). Influence of family life on the course of schizophrenic illness. *British Journal of Preventive & Social Medicine*, 16(2), 55–68.

Calvocoressi, L., Lewis, B., Harris, M., Trufan, S.J., Goodman, W.K., McDougle, C.J., & Price, L.H. (1995). Family accommodation in obsessive-compulsive disorder. *The American Journal of Psychiatry*, 152(3), 441–443. https://doi.org/10.1176/ajp.152.3.441.

Cardy, J.L., Waite, P., Cocks, F., & Creswell, C. (2020). A systematic review of parental involvement in cognitive behavioural therapy for adolescent anxiety disorders. *Clinical Child and Family Psychology Review*, 23(4), 483–509. https://doi.org/10.1007/s10567-020-00324-2.

Chambless, D.L., & Steketee, G. (1999). Expressed emotion and behavior therapy outcome: A prospective study with obsessive–compulsive and agoraphobic outpatients. *Journal of Consulting and Clinical Psychology*, 67, 658–665. https://doi.org/10.1037/0022-006X.67.5.658.

Cobham, V.E., Dadds, M.R., Spence, S.H., & McDermott, B. (2010). Parental anxiety in the treatment of childhood anxiety: A different story three years later. *Journal of Clinical Child & Adolescent Psychology, 39*(3), 410–420.

de Haan, E.D., Hoogduin, K.A.L., Buitelaar, J.K., & Keijsers, G.P.J. (1998). Behavior therapy versus clomipramine for the treatment of obsessive-compulsive disorder in children and adolescents. *Journal of the American Academy of Child & Adolescent Psychiatry, 37*(10), 1022–1029. https://doi.org/10.109 7/00004583-199810000-00011.

Dekel, I., Dorman-Ilan, S., Lang, C., Bar-David, E., Zilka, H., Shilton, T., Lebowitz, E.R., & Gothelf, D. (2021). The feasibility of a parent group treatment for youth with anxiety disorders and obsessive compulsive disorder. *Child Psychiatry and Human Development, 52*(6), 1044–1049. https://doi.org/10.1007/ s10578-020-01082-6.

Demaria, F., Pontillo, M., Tata, M.C., Gargiullo, P., Mancini, F., & Vicari, S. (2021). Psychoeducation focused on family accommodation: A practical intervention for parents of children and adolescents with obsessive-compulsive disorder. *Italian Journal of Pediatrics, 47*(1), 224. https://doi.org/10.1186/ s13052-021-01177-3.

Everett, Y., Martin, C.G., & Zalewski, M. (2021). A systematic review focusing on psychotherapeutic interventions that impact parental psychopathology, child psychopathology and parenting behavior. *Clinical Child and Family Psychology Review, 24*(3), 579–598. https://doi.org/10.1007/s10567-021-00355-3.

Freeman, J., Benito, K., Herren, J., Kemp, J., Sung, J., Georgiadis, C., Arora, A., Walther, M., & Garcia, A. (2018). Evidence base update of psychosocial treatments for pediatric obsessive-compulsive disorder: Evaluating, improving, and transporting what works. *Journal of Clinical Child & Adolescent Psychology, 47*(5), 669–698. https://doi.org/10.1080/15374416.2018.1496443.

Freeman, J.B., Garcia, A.M., Coyne, L., Ale, C., Przeworski, A., Himle, M., Compton, S., & Leonard, H.L. (2008). Early childhood OCD: Preliminary findings from a family-based cognitive-behavioral approach. *Journal of the American Academy of Child & Adolescent Psychiatry, 47*(5), 593–602. https:// doi.org/10.1097/CHI.0b013e31816765f9.

Freeman, J., Garcia, A., Frank, H., Benito, K., Conelea, C., Walther, M., & Edmunds, J. (2014a). Evidence base update for psychosocial treatments for pediatric obsessive-compulsive disorder. *Journal of Clinical Child & Adolescent Psychology, 43*(1), 7–26. https://doi.org/10.1080/15374416.2013.804386.

Freeman, J., Sapyta, J., Garcia, A., Compton, S., Khanna, M., Flessner, C., FitzGerald, D., Mauro, C., Dingfelder, R., Benito, K., Harrison, J., Curry, J., Foa, E., March, J., Moore, P., & Franklin, M. (2014b). Family-based treatment of early childhood obsessive-compulsive disorder: The Pediatric Obsessive-Compulsive Disorder Treatment Study for Young Children (POTS Jr)—a randomized clinical trial. *JAMA Psychiatry, 71*(6), 689–698. https://doi. org/10.1001/jamapsychiatry.2014.170.

Geller, D.A., & March, J. (2012). Practice parameter for the assessment and treatment of children and adolescents with obsessive-compulsive disorder. *Journal of the American Academy of Child & Adolescent Psychiatry, 51*(1), 98–113. https://doi.org/10.1016/j.jaac.2011.09.019.

Ginsburg, G.S., & Schlossberg, M.C. (2002). Family-based treatment of childhood anxiety disorders. *International Review of Psychiatry, 14*(2), 143–154. https:// doi.org/10.1080/09540260220132662.

Grunes, M.S., Neziroglu, F., & McKay, D. (2001). Family involvement in the behavioral treatment of obsessive-compulsive disorder: A preliminary investigation. *Behavior Therapy*, *32*(4), 803–820. https://doi.org/10.1016/S0005-7894(01)80022-8.

Hale, W.W., Raaijmakers, Q.A.W., van Hoof, A., & Meeus, W.H.J. (2011). The predictive capacity of perceived expressed emotion as a dynamic entity of adolescents from the general community. *Social Psychiatry and Psychiatric Epidemiology*, *46*(6), 507–515. https://doi.org/10.1007/s00127-010-0218-y.

Iniesta-Sepúlveda, M., Rosa-Alcázar, A.I., Sánchez-Meca, J., Parada-Navas, J.L., & Rosa-Alcázar, Á. (2017). Cognitive-behavioral high parental involvement treatments for pediatric obsessive-compulsive disorder: A meta-analysis. *Journal of Anxiety Disorders*, *49*, 53–64. https://doi.org/10.1016/j.janxdis.2017.03.010.

Kazdin, A.E., & Weisz, J.R. (1998). Identifying and developing empirically supported child and adolescent treatments. *Journal of Consulting and Clinical Psychology*, *66*(1), 19–36. https://doi.org/10.1037//0022-006x.66.1.19.

Koujalgi, S.R., Nayak, R.B., Patil, N.M., & Chate, S.S. (2014). Expressed emotions in patients with obsessive compulsive disorder: A case control study. *Indian Journal of Psychological Medicine*, *36*(2), 138–141. https://doi.org/10.4103/0253-7176.130972

Krypotos, A.M., Effting, M., Kindt, M., & Beckers, T. (2015). Avoidance learning: A review of theoretical models and recent developments. *Frontiers in Behavioral Neuroscience*, *9*, 189. https://doi.org/10.3389/fnbeh.2015.00189

Lebowitz, E. R. (2013). Parent-based treatment for childhood and adolescent OCD. *Journal of Obsessive-Compulsive and Related Disorders*, *2*(4), 425–431. https://doi.org/10.1016/j.jocrd.2013.08.004

Lebowitz, E.R., Marin, C., Martino, A., Shimshoni, Y., & Silverman, W.K. (2020). Parent-based treatment as efficacious as cognitive behavioral therapy for childhood anxiety: A randomized noninferiority study of supportive parenting for anxious childhood emotions. *Journal of the American Academy of Child and Adolescent Psychiatry*, S0890-8567(19)30173-X. https://doi.org/10.1016/j.jaac.2019.02.014.

Lebowitz, E.R., Omer, H., Hermes, H., & Scahill, L. (2014a). Parent training for childhood anxiety disorders: the SPACE program. *Cognitive and Behavioral Practice*, *21*(4), 456–469. https://doi.org/10.1586/ern.11.200.

Lebowitz, E.R., Panza, K.E., Su, J., & Bloch, M.H. (2012). Family accommodation in obsessive–compulsive disorder. *Expert Review of Neurotherapeutics*, *12*(2), 229–238.

Lebowitz, E.R., Scharfstein, L.A., & Jones, J. (2014b). Comparing family accommodation in pediatric obsessive-compulsive disorder, anxiety disorders, and nonanxious children. *Depression and Anxiety*, *31*(12), 1018–1025. https://doi.org/10.1002/da.22251.

Lebowitz, E.R., & Shimshoni, Y. (2018). The SPACE program, a parent-based treatment for childhood and adolescent OCD: The case of Jasmine. *Bulletin of the Menninger Clinic*, *82*(4), 266–287. https://doi.org/10.1521/bumc.2018.82.4.266.

Lewin, A.B., Park, J.M., Jones, A.M., Crawford, E.A., De Nadai, A.S., Menzel, J., Arnold, E.B., Murphy, T.K., & Storch, E.A. (2014). Family-based exposure and response prevention therapy for preschool-aged children with obsessive-compulsive disorder: A pilot randomized controlled trial. *Behaviour Research and Therapy*, *56*, 30–38. https://doi.org/10.1016/j.brat.2014.02.001.

Lin, S.Y., Schleider, J.L., & Eaton, N.R. (2021). Family processes and child psychopathology: A between- and within-family/child analysis. *Research on Child and Adolescent Psychopathology*, 49(3), 283–295. https://doi.org/10.1007/s10802-020-00749-x.

Marien, W.E., Storch, E.A., Geffken, G.R., & Murphy, T.K. (2009). Intensive family-based cognitive-behavioral therapy for pediatric obsessive-compulsive disorder: Applications for treatment of medication partial- or nonresponders. *Cognitive and Behavioral Practice*, 16(3), 10.1016/j.cbpra.2008.12.006. https://doi.org/10.1016/j.cbpra.2008.12.006.

Mash, E.J., & Barkley, R.A. (2014). *Child psychopathology* (3rd ed.) The Guilford Press.

McGuire, J.F., Piacentini, J., Lewin, A.B., Brennan, E.A., Murphy, T.K., & Storch, E.A. (2015). A meta-analysis of cognitive behavior therapy and medication for child obsessive compulsive disorder: Moderators of treatment efficacy, response, and remission. *Depression and Anxiety*, 32(8), 580–593. https://doi.org/10.1002/da.22389.

Miklowitz, D.J., Goldstein, M.J., Nuechterlein, K.H., Snyder, K.S., & Mintz, J. (1988). Family factors and the course of bipolar affective disorder. *Archives of General Psychiatry*, 45(3), 225–231. https://doi.org/10.1001/archpsyc.1988.01800270033004.

Monzani, B., Rijsdijk, F., Harris, J., & Mataix-Cols, D. (2014). The structure of genetic and environmental risk factors for dimensional representations of DSM-5 obsessive-compulsive spectrum disorders. *JAMA Psychiatry*, 71(2), 182–189. https://doi.org/10.1001/jamapsychiatry.2013.3524.

Mowrer, O.H. (1951). Two-factor learning theory: Summary and comment. *Psychological Review*, 58, 350–354. https://doi.org/10.1037/h0058956.

Nestadt, G., Grados, M., & Samuels, J.F. (2010). Genetics of OCD. *The Psychiatric Clinics of North America*, 33(1), 141–158. https://doi.org/10.1016/j.psc.2009.11.001.

Pediatric OCD Treatment Study (POTS) Team. (2004). Cognitive-behavior therapy, sertraline, and their combination for children and adolescents with obsessive-compulsive disorder: The Pediatric OCD Treatment Study (POTS) randomized controlled trial. *JAMA*, 292(16), 1969–1976. https://doi.org/10.1001/jama.292.16.1969.

Peris, T.S., & Miklowitz, D.J. (2015). Parental expressed emotion and youth psychopathology: New directions for an old construct. *Child Psychiatry & Human Development*, 46(6), 863–873. https://doi.org/10.1007/s10578-014-0526-7.

Peris, T.S., Rozenman, M.S., Sugar, C.A., McCracken, J.T., & Piacentini, J. (2017). Targeted family intervention for complex cases of pediatric obsessive-compulsive disorder: A randomized controlled trial. *Journal of the American Academy of Child and Adolescent Psychiatry*, 56(12), 1034–1042.e1. https://doi.org/10.1016/j.jaac.2017.10.008.

Peris, T.S., Sugar, C.A., Bergman, R.L., Chang, S., Langley, A., & Piacentini, J. (2012). Family factors predict treatment outcome for pediatric obsessive compulsive disorder. *Journal of Consulting and Clinical Psychology*, 80(2), 255–263. https://doi.org/10.1037/a0027084.

Piacentini, J., Bergman, R.L., Chang, S., Langley, A., Peris, T., Wood, J.J., & McCracken, J. (2011). Controlled comparison of family cognitive behavioral therapy and psychoeducation/relaxation training for child obsessive-compulsive disorder. *Journal of the American Academy of Child & Adolescent Psychiatry*, 50(11), 1149–1161. https://doi.org/10.1016/j.jaac.2011.08.003.

Przeworski, A., Zoellner, L.A., Franklin, M.E., Garcia, A., Freeman, J., March, J.S., & Foa, E.B. (2012). Maternal and child expressed emotion as predictors of treatment response in pediatric obsessive–compulsive disorder. *Child Psychiatry & Human Development*, 43(3), 337–353. https://doi.org/10.1007/s10578-011-0268-8.

Rosa-Alcázar, A.I., Sánchez-Meca, J., Rosa-Alcázar, Á., Iniesta-Sepúlveda, M., Olivares-Rodríguez, J., & Parada-Navas, J.L. (2015). Psychological treatment of obsessive-compulsive disorder in children and adolescents: A meta-analysis. *The Spanish Journal of Psychology*, 18, E20. https://doi.org/10.1017/sjp.2015.22.

Sanders, M.R. (1996). New directions in behavioral family intervention with children. In T. H. Ollendick & R. J. Prinz (Eds.), *Advances in Clinical Child Psychology* (pp. 283–330). Springer US. https://doi.org/10.1007/978-1-4613-0323-7_8.

Selles, R.R., Best, J.R., & Stewart, S.E. (2020). Family profiles in pediatric obsessive-compulsive disorder. *Journal of Obsessive-Compulsive and Related Disorders*, 27, 100588. https://doi.org/10.1016/j.jocrd.2020.100588.

Shimshoni, Y., Shrinivasa, B., Cherian, A.V., & Lebowitz, E.R. (2019). Family accommodation in psychopathology: A synthesized review. *Indian Journal of Psychiatry*, 61(Suppl 1), S93. https://doi.org/10.4103/psychiatry.Indian JPsychiatry_530_18.

Siqueland, L., Rynn, M., & Diamond, G.S. (2005). Cognitive behavioral and attachment based family therapy for anxious adolescents: Phase I and II studies. *Journal of Anxiety Disorders*, 19(4), 361–381.

Southam-Gerow, M.A., & Prinstein, M.J. (2014). Evidence base updates: The evolution of the evaluation of psychological treatments for children and adolescents. *Journal of Clinical Child & Adolescent Psychology*, 43(1), 1–6. https://doi.org/10.1080/15374416.2013.855128.

Stewart, S.E., Hu, Y.-P., Leung, A., Chan, E., Hezel, D.M., Lin, S.Y., Belschner, L., Walsh, C., Geller, D. A., & Pauls, D.L. (2017). A multisite study of family functioning impairment in pediatric obsessive-compulsive disorder. *Journal of the American Academy of Child & Adolescent Psychiatry*, 56(3), 241–249.e3. https://doi.org/10.1016/j.jaac.2016.12.012.

Storch, E.A., Geffken, G.R., Merlo, L.J., Mann, G., Duke, D., Munson, M., Adkins, J., Grabill, K.M., Murphy, T.K., & Goodman, W.K. (2007). Family-based cognitive-behavioral therapy for pediatric obsessive-compulsive disorder: Comparison of intensive and weekly approaches. *Journal of the American Academy of Child and Adolescent Psychiatry*, 46(4), 469–478. https://doi.org/10.1097/chi.0b013e31803062e7.

Storch, E.A., Lehmkuhl, H.D., Ricketts, E., Geffken, G.R., Marien, W., & Murphy, T.K. (2010). An open trial of intensive family based cognitive-behavioral therapy in youth with obsessive-compulsive disorder who are medication partial responders or nonresponders. *Journal of Clinical Child & Adolescent Psychology*, 39(2), 260–268. https://doi.org/10.1080/15374410903532676.

Van Leeuwen, W.A., Van Wingen, G.A., Luyten, P., Denys, D., & Van Marle, H.J.F. (2020). Attachment in OCD: A meta-analysis. *Journal of Anxiety Disorders*, 70, 102187. https://doi.org/10.1016/j.janxdis.2020.102187.

Van Noppen, B., Sassano-Higgins, S., Appasani, R., & Sapp, F. (2021). Cognitive-behavioral therapy for obsessive-compulsive disorder: 2021 update. *Focus (American Psychiatric Publishing)*, 19(4), 430–443. https://doi.org/10.1176/appi.focus.20210015.

Waters, T.L., & Barrett, P.M. (2000). The role of the family in childhood obsessive–compulsive disorder. *Clinical Child and Family Psychology Review*, 3(3), 173–184. https://doi.org/10.1023/A:1009551325629.

Wei, C., & Kendall, P.C. (2014). Parental involvement: Contribution to childhood anxiety and its treatment. *Clinical Child and Family Psychology Review*, 17(4), 319–339. https://doi.org/10.1007/s10567-014-0170-6.

8 Intensive Treatment of Childhood Obsessive-Compulsive Disorder

Megan A. Barthle-Herrera,[1]
Amanda Balkhi,[2] *Tannaz MirHosseini,*[1]
Melissa Munson,[1] *Ashley Ordway,*[1] *and*
Joseph P.H. McNamara[1]

[1] *Florida Exposure and Anxiety Research (FEAR)
Laboratory, University of Florida, Department of
Psychiatry, Gainesville, FL*

[2] *Balkhi Foundation, Palm Beach Gardens, FL*

For some children and families, barriers to the standard weekly delivery of cognitive-behavioral therapy with exposure and response prevention (CBT-E/RP) limit the effectiveness of this otherwise efficacious treatment of childhood obsessive-compulsive disorder (OCD). For children with refractory OCD (Lewin et al., 2005), comorbid presentations (Geller et al., 1998), or families who live within an area with limited availability of trained CBT-E/RP providers (Goodwin et al., 2002; Storch et al., 2003), a more intensive approach to treatment may be warranted. Typical pediatric intensive treatment approaches are composed of three or more treatment sessions per week and are usually comprised of 10–15 sessions (see Jónsson, Kristensen, & Arendt, 2015 for review), though episodes of care can often be extended based on clinical need, especially in a hospital intensive outpatient programs (IOP) setting. However, increasingly diverse methods of intensive treatment delivery have been trialed in recent years and will be reviewed in detail later in this chapter.

Broadly, intensive treatment for pediatric OCD is defined as treatment where both the frequency and duration of treatment sessions are increased as compared to standard once weekly treatment (Lewin et al., 2005). Intensive treatment has shown to have a slight advantage in initial treatment response as compared to standard weekly treatment, and it displays equivalent symptom maintenance at three months post treatment (Storch et al., 2007b; Storch et al., 2008). However, the unique experience of intensive treatment has additional benefits that must be considered when evaluating treatment options for childhood OCD.

DOI: 10.4324/9781003386278-8

A common barrier to traditional weekly treatment for children is lower insight into their OCD symptomatology, and worse insight is associated with increased OCD severity (Garcia et al., 2010; Selles et al., 2018). Fortunately, it has been shown that children's insight improved significantly following treatment with CBT-E/RP, though limited levels of a related variable, child impairment recognition relative to their caregivers, was associated with a reduced likelihood for treatment response (Selles et al., 2020). However, in intensive treatment, the experience of repeatedly challenging these thoughts more frequently can facilitate significant breakthroughs in OCD-related insight. Higher levels of care also allow the opportunity to correct mistakes in understanding quickly, as well as provide opportunities to repeatedly experience expectancy violations that promote inhibitory learning (Guzick et al., 2018) and challenge disgust sensitivity (Taboas, Ojserkis, & McKay, 2015). For many children, the necessity of staying away from home while accessing intensive treatment, such as in a hotel or residential facility, can also provide unique opportunities for exposure that would otherwise be out of reach in the home, such as engaging with shared restrooms, bedrooms, and kitchen areas.

Low motivation can also be a unique challenge for children with OCD symptomatology. Children's engagement in more frequent sessions can increase insight by allowing the child to see change more quickly over the course of days, rather than months. The increased frequency of intensive CBT-E/RP allows for treatment to be the primary focus for a specific period of time, rather than an event taking up a small portion of time during the week in once per week therapy. This increase in frequency and focus on treatment may encourage children to be more open to engaging in sessions (Foa & Steketee, 1987; Storch et al., 2003). Especially for children reluctant to engage in treatment, the compressed nature of sessions in an intensive course makes it easier to "see the finish line" than in a traditional weekly course spread over three to four months. More frequent sessions can also increase motivation to engage in more difficult exposures, as there is less ability for the child to escape the environment than in the home setting or to wait out the therapy team to avoid completing an exposure in a weekly hour-long session. Additionally, there is less time for the child to procrastinate on completing homework between sessions. As with weekly treatment, utilization of contingency management (i.e., rewards for engaging in exposures) can be given to increase engagement in treatment (Abramowitz et al., 2018) until insight is better developed and longer-term reduction in OCD symptoms becomes its own reinforcer for engaging in CBT-E/RP.

Another benefit of intensive treatment is the ability to adapt to target clinically significant comorbidities concurrently. Given the extended duration of intensive therapy sessions and the ability to see patients more than once a week, providers may be more comfortable delivering adjunctive interventions over the course of intensive treatment than in traditional weekly treatment. Anecdotally, providers may feel like they can more easily "maintain momentum" in OCD treatment, despite dedicating time to targeting these comorbidities, because of the frequency in which they see the patient. While research is limited, case reports suggest that intensive treatment for childhood OCD has been successfully integrated with treatment for misophonia (Reid et al., 2016), has benefits for childhood depression symptoms (Sperling, Boger, & Potter, 2020), and has been successfully adapted for use with children with comorbid autism (Merricks et al., 2017). Intensive treatment has also demonstrated effectiveness at increasing emotion regulation strategy use among adolescents; a skill which is potentially transferable to treatment of comorbid conditions (Wei et al., 2020).

Caregivers of children with OCD may also see benefits from the intensive treatment model, in which family participation is essential (Barrett, Healy-Farrell, & March, 2004; Knox, Albano, & Barlow, 1996). The longer duration and higher frequency of sessions allows for increased modeling of appropriate supportive behaviors for caregivers (Lewin et al., 2005). Caregivers and children (if developmentally able) should be included in the planning and execution of exposures early in the episode of care to increase autonomy. These collaborative treatment planning and exposure sessions also allow for the therapist to witness how the family is implementing exposures out of session. Therapists can then provide immediate feedback and guidance to ensure the family is conducting exposures properly, achieving appropriate approach behavior, and engaging in response prevention (Lewin et al., 2005). This immediate guidance can be especially helpful for caregivers who themselves exhibit anxious symptomatology or who are sensitive to the children's obsessional content, who otherwise may unintentionally encourage or exacerbate their child's symptoms with accommodation behaviors (Berman, Wilver, & Wilhelm, 2018; Mathieu et al., 2019).

Despite the efficacy of CBT-E/RP (McGuire et al., 2015), there is still a substantial lack of providers who are comfortable and competent in delivering CBT-E/RP to children with OCD or related disorders (Reid et al., 2018). As such, intensive treatment options can serve as an attractive mechanism to improve access to treatment for families who are not located near a treatment provider by limiting time spent in travel back and forth to treatment (Whiteside et al., 2017). Perhaps because of this reduced barrier to seeking treatment, intensive treatment has also demonstrated lower rates of attrition than weekly treatment sessions (Öst & Ollendick, 2017). This, coupled with the success of replicating intensive treatment internationally, makes intensive treatment a powerful tool to improve access to treatment for OCD (Wolters et al., 2021).

For the purposes of this chapter, childhood treatment is defined as care directed toward children aged six to seventeen. However, in many instances the skills and strategies that are effective for this age group can also be extended to younger children. The specific treatment recommendations and evidence for the treatment of younger children will be discussed in the following chapter. Similarly, in select cases young adults aged 18 to 21 years may benefit from the childhood strategies discussed here that integrate family involvement. While a full discussion of these cases is outside the scope of this handbook, patient factors such as intellectual functioning, poor insight, and severe functional impairment may indicate a young adult is better suited to a more traditional childhood approach. Additionally, family factors such as cultural norms that include extended cohabitation with one's parents or unique family dynamics may lead providers to consider treatment approaches akin to childhood treatment. Providers are encouraged to approach treatment decisions holistically and take into account each family's unique dynamic and culture.

Types of Intensive Treatment

Intensive treatment can be provided at varying levels of care, and it is not always easy for parents to know what level of services are needed for their child. While research around intensive CBT-E/RP is continually growing and changing as new programs are tested and evaluated, there are currently five levels of care that make up intensive treatment options.

Intensive Outpatient Programs

Intensive outpatient programs (IOP) are often structured similarly to weekly treatment, with sessions occurring at an increased frequency (usually five sessions per week) and often with increased duration of sessions (ranging from 50 minutes to approximately three hours). The number of sessions required varies by patient, but it is typically not less than 10–15 (see Jónsson, Kristensen, & Arendt, 2015 for review). IOPs housed in a hospital setting also usually occur five days per week and have an extended duration of interventions (four to eight weeks, three to four hours per day). These IOPs often include individual, group, and family components in their program. Intensive outpatient therapy for OCD has been shown to be as effective as weekly treatment (Jónsson, Kristensen, & Arendt, 2015; Storch et al., 2007b). Further, intensive outpatient treatment has been shown to be effective in youth with treatment refractory OCD (i.e. failed to respond to medication management; Storch et al., 2007a). Finally, IOPs typically involve the patient returning home between sessions or over the weekends, which may be beneficial for generalization of treatment gains and may make it easier to target context-specific symptoms (Veale et al., 2016).

Given that intensive CBT achieves results faster due to its increased frequency (Remmerswaal et al., 2021), patients with severe OCD symptomatology may find it preferable to weekly formats. Limited access to specialty clinics treating OCD necessitates intensive treatment options for families that are traveling to obtain the appropriate interventions in a time-limited way. IOPs can also be offered as part of a hospital tiered approach to facilitate step-down from a higher level of care as appropriate.

Partial Hospitalization Programs

Partial hospitalization programs (PHP) also utilize intensive treatment, with a format that is more intense than IOP where a significant portion of the day is spent in treatment-related activities. CBT with ERP is provided at a similar frequency to IOP by a trained mental health professional and the individual is also provided with approximately 20–30 hours per week of additional therapeutic activity, such as group therapy, art therapy, and family therapy. PHP has been found to have similar treatment gains to IOP, and while IOP was found to be slightly more cost effective (Gregory et al., 2020), the cost was also functionally very similar.

PHP is well suited to those individuals who have limited daytime support from caregivers, or who may need more time away from caregivers who are overly accommodating of the patient's OCD symptoms. Patients can also access additional support in the form of supplementary therapeutic activities to improve insight or to provide an appropriate environment to wait out the distress of exposures and to habituate over a longer period of time than allowed in a weekly or IOP intervention format. PHP day treatment also allows for increased frequency of medication monitoring including side effects and general effectiveness. This increased monitoring can aid in expediting medication titration, faster achievement of therapeutic doses, and prompt management of side effects, if present. Coupled with this support, as with IOP and weekly sessions, patients are still able to generalize skills to a non-therapeutic setting by practicing homework outside of the hospital overnight, or possibly over the weekends in the home setting if the patient is staying in local lodging during the week while attending PHP services.

Week-Long Day Camp

Currently there are many notable barriers to children and adolescents receiving treatment for OCD. Therapeutic camps focused on the treatment of OCD, anxiety, and related disorders may reduce many of these barriers by increasing access to treatment in an intensive format with providers who have received extensive training in CBT-E/RP. This shortens the time the patient is spending attending therapy, which in turn lessens the parental burden and reduces the cost associated with traditional weekly therapy.

Similarly to PHP, when attending a therapeutic camp, the patient may also have access to other types of providers that they may not have had previously. Common professionals include psychiatrists that have a focus in treating pediatric OCD and anxiety, occupational therapists who are trained in providing Comprehensive Behavior Intervention for Tics (CBIT), and Applied Behavior Analysis (ABA) therapists who are trained in providing treatment for children who have a comorbid diagnosis of autism. While research on therapeutic camps for OCD is still rapidly developing, the only existing efficacy study reported "highly successful" preliminary, qualitative results from this camp, including informal positive feedback from both parents and "almost all" of the participants as well as psychosocial benefits such as social skills, self-regulation, and generalized adaptability (Rice et al., 2017).

Fear Facers Summer Camp is a week-long day camp that is held at the University of Florida. The University of Florida has specialized in treating children with OCD, anxiety, and related disorders since 1991, and has offered treatment in a camp setting since 2017. During the week of the camp, the patients receive individual therapy, group therapy, and engage in a variety of activities that challenge a wide range of OCD and anxiety symptoms. While currently pending publication, data from the camp suggests that campers experience a significant decrease in OCD symptoms over the week-long camp and campers with a co-occurring depression diagnosis experience a significant decrease in symptoms (McCarty et al., 2023).

These studies provide preliminary evidence of the effectiveness of the summer-camp modality. However, at this time more extensive qualitative and quantitative research needs to be completed as we continue to understand the impact of attending a therapeutic camp on a patient's treatment trajectory.

Residential

Residential treatment programs for OCD offer patients with severe or treatment-refractory OCD similar treatment services to partial hospitalization programs, but patients live full time at the treatment facility for the duration of their treatment. Nursing support is not required, as patients at this level of care are generally able to engage in age-appropriate self-care and are not at increased risk of harming themselves or others (Veale et al., 2016). Treatment components can vary, but generally utilize multidisciplinary staff to provide individual therapy, medication management, group treatment, and staff support for response prevention during exposures outside of sessions (Brennan et al., 2014). Similarly to a therapeutic camp environment, individuals are encouraged to interact socially with their peers while seeking treatment.

This level of care may be appropriate for individuals that have not had appropriate response to treatment in lower levels of care. Common reasons for residential treatment include severity of OCD symptoms or comorbid conditions that make engaging in exposures without adequate support difficult, distance from intensive treatment services that makes travel back and forth cost prohibitive, and compulsions that put the patient at risk of harm or medical complications if not appropriately managed (e.g., readministering medication until it feels "just right" leading to possible overdose, harming self equally on each side of the body for symmetry, drinking bleach to kill internal contaminants). Outcomes are generally favorable, with most studies reporting a significant reduction of OCD symptoms from admission to discharge (see Veale et al., 2016 for a review). While many studies in this area focus on adults, there are also studies that demonstrate effectiveness in adolescent populations (Björgvinsson et al., 2008, Højgaard et al., 2020, Leonard et al., 2016, Schneider et al., 2018).

Inpatient

Inpatient treatment programs are the highest level of care. These programs add 24/7 monitoring of patients by nursing staff to the services offered at lower levels of care. This increased monitoring is appropriate for patients who are at risk of self-harm or suicide and/or have symptoms that severely impact self-care and medical stability. Treating OCD in a general inpatient unit may not be ideal due to the psychopathology of other patients on the unit and lack of training of the staff, though specialist inpatient services for OCD may be more beneficial (Veale et al., 2016, Balachander et al., 2020).

Patients that are appropriate for inpatient care are in crisis, have a high level of self-neglect, and have a high risk for medical and safety concerns. They may have not responded to lower levels of treatment despite full trials across those levels. Individuals in need of inpatient treatment have high levels of functional impairment, and caregivers may be unable to manage symptoms in the home setting (National Collaborating Centre for Mental Health, 2006). Goals during the initial stages of this treatment often focus on psychoeducation and stabilization of symptoms, as well as quickly titrating up medication and monitoring medication changes (Veale et al., 2016). Programs vary in therapeutic services offered at this level of care, with some providing similar services to residential treatment, and others providing stabilization and then transferring to residential treatment if needed. Even in hospitals that are not specifically offering ERP, the setting may engage patients in tolerating dimensions of OCD by nature of being housed in an inpatient unit in close quarters with other patients, limited privacy, and lack of access to excessive cleaning supplies or other self-soothing products. However, treatment with CBT-E/RP following discharge is essential to ensure that patients fully understand how to appropriately challenge their OCD.

Comparative Efficacy of Intensive Treatment Modalities

Approximately 50 percent of adolescents who undergo weekly CBT will experience symptom remission (Bloch & Storch, 2015), and given the burden of OCD on patients, families, and society, more effective treatments are needed. Oftentimes with intensive treatments more momentum and a quicker return to daily routines has been shown (Sperling, Boger, & Potter, 2020). Brief, intensive, or condensed formats of treatments have demonstrated efficacy for treating OCD (Ollendick, 2014; Öst & Ollendick, 2017), and noted similar effectiveness when compared to standard weekly treatments (Storch et al., 2007b; Chase et al., 2012). Additionally, the use of intensive CBT for pediatric OCD has shown lower rates of participant drop-out (Öst & Ollendick, 2017), and greater remission and improvement rates compared to weekly outpatient CBT (Storch et al., 2007b). Others have proposed that by decreasing the time between exposure sessions, one can improve the effectiveness of exposure therapy (Craske et al., 2012). One of the barriers to receiving quality treatment for OCD can be the limited number of specialty-care professionals for CBT-E/RP and a way to mitigate this is short-term intensive treatments. These types of treatments allow patients to be able to relocate for a short period of time, receive quality care, and return back to their normal routines in less than a month (Ehrenreich & Santucci, 2009; Ollendick, 2014). Researchers have found several predictors of intensive treatment such as more severe comorbid depression, use of psychotropic medication, low quality of life, and being single (du Mortier et al., 2021), as well as symptom severity and high family accommodation (Rudy et al., 2014).

While there is no research directly comparing the delivery of intensive treatments across settings (IOP, PHP, camp, residential, and inpatient), each individual treatment setting has been shown to substantially reduce OCD symptoms throughout the course of treatment. This is likely due to each setting's shared use of CBT-E/RP and implementation by trained providers. Compared to standard weekly treatment, intensive outpatient treatment, partial hospitalization treatment, and residential treatment have all proven to be at minimum equally effective in reducing childhood OCD symptoms (Chase et al., 2012; Leonard, et al., 2016; Storch et al., 2007b). Given the heterogeneous presentation of children with OCD and the lack of qualified treatment providers, a true comparison of effectiveness across settings may not be possible for some time.

Effective Modifications to Intensive Treatment

Telehealth

Given the impact of the COVID-19 pandemic on resources and treatment accessibility, recent efforts have shown a movement towards telehealth intensive treatments for OCD as well. Gittins Stone and colleagues (2023) at McLean Hospital and Harvard Medical School examined the effectiveness of an intensive group-based outpatient treatment targeting anxiety disorders and OCD in youth by delivering real-time treatment via video conferencing during the pandemic. Their study supported the effectiveness of telemental health-delivered treatment for pediatric anxiety and OCD and found reduction in functional impairment and anxiety symptoms comparative to in person CBT-E/RP.

Group Treatment

A hallmark of many PHP, residential, camp, and inpatient treatment programs is group therapy. The efficacy of individual versus group intensive treatment has been investigated for OCD. A comparison of individual and group CBT for OCD indicated that both were successful in decreasing OCD symptoms over both short and long periods (Cabedo et al., 2010). Both intensive individual and group cognitive behavioral therapies have been demonstrated as effective treatments for OCD (Taylor & Reeder, 2015). Group therapy as part of an intensive program has also been shown to be effective at both reducing OCD and depressive symptoms in children and improving daily functioning (Havnen et al., 2014; Sperling, Boger, & Potter, 2020).

Condensed Treatment Delivery

Given the limited availability of trained providers and the substantial burden to some families in traveling to a qualified treatment setting, some have proposed the exploration of short-term intensive treatments, typically defined as a five-day intensive outpatient experience. One such study is a five-day treatment focusing on children and their parents completing two sessions per day for five days (Whiteside, et al., 2008). Day one includes psychoeducation, days two to four include engagement in exposures with increased parent coaching and parent/patient autonomy conducting exposures, and day five consists of parent and child completing exposures independently from the therapy team and planning for maintenance of skills and treatment gains at home. This method has been shown to have good response from patients (Whiteside et al., 2008; Whiteside et al. 2014; Whiteside & Jacobsen, 2010). While more research is needed, these condensed treatment options may be an effective way for children and families to learn the essential skills of CBT-E/RP and experience an initial symptom reduction that then motivates the child and family to continue weekly sessions upon their return home. For children, these condensed treatment courses may be an especially helpful way to take advantage of school breaks to make gains in treatment.

Choosing the Right Level of Care

The level of care required for OCD treatment will vary depending on an individual's need and severity of symptoms. Choosing the appropriate level of care can be difficult for patients and their families. Among the numerous factors to consider are treatment dosage, academic or occupational responsibilities, comorbidity and medication management, location and duration of treatment, patient insight and awareness, family factors, patient motivation, and need for extended time to habituate to exposure stimuli (see Appendix A and Appendix B).

Treatment Dosage

The dosage of treatment, defined as frequency and duration of CBT-E/RP sessions, is important to consider. Individuals with severe symptoms impacting their functionality at home and at work will benefit from a higher level of care with a higher dosage of CBT-E/RP and support sessions such as residential programs and hospitalization (Grøtte et al., 2018).

Academic or Occupational Responsibilities

Alongside families, providers and patients should discuss the challenges that the child and family will face in intensive treatment as a result of being away from home. Anecdotally, lost wages and academic declines are two major concerns for families seeking an intensive treatment option. When thinking about the most cost-effective treatment, high-intensity multimodal therapy, such as that offered by a PHP, residential, or camp program, has been found to be the best option for treatment-refractory pediatric OCD patients (Gregory et al., 2020); however, this must be balanced with the family's ability to afford the time missed from school and work. School-break coordinated treatment options, condensed "spring break" treatment weeks, and residential programs that provide academic supports may help alleviate the concerns about missing school.

Comorbidity and Medication Management

When working with children with OCD, active management of comorbid conditions and liaising with a child's medication provider (if applicable) are critical. In cases where individuals' symptoms are extremely severe, there are signs that they may be a danger to themselves or others, and suicidality is in question, hospitalization will be the best option (Albert et al., 2019). Similarly, for complex cases with multiple comorbidities, a residential setting with intensive ERP (i.e., approximately 26.5 hours per week), additional cognitive behavioral therapy interventions, and medication management can be effective (Leonard et al., 2016). Family beliefs about medication management can also have an impact on the level of care. Families may pursue a higher level of care if they are struggling to tolerate medication, have a history of distressing side effects, experience medical comorbidities that impact medication metabolism, or do not want to take medication because of personal beliefs or fears related to contamination or poisoning. For these reasons, it is important that providers actively liaison with medication prescribers whenever feasible.

Location and Duration of Treatment

Unfortunately, many patients and their families do not have many, if any, local treatment options. Families that live at a substantial distance from intensive treatment clinics may consider undergoing a shorter course of IOP, PHP, or camp-based treatment to minimize the time spent traveling back and forth. Anecdotally, most families living more than three hours from care prefer to stay in a local accommodation over the course of treatment and often seek to maximize hands-on CBT-E/RP time while away from home. Families considering residential or inpatient treatment, where children are supervised throughout the entire day and night, may be more comfortable staying in their home despite the travel time to reduce the burden of finding local accommodations. Families who do not live close to weekly available services may benefit from the short-term intensive care of IOP, PHP, and residential services that makes treatment available while staying in the treatment location for a period of time.

Insight and Awareness

When patients and their families have a better understanding of the patient's OCD symptoms, they are better able to work with the treatment provider to develop an effective treatment intervention. However, not every patient has a good understanding of their symptoms, and some patients and families struggle to differentiate between their obsessions, personal moral beliefs, and their family's typical behaviors and obsessions. When this is the case, a higher level of care might be warranted. It is important to note that patients are frequently reluctant to share obsessions in the taboo domain (sexual or religious) because of a fear of judgment, rejection from the provider, or a concern about being reported to authorities (Belloch et al., 2008). This reluctance is not the same thing as poor insight into symptoms. An open and respectful relationship with both the child undergoing treatment and the family supporting them is essential, especially in intensive treatment options where the typical development of reciprocal trust between patient and provider must be accelerated.

Family Factors

Families and close friends can play a critical role in treatment success. Support and encouragement from loved ones can help a patient engage in treatment. However, family accommodation of OCD symptoms frequently leads to a significant worsening of symptoms over time because the patient's fears are reinforced by the accommodation (see Wu et al., 2016 for review). Effective treatment, regardless of the level of care, needs to work with the patient and family to change patterns of accommodation in and around the home environment. For families that struggle with accommodation, this may be done more effectively by engaging in PHP, camp, or residential services where changes in accommodation can occur more quickly due to the family's absence for a substantial part of the day. Caregiver psychopathology is another critical factor that providers must take into account when discussing potential levels of care. Families with caregivers who are less able to engage effectively in the family based IOP treatment sessions due to their own psychopathology may be better suited to a higher level of care where the child can work directly with providers prior to practicing skills at home. In some cases, a PHP-, camp-, or residential-based treatment setting allows for the caregiver to receive their own treatment to reduce the impact of caregiver psychology on the family system.

Patient Motivation

Patients' motivation for treatment can vary significantly. The higher a patient's motivation for treatment, the more likely they are to engage in homework outside of session. This increased adherence to treatment protocols allows for a broader range of effective treatment options. With patients that are less motivated for treatment, higher levels of care may be necessary to offset the loss of therapeutic practice outside of session.

Habituation and Inhibitory Learning

In some cases, children may be willing to engage in treatment but find themselves unable to adequately complete exposures in the time allotted in a typical weekly outpatient setting. They may have difficulty habituating down to a functional level in relation to the anxiety producing stimulus, or they may have an OCD fear expectation which outlasts the session time. For example, a patient may have the belief that they could resist harming someone for an hour, but that they would harm someone eventually if given more time with them. Likewise, obsessions that are tied to a long-lasting process (e.g., food digestion, illness incubation periods, sunrise or sunset, etc.) may enable patients to resist compulsions during the session, though these patients may engage in the neutralizing response when they are alone without the direct support of the treatment team. For these patients, a level of care that allows for extended time to violate OCD expectances, increase habituation, and to resist the neutralizing behavior response may be most beneficial.

Intensive treatment settings also allow for patient engagement in unexpected exposures due to change in setting and more direct interaction with others who are not accommodating their compulsive behaviors. Patients may also be more willing to engage in exposures of varying difficulty when they have limited ability to escape the feared situation and when they have added support and motivation from their treatment team for an extended period of time. Overall, in addition to extended time for habituation, intensive treatment settings are an appropriate setting to engage in inhibitory learning principles such as distress tolerance, expectancy violation, unexpected exposures, and variable difficulty of exposures (see Jacoby & Abramowitz, 2016 and McGuire & Storch, 2019 for review).

Guidance to Providers

Amongst the many effective intensive treatments for OCD, it can be difficult for families to choose the right treatment for their child. As providers, it is critical to assess with the family what the child's needs are, as well as what family strengths and challenges may contribute to success in treatment.

For patients with good insight, limited burden reaching a treatment clinic, low to moderate symptom severity, and a preference for extended time to practice outside of the treatment session, traditional weekly treatment may be ideal. PHP and residential care may be more appropriate for individuals with more severe symptoms or who require a higher level of care, while IOP may be a better fit for those with less severe symptoms or who need more flexibility in their treatment schedule. For individuals with medication-resistant, severe, and chronic OCD, undergoing residential treatment has proven to be an effective form of treatment (Nanjundaswamy et al., 2020). Providers may find that using Appendix A to compare treatment options is helpful in guiding conversations around treatment choice. While providers are encouraged to guide patients in choosing the most appropriate treatment setting based on their needs, the authors recognize that due to access issues, treatment may be determined by availability rather than best fit (National Collaborating Centre for Mental Health, 2006).

Providers are encouraged to remember that many families struggle with reaching out and receiving timely help (Ziegler et al., 2021). OCD is a debilitating disorder that can impact all areas of a child's life and their family's life, and feelings of shame or embarrassment are common among caregivers (Torres et al., 2012). Finding effective treatment and working together with providers can help children and their families feel like they have their lives back, and providers should continue to emphasize with patients and families the potential for major improvements in function in life after treatment. Treatment can be challenging and at times unpredictable. Providers are encouraged to share with patients that there is not a magic pill, but effective treatments exist that lead to a significant reduction in symptoms and improved quality of life. The authors often tell our patients that it takes bravery to take on OCD, but the investment is worth it.

Conclusion

In summary, intensive treatment options have distinct advantages for children with OCD and their families. Intensive treatment may be especially powerful for children with low insight or motivation for treatment or children with significant challenges due to other co-occurring conditions. For families, intensive treatment can allow for intensive modeling of appropriate behavior and the opportunity to receive evidence-based treatment that is otherwise unattainable in the family's local area. For caregivers of children with OCD who themselves struggle with the exposure stimuli or have poor insight into their child's unique OCD presentation, intensive treatment can serve as a powerful tool for improving their insight while prioritizing the child's treatment.

As research into adaptations of intensive treatment continues, families and providers are presented with a number of treatment options that vary in duration, location, and intensity. The authors recommend that families and providers work in concert using the provided decision table to determine which intensive treatment option may work best for a given family. However, providers are cautioned to take financial and access restrictions into account as cost, insurance coverage, and availability of providers vary substantially. Regardless of what treatment option families pursue, ongoing communication and cooperation between a patient's primary provider and the intensive treatment provider (if they differ) is essential to ensure treatment gains are maintained following intensive treatment.

References

Abramowitz, J.S., Blakey, S.M., Reuman, L., & Buchholz, J.L. (2018). New directions in the cognitive-behavioral treatment of OCD: Theory, research, and practice. *Behavior Therapy*, 49(3), 311–322. https://doi.org/10.1016/j.beth.2017.09.002.

Albert, U., De Ronchi, D., Maina, G., & Pompili, M. (2019). Suicide risk in obsessive-compulsive disorder and exploration of risk factors: A systematic review. *Current Neuropharmacology*, 16(8). https://doi.org/10.2174/1570159x16666180620155941.

Balachander, S., Bajaj, A., Hazari, N., Kumar, A., Anand, N., Manjula, M., Sudhir, P.M., Cherian, A.V., Narayanaswamy, J.C., Jaisoorya, T.S., Math, S.B., Kandavel, T., Arumugham, S.S., & Janardhan Reddy, Y.C. (2020). Long-term outcomes of intensive inpatient care for severe, resistant obsessive-compulsive disorder: Résultats à long terme de soins intensifs à des patients hospitalisés pour un trouble obsessionnel-compulsif grave et résistant. *The Canadian Journal of Psychiatry*, 65(11), 779–789. https://doi.org/10.1177/0706743720927830.

Barrett, P., Healy-Farrell, L., & March, J.S. (2004). Cognitive-behavioral family treatment of childhood obsessive-compulsive disorder: A controlled trial. *Journal of the American Academy of Child & Adolescent Psychiatry*, 43(1), 46–62. https://doi.org/10.1097/00004583-200401000-00014.

Belloch, A., del Valle, G., Morillo, C., Carrió, C., & Cabedo, E. (2008). To seek advice or not to seek advice about the problem: The help-seeking dilemma for obsessive-compulsive disorder. *Social Psychiatry and Psychiatric Epidemiology*, 44(4), 257–264. https://doi.org/10.1007/s00127-008-0423-0.

Berman, N.C., Wilver, N.L., & Wilhelm, S. (2018). My child's thoughts frighten me: Maladaptive effects associated with parents' interpretation and management of children's intrusive thoughts. *Journal of Behavior Therapy and Experimental Psychiatry*, 61, 87–96. https://doi.org/10.1016/j.jbtep.2018.06.007.

Björgvinsson, T., Wetterneck, C.T., Powell, D.M., Chasson, G.S., Webb, S.A., Hart, J., Heffelfinger, S., Azzouz, R., Entricht, T.L., Davidson, J.E., & Stanley, M.A. (2008). Treatment outcome for adolescent obsessive-compulsive disorder in a specialized hospital setting. *Journal of Psychiatric Practice*, 14(3), 137–145. https://doi.org/10.1097/01.pra.0000320112.36648.3e.

Bloch, M.H., & Storch, E.A. (2015). Assessment and management of treatment-refractory obsessive-compulsive disorder in children. *Journal of the American Academy of Child and Adolescent Psychiatry*, 54(4), 251–262. https://doi.org/10.1016/j.jaac.2015.01.011.

Brennan, B.P., Lee, C., Elias, J.A., Crosby, J.M., Mathes, B.M., Andre, M.-C., Gironda, C.M., Pope, H.G., Jenike, M.A., Fitzmaurice, G.M., & Hudson, J.I. (2014). Intensive residential treatment for severe obsessive-compulsive disorder: Characterizing treatment course and predictors of response. *Journal of Psychiatric Research*, 56, 98–105. https://doi.org/10.1016/j.jpsychires.2014.05.008.

Cabedo, E., Belloch, A., Carrió, C., Larsson, C., Fernández-Alvarez, H., & García, F. (2010). Group versus individual cognitive treatment for obsessive-compulsive disorder: Changes in severity at post-treatment and one-year follow-up. *Behavioural and Cognitive Psychotherapy*, 38(2), 227–232. https://doi.org/10.1017/s135246580999066x.

Chase, R.M., Whitton, S.W., & Pincus, D.B. (2012). Treatment of adolescent panic disorder: A nonrandomized comparison of intensive versus weekly CBT. *Child & Family Behavior Therapy*, 34(4), 305–323. https://doi.org/10.1080/0731710 7.2012.732873.

Craske, M.G., Liao, B., Brown, L., & Vervliet, B. (2012). Role of inhibition in exposure therapy. *Journal of Experimental Psychopathology*, 3(3), 322–345. https://doi.org/10.5127/jep.026511.

du Mortier, J.A.M., Remmerswaal, K.C.P., Batelaan, N.M., Visser, H.A.D., Twisk, J.W.R., van Oppen, P., & van Balkom, A.J.L.M. (2021). Predictors of intensive treatment in patients with obsessive-compulsive disorder. *Frontiers in Psychiatry*, 12, 659401. https://doi.org/10.3389/fpsyt.2021.659401.

Ehrenreich, J.T., & Santucci, L.C. (2009). SPECIAL SERIES: Intensive cognitive-behavioral treatments for child and adolescent anxiety disorders. *Cognitive and Behavioral Practice*, 16(3), 290–293. https://doi.org/10.1016/j.cbpra.2009.04.001.

Foa, E.B., & Steketee, G. (1987). Behavioral treatment of phobics and obsessive-compulsives. In N.S. Jacobson (Ed.), *Psychotherapists in clinical practice: Cognitive and behavioral perspectives* (pp. 78–120). Guilford Press.

Garcia, A.M., Sapyta, J.J., Moore, P.S., Freeman, J.B., Franklin, M.E., March, J.S., & Foa, E.B. (2010). Predictors and moderators of treatment outcome in the pediatric obsessive compulsive treatment study (POTS I). *Journal of the American Academy of Child & Adolescent Psychiatry*, 49(10), 1024–1033. https://doi.org/10.1016/j.jaac.2010.06.013.

Geller, D.A., Biederman, J., Jones, J., Shapiro, S., Schwartz, S., & Park, K.S. (1998). Obsessive-compulsive disorder in children and adolescents: A review. *Harvard Review of Psychiatry*, 5(5), 260–273. https://doi.org/10.3109/10673229809000309.

Gittins Stone, D.I., Elkins, R.M., Gardner, M., Boger, K., & Sperling, J. (2023). Examining the effectiveness of an intensive telemental health treatment for pediatric anxiety and OCD during the COVID-19 pandemic and pediatric mental health crisis. *Child Psychiatry & Human Development*. https://doi.org/10.1007/s10578-023-01500-5.

Goodwin, R., Koenen, K.C., Hellman, F., Guardino, M., & Struening, E. (2002). Helpseeking and access to mental health treatment for obsessive-compulsive disorder. *Acta Psychiatrica Scandinavica*, 106(2), 143–149. https://doi.org/10.1034/j.1600-0447.2002.01221.x.

Gregory, S.T., Kay, B., Riemann, B.C., Goodman, W.K., & Storch, E.A. (2020). Cost-effectiveness of treatment alternatives for treatment-refractory pediatric obsessive-compulsive disorder. *Journal of Anxiety Disorders*, 69, 102151. https://doi.org/10.1016/j.janxdis.2019.102151.

Grøtte, T., Hansen, B., Haseth, S., Vogel, P.A., Guzey, I.C., & Solem, S. (2018). Three-week inpatient treatment of obsessive-compulsive disorder: A 6-month follow-up study. *Frontiers in Psychology*, 9, 620. https://doi.org/10.3389/fpsyg.2018.00620.

Guzick, A.G., Reid, A.M., Balkhi, A.M., Geffken, G.R., & McNamara, J.P.H. (2018). That was easy! Expectancy violations during exposure and response prevention for childhood obsessive-compulsive disorder. *Behavior Modification*, 44(3), 319–342. https://doi.org/10.1177/0145445518813624.

Havnen, A., Hansen, B., Öst, L.-G., & Kvale, G. (2014). Concentrated ERP delivered in a group setting: An effectiveness study. *Journal of Obsessive-Compulsive and Related Disorders*, 3(4), 319–324. https://doi.org/10.1016/j.jocrd.2014.08.002.

Højgaard, D.R.M.A., Schneider, S.C., La Buissonnière-Ariza, V., Kay, B., Riemann, B.C., Jacobi, D., Eken, S., Lake, P., Nadeau, J., Goodman, W.K., McIngvale, E., & Storch, E.A. (2020). Predictors of treatment outcome for youth receiving intensive residential treatment for obsessive–compulsive disorder (OCD). *Cognitive Behaviour Therapy*, 49(4), 294–306. https://doi.org/10.1080/16506073.2019.1614977.

Jacoby, R.J., & Abramowitz, J.S. (2016). Inhibitory learning approaches to exposure therapy: A critical review and translation to obsessive-compulsive disorder. *Clinical Psychology Review*, 49, 28–40. https://doi.org/10.1016/j.cpr.2016.07.001.

Jónsson, H., Kristensen, M., & Arendt, M. (2015). Intensive cognitive behavioural therapy for obsessive-compulsive disorder: A systematic review and meta-analysis. *Journal of Obsessive-Compulsive and Related Disorders*, 6, 83–96. https://doi.org/10.1016/j.jocrd.2015.04.004.

Knox, L.S., Albano, A.M., & Barlow, D.H. (1996). Parental involvement in the treatment of childhood obsessive compulsive disorder: A multiple-baseline examination incorporating parents. *Behavior Therapy*, 27(1), 93–114. https://doi.org/10.1016/s0005-7894(96)80038-4.

Leonard, R.C., Franklin, M.F., Wetterneck, C.T., Riemann, B.C., Simpson, H.B., Kinnear, K., Cahill, S.P., & Lake, P.M. (2016). Residential treatment outcomes for adolescents with obsessive-compulsive disorder. *Psychotherapy Research*, 26(6), 727–736. https://doi.org/10.1080/10503307.2015.1065022.

Lewin, A.B., Storch, E.A., Merlo, L.J., Adkins, J.W., Murphy, T., & Geffken, G.A. (2005). Intensive cognitive behavioral therapy for pediatric obsessive compulsive disorder: A treatment protocol for mental health providers. *Psychological Services, 2*(2), 91–104. https://doi.org/10.1037/1541-1559.2.2.91.

Mathieu, S.L., Conlon, E.G., Waters, A.M., McKenzie, M.L., & Farrell, L.J. (2019). Inflated responsibility beliefs in paediatric OCD: Exploring the role of parental rearing and child age. *Child Psychiatry & Human Development, 51*(4), 552–562. https://doi.org/10.1007/s10578-019-00938-w.

McCarty, R.J., Downing, S.T., Guastello, A.D., Lazaroe, L.M., Ordway, A.R., Mirhosseini, T., Barthle-Herrera, M.A., Cooke, D.L., Mathews, C.A., & McNamara, J.P.H. (2023). *Implementation and preliminary data of an exposure-based summer camp for pediatric OCD and anxiety.* [Manuscript submitted for publication]. Department of Psychiatry, University of Florida.

McGuire, J.F., Piacentini, J., Lewin, A.B., Brennan, E.A., Murphy, T.K., & Storch, E.A. (2015). A meta-analysis of cognitive behavior therapy and medication for child obsessive-compulsive disorder: Moderators of treatment efficacy, response, and remission. *Depression and Anxiety, 32*(8), 580–593. https://doi.org/10.1002/da.22389.

McGuire, J.F., & Storch, E.A. (2019). An inhibitory learning approach to cognitive-behavioral therapy for children and adolescents. *Cognitive and Behavioral Practice, 26*(1), 214–224. https://doi.org/10.1016/j.cbpra.2017.12.003.

Merricks, K.L., Nadeau, J.M., Ramos, A., & Storch, E.A. (2017). A case report of intensive exposure-based cognitive behavioral therapy for a child with comorbid autism spectrum disorder and obsessive-compulsive disorder. *Journal of Cognitive Psychotherapy, 31*(2), 118–123. https://doi.org/10.1891/0889-8391.31.2.118.

Nanjundaswamy, M.H., Arumugham, S.S., Narayanaswamy, J.C., & Reddy, Y.C.J. (2020). A prospective study of intensive in-patient treatment for obsessive-compulsive disorder. *Psychiatry Research, 291*, 113303. https://doi.org/10.1016/j.psychres.2020.113303.

National Collaborating Centre for Mental Health (UK) (2006). *Obsessive-compulsive disorder: Core interventions in the treatment of obsessive-compulsive disorder and body dysmorphic disorder.* British Psychological Society (UK).

Ollendick, T.H. (2014). Brief, high intensity interventions with children and adolescents with anxiety disorders: Introductory comments. *Psychopathology Review, a1*(1), 169–174. https://doi.org/10.5127/pr.034813.

Öst, L.-G., & Ollendick, T.H. (2017). Brief, intensive and concentrated cognitive behavioral treatments for anxiety disorders in children: A systematic review and meta-analysis. *Behaviour Research and Therapy, 97*, 134–145. https://doi.org/10.1016/j.brat.2017.07.008.

Reid, A.M., Guzick, A.G., Fernandez, A.G., Deacon, B., McNamara, J.P.H., Geffken, G.R., McCarty, R., & Striley, C.W. (2018). Exposure therapy for youth with anxiety: Utilization rates and predictors of implementation in a sample of practicing clinicians from across the United States. *Journal of Anxiety Disorders, 58*, 8–17. https://doi.org/10.1016/j.janxdis.2018.06.002.

Reid, A.M., Guzick, A.G., Gernand, A., & Olsen, B. (2016). Intensive cognitive-behavioral therapy for comorbid misophonic and obsessive-compulsive symptoms: A systematic case study. *Journal of Obsessive-Compulsive and Related Disorders, 10*, 1–9. https://doi.org/10.1016/j.jocrd.2016.04.009.

Remmerswaal, K.C.P., Lans, L., Seldenrijk, A., Hoogendoorn, A.W., van Balkom, A.J.L.M., & Batelaan, N.M. (2021). Effectiveness and feasibility of intensive versus regular cognitive behaviour therapy in patients with anxiety and obsessive-compulsive disorders: A meta-analysis. *Journal of Affective Disorders Reports*, 6, 100267. https://doi.org/10.1016/j.jadr.2021.100267.

Rice, T.R., Kostek, N.T., Gair, S.L., & Rojas, A. (2017). Summer camp program for children with obsessive–compulsive disorder: Description and preliminary observations. *Cognitive and Behavioral Practice*, 24(2), 142–151. https://doi.org/10.1016/j.cbpra.2016.03.006.

Rudy, B.M., Lewin, A.B., Geffken, G.R., Murphy, T.K., & Storch, E.A. (2014). Predictors of treatment response to intensive cognitive-behavioral therapy for pediatric obsessive-compulsive disorder. *Psychiatry Research*, 220(1–2), 433–440. https://doi.org/10.1016/j.psychres.2014.08.002.

Schneider, S.C., La Buissonnière-Ariza, V., Højgaard, D.R.M.A., Kay, B.S., Riemann, B.C., Eken, S.C., Lake, P., Nadeau, J.M., & Storch, E.A. (2018). Multimodal residential treatment for adolescent anxiety: Outcome and associations with pre-treatment variables. *Child Psychiatry & Human Development*, 49, 434–442. https://doi.org/10.1007/s10578-017-0762-8.

Selles, R.R., Højgaard, D.R.M.A., Ivarsson, T., Thomsen, P.H., McBride, N., Storch, E.A., Geller, D., Wilhelm, S., Farrell, L.J., Waters, A.M., Mathieu, S., Lebowitz, E., Elgie, M., Soreni, N., & Stewart, S.E. (2018). Symptom insight in pediatric obsessive-compulsive disorder: Outcomes of an international aggregated cross-sectional sample. *Journal of the American Academy of Child & Adolescent Psychiatry*, 57(8), 615–619.e5. https://doi.org/10.1016/j.jaac.2018.04.012.

Selles, R.R., Højgaard, D.R.M.A., Ivarsson, T., Thomsen, P.H., McBride, N.M., Storch, E.A., Geller, D., Wilhelm, S., Farrell, L.J., Waters, A.M., Mathieu, S., & Stewart, S.E. (2020). Avoidance, insight, impairment recognition concordance, and cognitive-behavioral therapy outcomes in pediatric obsessive-compulsive disorder. *Journal of the American Academy of Child & Adolescent Psychiatry*, 59(5), 650–659. https://doi.org/10.1016/j.jaac.2019.05.030.

Sperling, J., Boger, K., & Potter, M. (2020). The impact of intensive treatment for pediatric anxiety and obsessive-compulsive disorder on daily functioning. *Clinical Child Psychology and Psychiatry*, 25(1), 133–140. https://doi.org/10.1177/1359104519871338.

Storch, E.A., Bagner, D.M., Geffken, G.R., Adkins, J.W., Murphy, T.K., & Goodman, W.K. (2007a). Sequential cognitive-behavioral therapy for children with obsessive–compulsive disorder with an inadequate medication response: A case series of five patients. *Depression and Anxiety*, 24(6), 375–381. https://doi.org/10.1002/da.20260.

Storch, E.A., Geffken, G.R., Merlo, L.J., Mann, G., Duke, D., Munson, M., Adkins, J., Grabill, K.M., Murphy, T.K., & Goodman, W.K. (2007b). Family-based cognitive-behavioral therapy for pediatric obsessive-compulsive disorder. *Journal of the American Academy of Child & Adolescent Psychiatry*, 46(4), 469–478. https://doi.org/10.1097/chi.0b013e31803062e7.

Storch, E.A., Gelfand, K.M., Geffken, G.R., & Goodman, W.K. (2003). An intensive outpatient approach to the treatment of obsessive-compulsive disorder: Case exemplars. *Annals of the American Psychotherapy Association*, 6(4), 14–20. https://go.gale.com/ps/i.do?id=GALE%7CA112984666&sid=googleScholar&v=2.1&it=r&linkaccess=abs&issn=15354075&p=AONE&sw=w&userGroupName=anon%7Eec9e4c04.

Storch, E.A., Merlo, L.J., Lehmkuhl, H., Geffken, G.R., Jacob, M., Ricketts, E., Murphy, T.K., & Goodman, W.K. (2008). Cognitive-behavioral therapy for obsessive–compulsive disorder: A non-randomized comparison of intensive and weekly approaches. *Journal of Anxiety Disorders*, 22(7), 1146–1158. https://doi.org/10.1016/j.janxdis.2007.12.001.

Taboas, W., Ojserkis, R., & McKay, D. (2015). Change in disgust reactions following cognitive-behavioral therapy for childhood anxiety disorders. *International Journal of Clinical and Health Psychology*, 15(1), 1–7. https://doi.org/10.1016/j.ijchp.2014.06.002.

Taylor, R., & Reeder, C. (2015). Intensive individual and group cognitive behavioural therapy for obsessive-compulsive disorder. *American Journal of Psychotherapy*, 69(3), 269–284. https://doi.org/10.1176/appi.psychotherapy.2015.69.3.269.

Torres, A.R., Hoff, N.T., Padovani, C.R., & Ramos-Cerqueira, A.T. de A. (2012). Dimensional analysis of burden in family caregivers of patients with obsessive-compulsive disorder. *Psychiatry and Clinical Neurosciences*, 66(5), 432–441. https://doi.org/10.1111/j.1440-1819.2012.02365.x.

Veale, D., Naismith, I., Miles, S., Gledhill, L.J., Stewart, G., & Hodsoll, J. (2016). Outcomes for residential or inpatient intensive treatment of obsessive–compulsive disorder: A systematic review and meta-analysis. *Journal of Obsessive-Compulsive and Related Disorders*, 8, 38–49. https://doi.org/10.1016/j.jocrd.2015.11.005.

Wei, M.A., Van Kirk, N., Reid, A.M., Garner, L.E., Krompinger, J.W., Crosby, J.M., Elias, J.A., & Weisz, J.R. (2020). Emotion regulation strategy use and symptom change during intensive treatment of transitional age youth patients with obsessive compulsive disorder. *Journal of Behavioral and Cognitive Therapy*, 30(2), 95–102. https://doi.org/10.1016/j.jbct.2020.03.009.

Whiteside, S.P., Brown, A.M., & Abramowitz, J.S. (2008). Five-day intensive treatment for adolescent OCD: A case series. *Journal of Anxiety Disorders*, 22(3), 495–504. https://doi.org/10.1016/j.janxdis.2007.05.001.

Whiteside, S.P., Dammann, J.E., Tiede, M.S., Biggs, B.K., & Hillson Jensen, A. (2017). Increasing availability of exposure therapy through intensive group treatment for childhood anxiety and OCD. *Behavior Modification*, 42(5), 707–728. https://doi.org/10.1177/0145445517730831.

Whiteside, S.P., & Jacobsen, A.B. (2010). An uncontrolled examination of a 5-day intensive treatment for pediatric OCD. *Behavior Therapy*, 41(3), 414–422. https://doi.org/10.1016/j.beth.2009.11.003.

Whiteside, S.P., McKay, D., De Nadai, A.S., Tiede, M.S., Ale, C.M., & Storch, E.A. (2014). A baseline controlled examination of a 5-day intensive treatment for pediatric obsessive-compulsive disorder. *Psychiatry Research*, 220(1–2), 441–446. https://doi.org/10.1016/j.psychres.2014.07.006.

Wolters, L.H., Ball, J., Brezinka, V., Bus, M., Huyser, C., & Utens, E. (2021). Brief intensive cognitive behavioral therapy for children and adolescents with OCD: Two international pilot studies. *Journal of Obsessive-Compulsive and Related Disorders*, 29, 100645. https://doi.org/10.1016/j.jocrd.2021.100645.

Wu, M.S., McGuire, J.F., Martino, C., Phares, V., Selles, R.R., & Storch, E.A. (2016). A meta-analysis of family accommodation and OCD symptom severity. *Clinical Psychology Review*, 45, 34–44. https://doi.org/10.1016/j.cpr.2016.03.003.

Ziegler, S., Bednasch, K., Baldofski, S., & Rummel-Kluge, C. (2021). Long durations from symptom onset to diagnosis and from diagnosis to treatment in obsessive-compulsive disorder: A retrospective self-report study. *PLoS ONE*, 16(12), e0261169. https://doi.org/10.1371/journal.pone.0261169.

APPENDIX A

Patient Factors Best Suited for Alternatives to Weekly Outpatient Treatment

	IOP Outpatient	IOP Hospital	PHP	Therapeutic Camp	Residential Treatment	Inpatient Treatment
Caregiver Availability	Patients participate in sessions with caregiver	Patients in partial day treatment with limited caregiver involvement; possible option of family sessions		Patients in drop-off day program without caregiver	Patients housed for treatment without caregiver; possible option of family sessions	
Challenges with Insight or Motivation	Multisession delivery assists in challenging poor insight	Opportunity to be surrounded by peers engaging in similar tasks to incentivize participation and challenge poor insight				Short duration and full-time supervision to ensure safety despite challenges with insight or motivation
Overcoming Environmental Accommodations	Limited treatment team impact on environment outside of session	Extended time in therapeutic environment with limited treatment team impact outside of session			Full time residence in therapeutic environment	
Caregiver Psychopathology/Limitation of Support	Caregiver is safely able to participate in outpatient treatment and treatment homework	Caregiver is able to safely participate in treatment homework and receive psychoeducation from treatment team; caregiver's psychopathology may inhibit treatment			Caregiver is unable to safely participate in direct treatment or treatment homework	

Patient Factors Best Suited for Alternatives to Weekly Outpatient Treatment

| | IOP | | PHP | Therapeutic Camp | Residential Treatment | Inpatient Treatment |
	Outpatient	Hospital				
Comorbidity Management	Can integrate treatment for comorbidities		Comorbidity treatment integrated into OCD care and patient can participate in standalone sessions for comorbidity treatment as time allows	Limited opportunity to customize for comorbidity	Comorbidity treatment integrated into OCD care and patient can participate in standalone sessions for comorbidity treatment as time allows	Manage existing psychiatric disorder(s) or acute suicidality
Average Duration of Treatment	Generally one to three weeks		Dependent on program and progress	Week-long sessions offered	Generally 30–90 days	One to seven days for stabilization
Need for Academic Support During Treatment	Focused on OCD treatment without academic oversight unless it is an area of OCD symptomatology				Some programs offer academic support time	Focus on crisis stabilization, not academic support

Note. Recommendations suggested based on existing research, current treatment facility standards, and clinical experience.

APPENDIX B

Comparison of Typical Offerings by Treatment Setting

	Weekly Treatment	Outpatient IOP	Hospital IOP	PHP	Therapeutic Camp	Residential Treatment	Inpatient Treatment
Evidence-Based Treatment	X	X	X	X	X	X	X
Integrated Medication Management	X	X	X	X	X	X	X
Multiple Sessions a Week		X	X	X	X	X	X
Extended Session Duration (Over 1.5 Hours)			X	X	X	X	X
Group and Individual Treatment			X	X	X	X	X
24/7 Controlled Environment						X	X
Acute Crisis Stabilization							X

9 Treatment of Young Children with Obsessive-Compulsive Disorder

Ana I. Rosa-Alcázar,[1] Ángel Rosa-Alcázar,[1] Cristina Bernal-Ruiz,[1] and Cynthia Onyeka[2]

[1] *Department of Personality, Assessment, and Psychological Treatment, University of Murcia, Murcia, Spain*

[2] *Department of Psychiatry and Behavioral Sciences, Baylor College of Medicine, Houston, TX, USA*

In recent years, increased interest in early-onset obsessive-compulsive disorder (OCD) has ushered in significant improvement in evidence-based assessment instruments and an increase in psychological and pharmacological therapeutic interventions for this population. In the present chapter, we offer a review of the recent advancements in this area, focusing on the assessment and psychological treatment of young children (roughly three to eight years-old) with OCD.

I. Clinical Characteristics of Young Children with Obsessive-Compulsive Disorder and Comorbidity

OCD is characterized by the presence of intrusive thoughts or images (i.e., obsessions) and the performance of repetitive or ritual tasks (i.e., compulsions). Childhood OCD, however, is unique in that the obsession may not be present, but the need to conduct the compulsion is. Children may try to hide obsessions or justify themselves with simple reasoning. Parents may also participate in rituals (also known as family accommodation, discussed in Section 3.2.

It is important to note that most children go through a sequelae of developmental stages where patterns of behavior and rituals are common (e.g., asking parents to leave the light on before bed in early childhood). However, in order to differentiate OCD from normative conduct, the behaviors must be distinguished from evolutionarily adaptive rituals (i.e., ego-syntonic and developmentally appropriate behaviors). Differences between psychopathological and evolutionarily adaptive rituals are shown in Table 9.1.

DOI: 10.4324/9781003386278-9

Table 9.1 Differences between pathological and evolutionary rituals (Modified from Toro, 2006)

	EVOLUTIONARILY ADAPTIVE RITUALS	*COMPULSIONS*
Emotion	Pleasant	Unpleasant
Consequences at the end of the ritual	No anxiety	Temporary relief; anxiety and aggressiveness in the longer-term
Interference	None	High
Purpose of ritual	Adaptive	Eliminate anxiety
Parental behavior	Calm	Worry about excessive participation in exaggerated rituals

Three components or responses participate in childhood OCD (Rosa-Alcázar et al., 2022).

(i) *Cognitions*. Cognitions consist of obsessive thoughts, images, or impulses (with thoughts as the most frequent). Obsessions interfere with daily activity. When obsessions are perceived as images, they tend to be repulsive and intrusive. Children may constantly feel the impulse to perform an action that could cause harm to themself or others. Young children may not recognize what obsessions consist of, or even not have them. Compulsions can also appear as cognitive responses (i.e., mental rituals). Mental rituals are intended to neutralize discomfort caused by obsessions. Examples include silently praying, counting, or repeating phrases and words.

(ii) *Motor responses*. The motor responses related to childhood OCD (e.g., compulsions or rituals) often demonstrate significant impairment. Compulsions such as checking and ordering present a host of challenges and hinder conducting daily childhood activities, and are often unknowingly maintained by caregivers. For example, a child with OCD may be late for school due to repeatedly checking they have everything in their schoolbag or by having to dress and undress several times. They may also spend considerable time arranging toys and objects in their room. These behaviors impede them from doing homework or establishing relationships with peers. Avoidance is another characteristic response of OCD, where a child may avoid situations that cause fear or anxiety, usually related to the obsessive subject. Regarding contamination obsessions, it is common to avoid touching objects that have been in contact with other people or avoid places with perceived germs (e.g., hospitals, places with animals, etc.). Children will often want their parents to act similarly (i.e., accommodate) to protect them from their own fears. This often causes conflict at home if parents refuse to comply. As a result, family members may experience frustration, confusion, or even anger in response to their child's behavior.

(iii) *Psychophysiological and physical responses.* Children with OCD may experience psychophysiological responses, either related to the distress associated with the cognitive response or when the motor response is prevented. Example physical responses include sweating, tachycardia, accelerated respiratory rate, headache and stomachache, dullness, fatigue, muscle tension, etc. These responses may result in functional impairment in the child's daily work (academic, social, family, school, etc.).

The most common obsessions observed in clinical practice are contamination, disease, and accidents (McKay et al., 2003). Relatedly, the most frequent compulsions are cleaning, checking, repeating, and counting. When OCD begins at an early age, the most frequent associated disorders are anxiety, tics and Tourette's syndrome, attention deficit hyperactivity, disruptive behavior, and autism spectrum disorders (Lavell et al., 2016; Mathes et al., 2019; Murray et al., 2015; Storch et al., 2010).

II.   Evaluation

2.1.   *Preliminary Considerations*

When assessing for OCD, the primary goal is to identify obsessions and compulsions, which involves an analysis of cognitive responses (i.e., beliefs, images, attributions, expectations, self-verbalizations), psychophysiological responses, and motor responses (overt or covert rituals) relevant to both obsessions and compulsions. Doing so calls for a multidimensional, multi-informant evaluation while utilizing a biopsychosocial approach.

According to the cognitive-behavioral model of OCD, a comprehensive assessment of OCD should consider the following:

  i. The topography of the anxiety response system (cognitive, physiological, and motor).
 ii. The variables that precede these responses, including external factors (e.g., environmental), internal factors (i.e., thoughts, images, attributions, expectations), and psychophysiological reactions.
iii. The responses of organs, systems, and biological factors related to the child.
 iv. The contingencies following obsessive-compulsive responses, whether facilitated by adults significant to the child or their peers, or due to an internal effect consequent to avoidance/escape responses.
  v. Other influencing variables such as the occurrence of previous psychological treatment and attitude of family members towards OCD.

The following are the most relevant responses, which can occur in the context of obsessions and/or compulsions.

Cognitive responses. The cognitive responses consist of thoughts, images, and impulses which trigger the need to perform rituals and mental rituals to neutralize obsessions. When assessing cognitive responses, it is important to record the frequency, duration or intensity, and contingencies or reinforcements that maintain or facilitate behavior offered by the parent. Positive reinforcements include encouragement, consolation, of behaviors or negative reinforcements.

Motor responses. The compulsions or rituals precursing the stimulus (internal or external) that elicits anxiety make up the motor responses. From these responses, parameters mentioned in the cognitive responses must be recorded, such as avoidance responses and anxiety responses linked to the situation (e.g., crying, scratching, clenching fists, biting nails, kicking, yelling at parents, etc.). In addition, it is imperative to analyze responses of parents or relatives regarding whether they collaborate in performance of rituals.

Psychophysiological responses. When applicable (and not intrusive to the child), psychophysiological responses may be assessed. Example variables include muscle tension, heart and respiratory rate, sweating, and redness of skin. Some responses can be quantified by behavioral observation.

Environmental variables. There are several environmental variables which can influence OCD symptom initiation, development, and maintenance. Example variables include self-care responses developed by the child (e.g., grooming, dressing, toilet control, etc.), the behavior of parents/caregivers regarding the child (e.g., overprotection, criticism, fear), stressful situations for the child (e.g., change of school, hospitalization), educational style of parents and teachers/caregivers, other family members who have suffered the same problem or other pathologies, adaptive, social, and school behavior, and interpersonal relationships with siblings or peers.

Biomedical variables. A biomedical examination can be conducted to analyze streptococcal infections, tics, etc., in addition to indicating the presence of an associated psychopathology (attention-deficit hyperactivity disorder [ADHD], learning problems, etc.)

2.2. *Relevant Questionnaires*

2.2.1. *Obsessive-Compulsive Disorder Symptom and Severity*

In a systematic review of the literature, Iniesta-Sepúlveda and colleagues (2014) identified several evidence-based assessments (EBAs) to assess OCD symptom and severity. The authors specify the three levels of empirical support utilized to define a measure as an EBA: well-established assessment, approaching well-established assessment, and promising assessment (Cohen et al., 2008; Iniesta-Sepúlveda et al., 2014).

Well-established assessment. Measures that meet criteria as a well-established assessment must demonstrate reliability and validity in two published, empirical studies by at least two research teams. The Children's Yale-Brown Obsessive-Compulsive Scale (CY-BOCS; Scahill et al., 1997) is the only EBA classified as a well-established assessment to measure OCD symptom presence and severity. Given its excellent psychometric properties (see Iniesta-Sepúlveda et al., 2014; McKay et al., 2003; Storch et al., 2005), the CY-BOCS is the gold-standard and most widely used assessment for pediatric OCD (Storch et al., 2019). The semi-structured interview consists of two sections: a symptom checklist containing common obsessions and compulsions (62 in total grouped into 17 categories) and a severity score measuring frequency, interference, distress, and control of symptoms (Iniesta-Sepúlveda et al., 2014; Scahill et al., 1997). Moreover, Storch and colleagues (2006) developed self-report and parent-report versions of the measure for clinical populations, which demonstrated strong and significant associations with the clinician-rated measure. Cook et al. (2015) evaluated the psychometric properties of the CY-BOCS for assessing young children, aged five to eight years. The CY-BOCS Total score demonstrated adequate internal consistency, although at a lower level than is typically reported in studies of older children. Internal consistency of the Obsessions and Compulsions subscales was poor. The Total and subscale scores demonstrated good temporal stability over five weeks. Agreement between clinician and parent versions was poor at baseline but improved substantially throughout the course of the trial. Although there appears to be room for improvement, the CY-BOCS remains the most well-tested assessment of OCD in this younger age group.

The CY-BOCS was recently revised (Children's Yale-Brown Obsessive-Compulsive Scale II (CY-BOCS II; Storch et al., 2019) and demonstrates similar psychometric properties. The measure consists of five items that assess severity of obsessions, and five items that assess compulsions. All items have a Likert-type scale scored from zero (none) to four (extreme), resulting in a total score by adding the ten items (range = 0–40). In addition to the total score, specific scores for obsessive and compulsive subscales (range = 0–20) are generated (Storch et al., 2019).

Approaching well-established assessment. Assessments that satisfy approaching well-established assessment criteria either have validity and reliability demonstrated in at least two empirical studies by one research team or two research teams publishing studies suggesting mixed psychometric results (Cohen et al., 2008). That said, with the exception of the CY-BOCS-II, there have been minimal psychometric studies of OCD assessments with young children. The Obsessive-Compulsive Inventory-Child Version (OCI-CV; Foa et al., 2010) is the only OCD measure that meets criteria in this domain. The self-report measure assesses symptom presence and dimensionality in children and adolescents. The 21-item measure demonstrated good psychometric properties and yielded a six-factor solution following exploratory factor analysis (EFA): Doubt/Checking, Obsessions, Hoarding, Washing, Neutralizing, and Ordering (Foa et al., 2010; Jones et al., 2013).

Promising assessment. Several measures were determined to satisfy promising assessment criteria, where reliability and validity was demonstrated in at least one empirical study (Cohen et al., 2008).

The Children's Florida Obsessive-Compulsive Inventory (C-FOCI; Storch et al., 2009), assesses the presence and severity of obsessive-compulsive symptoms in children and adolescents. The measure consists of two sections. The first section contains 17 items on symptoms (obsessions and compulsions) experienced in the last month. The second section includes a severity scale with five items designed to assess symptom severity for both obsessions and compulsions. The C-FOCI demonstrates good psychometric properties and internal consistency (Storch et al., 2009).

The Children's Obsessional Compulsive Inventory (CHOCI; Shafran et al., 2003) is a comprehensive self-report measure assessing OCD symptoms and related impairment. The 19-item measure consists of items specifying obsessions and compulsions on a 3-point Likert scale (*Not at all* to *A lot*). With both parent-report and child-report, the measure demonstrates good internal consistency, convergent validity, and discriminant validity (Iniesta-Sepúlveda et al., 2014; Shafran et al., 2003).

Additional measures, such as the Leyton Obsessional Inventory-Child Version Survey Form (LOI-CV; Berg et al., 1986), do not presently meet criteria as an EBA (i.e., are insufficiently tested), but have been assessed among community samples. The 20-item measure assesses the presence and frequency of OCD symptoms across a four-factor model, as evidenced by factor analysis: General/Obsessive, Dirt/Contamination, Numbers/Look, and School Factors (Berg et al., 1986. However, across studies (Stewart et al., 2005; Storch et al., 2011) the measure demonstrates mixed psychometric properties, namely concerns regarding sensitivity and specificity (Iniesta-Sepúlveda et al., 2014). As such, clinicians should proceed with caution when selecting the LOI-CV for clinical use for screening or assessment (Storch et al., 2011).

2.2.2. *Obsessive-Compulsive-Disorder-Related Impairment and Family Functioning*

In addition to measures assessing symptom presence and severity, several measures have been identified to examine related responses and impacts of OCD among children and adolescents.

The Child Obsessive-Compulsive Impact Scale (COIS-C; Piacentini & Jaffer, 1999) is a self-report measure evaluating the effect of obsessive-compulsive responses on psychosocial functioning in children and adolescents with OCD. Consisting of corresponding child-report and parent-report forms, the measure contains 56 items assessing impairment at family, academic, and social levels (Piacentini & Jaffer, 1999). However, a four-factor structure was established in a later study in the parent-report measure consisting of Social Activities, School Activities, Living Skills, and Family Activities (Piacentini et al., 2007). Both the original and revised versiona of the measure demonstrate adequate to good psychometric properties (Piacentini et al., 2007). Presently, the COIS-C meets criteria as an approaching well-established assessment (Iniesta-Sepúlveda et al., 2014).

The Family Accommodation Scale for Obsessive-Compulsive Disorder (FAS) (Calvocoressi et al., 1995) is a measure that evaluates the degree of family accommodation, as well as the degree of discomfort and level of dysfunction brought about by OCD in family members. Family accommodation refers to the way caregivers modify or alter their behaviors to help their child reduce or avoid distress caused by a disorder, namely in OCD (Lebowitz et al., 2012). The measure consists of two sections: an OCD symptom checklist and a semi-structured interview detailing accommodation behaviors and the level of distress associated with accommodation (Calvocoressi et al., 1995). Self-report versions for both child (Family Accommodation Scale – Self Rated version [FAS-SR]) and parent (Family Accommodation Scale – Parent Report [FAS-PR]) have been developed and demonstrate good psychometric properties (Calvocoressi et al., 1999). The measure currently meets criteria as an approaching well-established assessment (Iniesta-Sepúlveda et al., 2014).

III.   Treatments

According to the current evidence base, the empirically supported treatment options for children with OCD include cognitive behavioral therapy (CBT), pharmacotherapy, or both (Freeman et al., 2018; Geller & March, 2012; Selles et al., 2018). Please see Chapters 3 and 11 for more details. The American Academy of Child and Adolescent Psychiatry Committee on Quality Issues (2012) reports that the standard of care in very young children with OCD is family-based CBT, which includes the same core components of CBT with significant family involvement.

3.1.   Psychological Treatments

Exposure with response prevention (ERP) is the main component of CBT for OCD, either applied alone or with other techniques in both adults and children (McGuire et al., 2015; Rosa-Alcázar et al., 2008; Rosa-Alcázar et al., 2015). As the intervention gold standard, ERP has shown superiority over pharmacological treatment (Sánchez-Meca et al., 2014) and other active psychotherapies, such as relaxation (Freeman et al., 2014; Piacentini et al., 2011).

The first-choice intervention modality for treatment of young children with OCD is family-involved or family-based CBT. This includes ERP as well as psychoeducation, cognitive therapy, and relapse prevention along with operant techniques and problem-solving. The focus of treatment is on the child and family system, where at least one parent is required to attend treatment (Freeman et al., 2014; Geller & March, 2012).

The participation of parents of children and adolescents with OCD is crucial for several reasons (please see Chapter 6 and Chapter 7 for more details on family involvement in childhood obsessive-compulsive and related disorders (OCRDs) treatment more broadly). First, poor functioning, high distress levels, conflict, and anxiety have been observed in relatives of OCD symptomatic children. Family-based CBT may help caregivers identify and manage these parent-level factors. Second, parents can participate in evaluation and can report objective data to the therapist. Lastly, family accommodation behaviors have key consequences throughout the course and maintenance of a child's OCD.

Meta-analytic studies reported greater effect sizes for studies that included family in the intervention (parents were trained to assist ERP and to manage problematic behavior) explaining 25–65 percent of variance (Barrett, Healy-Farrell, & March, 2004; Farrell, Schlup, & Boschen, 2010; Piacentini & Langley, 2004; Rosa-Alcázar et al., 2015; Scahill et al., 1996; Valderhaug et al., 2007; Waters, Barrett, & March, 2001).

Family-based CBT for OCD includes parent-focused techniques such as psychoeducation, problem solving, instructions on targeting accommodation, training in contingency management, and parent training to create co-therapists at home.

Table 9.2 Problems and Solutions

Problems	Mode of action
Child refuses to perform ERP	The therapist should start with stimuli that elicit minimal anxiety and/or add other behavioral techniques such as the reward program or the cost of response.
Child has covert rituals	The therapist should implement a motivational program before starting ERP.
Child seeks reinsurance	Parents and therapist should not provide reassurance to the child especially during exposure exercises as the child may use reassurance seeking as a means of reducing anxiety caused by ERP exercises. Extinction is the most appropriate procedure to eliminate these behaviors.

Several issues may arise during treatment on behalf of the child, the caregiver, or both. Table 9.2 presents some problems that may arise in the treatment of young children.

3.2.   Treatment Studies in Very Young Children

Whilst family-based CBT for OCD stands as the gold-standard treatment, there are a few adaptations to consider when applied to young children. According to Ginsburg and colleagues (2011), three main principles should be considered when working with younger children in treatment:

i. Modifying core CBT/ERP strategies for younger children.
ii. Addressing anxiogenic parent behaviors (e.g., expressed emotion, family accommodation, family dysfunction) within treatment.
iii. Strengthening the parent-child relationship to reduce incidence of child behavior problems to promote implementation of skills and generalize treatment gains.

Many interventions developed for younger children include these principles (e.g., Freeman et al., 2008; Freeman et al., 2014; Lewin et al., 2014; Storch et al., 2006; Storch et al., 2007). As such, several research studies examining the efficacy and effectiveness of OCD treatment for youth children have emerged in the last two decades. Table 9.3 presents characteristics of relevant studies.

Freeman and colleagues (2008) conducted the first randomized clinical trial (RCT) focused exclusively on young children with OCD (four to eight years). Researchers compared the relative efficacy of family-based CBT versus a comparable relaxation treatment. The treatment (Family Treatment Protocol; Freeman & Garcia, 2008) was comprised of 12 family CBT sessions over 14 weeks, including psychoeducation, ERP with cognitive techniques and instructions to reduce accommodation, ERP training to perform at home, operant techniques, and problem solving. The first two 90-minute sessions were only with parents, while other sessions with parents and children lasted 60 minutes. Findings revealed that the intervention proved more effective than relaxation techniques. The effect size for children completing treatment was high ($d = .85$).

Similarly, Freeman et al. (2014) conducted a new RCT utilizing the same protocol with 127 children (four to eight years). Study findings suggested that CBT with family involvement was superior to family relaxation training ($d = .84$). The percentage of clinical improvement for the group treated in family CBT was 72 percent versus 41 percent for family relaxation.

Lewin et al. (2014) examined the efficacy of family CBT with children aged three to eight years, focusing more on ERP at an increased intensity. Using a modified ERP protocol (Freeman et al., 2008), the intervention comprised 12 sessions, lasting 60 minutes, twice a week over six weeks. The twice-weekly format was to provide more frequent contact and thus reduce attrition. All treatment sessions were conducted with the child and at least one primary caregiver. Treatment included parent-child psychoeducation (allying against "OCD", introducing developmentally appropriate metaphors or examples), parenting tools (reward program, differential reinforcement, extinction, and modeling), ERP, and relapse prevention planning. The effect size achieved was high ($d = 1.8$), with 58.8 percent clinical remission (mean CY-BOCS ≤ 12) in the family treatment condition. Improvements were obtained in other secondary measures as well (symptom severity, accommodation, and parental anxiety).

Several single-case studies have been conducted as well, obtaining salutary results in young children (Comer et al. 2014; Ginsburg et al., 2011). Similar findings were demonstrated with online (i.e., internet-delivered, video teleconferencing [VTC]) methods. Comer and colleagues (2017) examined the efficacy of family CBT treatment presented in an online format when compared to traditional clinic-based family CBT. Based upon an established protocol (Freeman & Garcia, 2008), the RCT consisted of a 14-week treatment consisting of ERP specifically tailored for young children (four to eight years). Caregivers were trained as co-therapists to ensure adherence and motivation. As such, parents learned differential attention techniques, modeling, and how to manage the child's symptoms. Study findings revealed that online family-based CBT therapy was efficient, showing results like those achieved in the clinic.

The degree to which parents are involved also may vary. Rosa-Alcázar et al. (2017) examined the efficacy of two modes of intervention (parent only and parent-child dyad) of a program developed for and adapted to young children based on several programs (Choate-Sumers et al., 2008; Freeman & Garcia, 2008; March & Mulle, 1998). Both modalities demonstrated high effect sizes ($d = 3.710$ and $d = 2.285$, respectively). A better result was obtained in the group where mothers and children had been trained together. Some limitations of this study were its reduced sample size ($n = 10$), the need to increase exposure sessions, and failure to include measures to evaluate accommodation of both parents.

To address the previous studies limitations, the authors conducted a new study with young children with OCD (Rosa-Alcázar et al., 2019). The differential efficacy of three experimental conditions was analyzed:

a) Treatment of parents and child. Two parents and the child were involved in sessions. Exposure tasks at home had to be guided and supervised by multiple parents. Parents were encouraged to reinforce the achievements of the child.
b) Treatment of mother and child. In this condition, all parent participants were mothers. The mother and child participated in the sessions.

ERP at home was guided and supervised by the mother. The father was required to read the workbooks with the aim of being able to collaborate in the reduction of family accommodation, the control of problems at home, and the reinforcement of exposure to fear stimulus, or in the worst case not to obstruct the changes the mother was making.

c) Treatment of mother. All participants were mothers. They attended 12 weekly sessions with the psychologist. Treatment was the same but the time invested in the child instead focused on instructing and training the mother on what was to be done at home with the child (e.g., via role-play, as in consultation). The treatment program was comprised of two manuals: one for parents and another for children. The child workbook consisted of developmentally appropriate examples (e.g., OCD represented as an annoying ball that the child tries to throw away, but which repeatedly comes back). Relatedly, the parent workbook included psychoeducation, cognitive training to externalize OCD and reduce family accommodation, ERP training, management of problem-behaviors (Reinforcement, Extinction, Stimulus Control, Token Economy, Problem Solving Skills, and Relaxation Training), relapse prevention, and reinforcement (Rosa-Alcázar et al., 2019).

The three conditions produced clinical improvements in post-test and follow-up in the primary (symptom severity OCD) and secondary outcomes. The results showed no intergroup differences in variables related to OCD symptom severity, although statistically significant differences were found in groups regarding Internalizing and Externalizing problems, or mother and father accommodation. The most efficient condition was including a greater number of family members even when there was high family accommodation. The direct involvement of the child in the psychological treatment was important in achieving better results.

Despite the effectiveness of these interventions, some patients may not respond well to treatment. As such, it is necessary to identify relevant variables that may influence both severity of disorder and resistance to treatment. Several studies suggest the importance of understanding risk factors that may be influential in the development of the disorder (Eisen et al., 2010; Tibi et al., 2020). Others have focused on specific variables that may impact the course and maintenance of symptoms and/or hinder treatment effectiveness (Marcks et al., 2011; Reuman et al., 2018; Sharma & Math, 2019). Example variables include comorbidity, insight, family accommodation, family psychopathology, type of obsession or compulsion, personality, and neuropsychological and sociodemographic variable (De Avila et al., 2019; Du Mortier et al., 2021; Lebowitz, 2016; McGuire et al., 2015; Olatunji et al., 2013; Wu & Storch, 2016).

Table 9.3 Characteristics of representative studies

Authors	Mean age	Male (%)	Protocol	
Comer et al. (2014)	6.5	100	Family-Based CBT for Early Childhood OCD (Freeman & Garcia, 2008)	• 14 weeks of treatment • Parents participate in a structured way • Training parents as coaches of their children • Adaptation of parents to symptoms • Exposing parents to tolerate distress
Comer et al. (2017)	6.65	59.1%	Family-Based CBT for Early Childhood OCD (Freeman & Garcia, 2008)	• 14 weeks of treatment • Exposure and prevention of response adapted to children • Training parents for adherence and motivation, differential attention, modeling, and scaffolding • Children learn to externalize symptoms
Freeman et al. (2012)	5–8 (range)	47%	Pediatric Obsessive-Compulsive Disorder Treatment Study for Young Children (POTS jr) (Freeman et al., 2014)	• 14 weeks of treatment • Family-based CBT: psychoeducation, training in behavior management skills, externalizing OCD, ERP, and components of the family process • Family-based relaxation: psychoeducation, affective education, and relaxation training
Freeman et al. (2014)	7.2	47.2%	Pediatric Obsessive-Compulsive Disorder Treatment Study for Young Children (POTS jr) (Freeman et al., 2014)	• 14 weeks of treatment Family-based CBT: psychoeducation, training in behavior management skills (tools for parents), externalizing OCD and exposure with response prevention (tools for children), and components of the family process • Family-based relaxation: psychoeducation, affective education, and relaxation training

(Continued)

Table 9.3 (Continued)

Authors	Mean age	Male (%)	Protocol	
Lewin et al. (2014)	5.8	71%	Family-Based CBT for Early Childhood OCD (Freeman & Garcia, 2008)	• 12 sessions developed in 14 weeks • Sessions always developed with children and parent • ERP adapted in the manual for children with OCD • Psychoeducation for parents and children • Development of tools for parents • Relapse prevention program
Rosa-Alcázar et al. (2017)	6.6	65%	Cognitive Behavior Treatment Family (CBTF; annoying ball)	• 14 weeks of treatment • First 30 minutes with mothers and children (psychoeducation, cognitive training to outsource OCD, ERP graduated to feared situations and relapse prevention) • 30 minutes remaining mothers only (psychoeducation, family accommodation, outsourcing, contingency management, training for ERP exercises, reinforcing parenting skills and relapse prevention)
Rosa-Alcázar et al. (2019)	6.7	G1: 78.6% males G2: 73.3% G3: 73.3%	CBTF (annoying ball)	• 12 weeks of treatment • G1: Treatment for parents and children • G2: Treatment of mothers and children • G3: Treatment of mother only

Note. Family accommodation, relevant variables in treatment of young children.

For younger children with OCD, family accommodation is a common variable examined and addressed in treatment. As discussed earlier, family accommodation refers to the caregiver behaviors that aim to limit symptom-related distress (e.g., actions that facilitate rituals, participate in child's demands, provide reassurance, modify routines) with good intention, but result in greater impairment and symptom severity (Storch et al., 2007). Family accommodation has been analyzed as a predictor of both severity of the disorder (Strauss, Hale, & Stobie, 2015; Wu & Storch, 2016) and poor response to treatment (García et al., 2010; Iniesta-Sepúlveda et al., 2017; McGrath & Abbott, 2019; Rosa-Alcázar et al., 2015; Rudy et al., 2014; Torp et al. 2015).

Piacentini et al. (2011) indicated that one way to improve treatment was to intervene in family behaviors and processes which might lie at the root of maintenance of the problem. Sukhodolsky and colleagues (2013) assessed the importance of training parents in management of disruptive behaviors together with ERP, demonstrating greater improvement when both strategies were combined in children with a secondary diagnosis of behavioral problems. Relatedly, Rudy et al. (2014) highlighted the importance of family accommodation, sex, and severity as predictors of the efficacy of intensive CBT, requiring family involvement as a part of treatment. Study results were consistent with literature centered on developing interventions to help parents reduce accommodation (Lebowitz, 2016; Liebowitz et al., 2012). Rosa-Alcázar et al. (2021) analyzed predictors of family accommodation in 56 children with early-onset OCD. Results of the study indicated a high correlation between obsessive-compulsive symptom severity and parent-report accommodation.

In contrast, Öst et al. (2016) concluded that parental involvement of CBT was not a crucial factor for treatment effects. Riise et al. (2019) also found that this variable did not predict outcome after treatment and follow-up.

In summary, parental involvement in the treatment of young children with OCD is critically important for several reasons. First, young children demonstrate limited introspection and insight regarding their obsessions and compulsions which hinders their involvement in treatment and in motivation for change (Bornas et al., 2017; Chou et al., 2017). Second, elevated levels of distress, anxiety, and conflict have been observed in relatives of children with OCD (Flessner et al., 2009; Ho et al., 2018. Third, behavioral family accommodation can have important implications in the course and maintenance of a child's OCD (Calvocoressi et al., 1999; Lebowitz, 2016; Wu & Storch, 2016). Finally, the fact that parents participate as co-therapists and perform exposure tasks at home contributes to both generalizing and maintaining achievements (Choate-Summers et al., 2008; Freeman et al., 2003; Storch et al., 2013).

Conclusion

The chapter presents the main advances in evaluation and treatment of young children with OCD. It begins with the clinical characterization and epidemiological data of the problem to focus on the evaluation, highlighting the most relevant questionnaires. We conclude with the section on treatments, focusing especially on studies carried out on younger children and the importance of family accommodation.

References

American Academy of Child and Adolescent Psychiatry Committee on Quality Issues. (2012). Practice parameter for the assessment and treatment of children and adolescents with obsessive-compulsive disorder. *Journal of the American Academy of Child and Adolescent Psychiatry, 51*, 98–113.

Barrett, P., Healy-Farrell, L., & March, J.S. (2004). Cognitive-behavioral family treatment of childhood obsessive compulsive disorder: A controlled trial. *Journal of the American Academy of Child and Adolescent Psychiatry, 43*, 46–62.

Berg, C.J., Rapoport, J.L., & Flament, M. (1986). The Leyton obsessional inventory-child version. *Journal of the American Academy of Child Psychiatry, 25*(1), 84–91.

Bornas, X., Torre-Luque, A., Fiol-Veny, A., & Balle, M. (2017). Trajectories of anxiety symptoms in adolescents: Testing the model of emotional inertia. *International Journal of Clinical and Health Psychology, 17*, 192–196.

Calvocoressi, L., Lewis, B., Harris, M., Trufan, S.J., Goodman, W.K., McDougle, C.J., & Price, L.H. (1995). Family accommodation in obsessive-compulsive disorder. *The American Journal of Psychiatry, 152*(3), 441–443. https://doi.org/10.1176/ajp.152.3.441.

Calvocoressi, L., Mazure, C.M., Kasl, S.V., Skolnick, J., Fisk, D., Vegso, S.J., Van Oppen, B., & Precio, L.H. (1999). Family accommodation of obsessive-compulsive symptoms: Instrument development and assessment of family behavior. *The Journal of Nervous and Mental Disease, 187*, 636–642.

Choate-Summers, M.L., Freeman, J.B., Garcia, A.M., Coyne, L., Przeworski, A., & Leonard, H.L. (2008). Clinical considerations when tailoring cognitive behavioral treatment for young children with obsessive compulsive disorder. *Education and Treatment of Children, 31*, 395–416.

Chou, T., DeSerisy, M., Garcia, A.M., Freeman, J.B., & Comer, J.S. (2017). Obsessive-compulsive problems in very young children. In S. Abramowitz, D. McKay, & E.A. Storch (Eds.), *The Wiley Handbook of Obsessive Compulsive Disorders* (pp. 474–491). John Wiley & Sons Ltd.

Cohen, L.L., La Greca, A.M., Blount, R.L., Kazak, A.E., Holmbeck, G.N., & Lemanek, K.L. (2008). Introduction to special issue: Evidence-based assessment in pediatric psychology. *Journal of Pediatric Psychology, 33*(9), 911–915. https://doi.org/10.1093/jpepsy/jsj115.

Comer, J.S., Furr, J.M., Cooper-Vince, C.E., Kerns, C.E., Chan, P.T., Edson, A.L., Khanna, M., Franklin, M., Garcia, A., & Freeman, J.B. (2014). Internet-delivered, family-based treatment for early-onset OCD: A preliminary case series. *Journal of Clinical Child and Adolescent Psychology, 43*, 74–87.

Comer, J.S., Furr, J.M., Kerns, C.E., Miguel, E., Coxe, S., Elkins, R.M., Carpenter, A.L., Cornacchio, D., Cooper-Vince, C.E., DeSerisy, M., Chou, T.,

Sanchez, A.L., Khanna, M., Franklin, M.E., Garcia, A.M., & Freeman, J.B. (2017). Internet-delivered, family-based treatment for early-onset OCD: A pilot randomized trial. *Journal of Consulting and Clinical Psychology, 85*(2), 178–186.

Cook, N.E., Freeman, J.B., Garcia, A.M., Sapyta, J., & Franklin, M. (2015). Assessment of obsessive compulsive disorder in young children: Psychometric properties of the Children's Yale-Brown Obsessive Compulsive Scale. *Journal Psychopatholy Behavioral Assessment, 37*, 432–441.

De Avila, R.C.S., Do Nascimento, L.G., Porto, R.L.D.M., Fontenelle, L., Filho, E.C.M., Brakoulias, V., & Ferrão, Y.A. (2019). Level of insight in patients with obsessive–compulsive disorder: An exploratory comparative study between patients with "good insight" and "poor insight." *Frontiers in Psychiatry, 10*, 413.

Du Mortier, J.A., Remmerswaal, K.C., Batelaan, N.M., Visser, H.A., Twisk, J.W., Van Oppen, P., & Van Balkom, A.J. (2021). Predictors of Intensive treatment in patients with obsessive-compulsive disorder. *Frontiers in Psychiatry, 12*, 659401.

Eisen, J.L., Pinto, A., Mancebo, M.C., Dyck, I.R., Orlando, M.E., & Rasmussen, S.A. (2010). A 2-year prospective follow-up study of the course of obsessive-compulsive disorder. *The Journal of Clinical Psychiatry, 71*(8), 15786.

Farrell, L.J., Schlup, B., & Boschen, M.J. (2010). Cognitive–behavioral treatment of childhood obsessive–compulsive disorder in community-based clinical practice: Clinical significance and benchmarking against efficacy. *Behavior Research and Therapy, 48*, 409–417.

Flessner, C.A., Berman, N., Garcia, A., Freeman, J.B., & Leonard, H.L. (2009). Symptom profiles in pediatric obsessive-compulsive disorder (OCD): The effects of comorbid grooming conditions. *Journal of Anxiety Disorders, 23*(6), 753–759.

Foa, E.B., Coles, M., Huppert, J.D., Pasupuleti, R.V., Franklin, M.E., & March, J. (2010). Development and validation of a child version of the obsessive compulsive inventory. *Behavior Therapy, 41*(1), 121–132.

Freeman, J., Benito, K., Herren, J., Kemp, J., Sung, J., Georgiadis, C., Arora, A., Walther, M., & Garcia, A. (2018). Evidence base update of psychosocial treatments for pediatric obsessive-compulsive disorder: Evaluating, improving, and transporting what works. *Journal of Clinical Child & Adolescent Psychology, 47*(5), 669–698. https://doi.org/10.1080/15374416.2018.1496443.

Freeman, J., & Garcia, A.M. (2008). *Family-based treatment for young children with OCD: Therapist guide.* New York: Oxford University Press.

Freeman, J., Garcia, A., Benito, K., Conelea, C., Sapyta, J., Khanna, M., March, J., & Franklin, M. (2012). The pediatric obsessive compulsive disorder treatment study for young children (POTS jr): Developmental considerations in the rationale, design, and methods. *Journal of Obsessive-Compulsive and Related Disorders, 1*(4), 294–300.

Freeman, J.B., Garcia, A.M., Coyne, L., Ale, C., Przeworski, A., Himle, M., Compton, S., & Leonard, H.L. (2008). Early childhood OCD: Preliminary findings from a family-based cognitive-behavioral approach. *Journal of the American Academy of Child and Adolescent Psychiatry, 47*, 593–602.

Freeman, J.B., Garcia, A.M., Fucci, C., Karitani, M., Miller, L., & Leonard, H.L. (2003). Family-based treatment of early-onset obsessive-compulsive disorder. *Journal of Child and Adolescent Psychopharmacology, 13*, 71–80.

Freeman, J.B., Sapyta, J., Garcia, A.M., Compton, S., Khanna, M., Flessner, C., FitzGerald, D., Mauro, C., Dingfelder, R., Benito, K., Harrison. J., Curry, J., Foa, E. Marzo, J., Mooore, P., & Franklin, M. (2014). Family-based treatment of early childhood obsessive-compulsive disorder: The Pediatric Obsessive-Compulsive

Disorder Treatment Study for Young Children (POTS Jr) a randomized clinical trial. *JAMA Psychiatry, 71*, 689–698.

Garcia, A.M., Sapyta, J.J., Moore, P.S., Freeman, J.B., Franklin, M.E., March, J.S. & Foa, E.B. (2010). Predictors and moderators of treatment outcome in the Pediatric Obsessive Compulsive Treatment Study (POTS I). *Journal of the American Academy of Child & Adolescent Psychiatry, 49*(10), 1024–1033.

Geller, D.A., & March, J. (2012). Practice parameter for the assessment and treatment of children and adolescents with obsessive-compulsive disorder. *Focus, 10*, 360–373.

Ginsburg, G.S., Burstein, M., Becker, K.D., & Drake, K.L. (2011). Treatment of obsessive compulsive disorder in young children: An intervention model and case series. *Child & Family Behavior Therapy, 33*(2), 97–122. https://doi.org/10.108 0/07317107.2011.571130.

Ho, S.M., Dai, D., Mak, C., & Liu, K. (2018). Cognitive factors associated with depression and anxiety in adolescents: A two-year longitudinal study. *International Journal of Clinical and Health Psychology, 18*, 227–234.

Iniesta-Sepúlveda, M., Rosa-Alcázar, A.I., Rosa-Alcázar, Á. & Storch, E.A. (2014). Evidence-based assessment in children and adolescents with obsessive–compulsive disorder. *Journal of Child and Family Studies, 23*, 1455–1470.

Iniesta-Sepúlveda, M., Rosa-Alcázar, A.I., Sánchez-Meca, J., Parada-Navas, J.L., & Rosa-Alcázar, Á. (2017). Cognitive-behavioral high parental involvement treatments for pediatric obsessive-compulsive disorder: A meta-analysis. *Journal of Anxiety Disorders, 49*, 53–64.

Jones, A.M., De Nadai, A.S., Arnold, E.B., McGuire, J.F., Lewin, A.B., Murphy, T.K., & Storch, E.A. (2013). Psychometric properties of the obsessive compulsive inventory: Child version in children and adolescents with obsessive-compulsive disorder. *Child Psychiatry and Human Development, 44*(1), 137–151. https://doi.org/10.1007/s10578-012-0315-0.

Lavell, C.H., Farrell, L.J., Waters, A.M., & Cadman, J. (2016). Predictors of treatment response to group cognitive behavioural therapy for pediatric obsessive-compulsive disorder. *Psychiatry Research, 245*, 186–193.

Lebowitz E.R. (2016). Treatment of extreme family accommodation in a youth with obsessive-compulsive disorder. In A.E. Storch & A.B Lewin (Eds), *Clinical handbook of obsessive-compulsive and related disorders* (pp. 321–335). Sprinter International Publishing Switzerland.

Lebowitz, E. R., Panza, K. E., Su, J., & Bloch, M. H. (2012). Family accommodation in obsessive–compulsive disorder. *Expert Review of Neurotherapeutics, 12*(2), 229–238.

Lewin, A. B., Park, J. M., Jones, A. M., Crawford, E. A., De Nadai, A. S., Menzel, J., Arnold, E., Murphy, T., & Storch, E. A. (2014). Family-based exposure and response prevention therapy for preschool-aged children with obsessive-compulsive disorder: A pilot randomized controlled trial. *Behaviour Research and Therapy, 56*, 30–38.

Locher, C., Koechlin, H., Zion, S. R., Werner, C., Pine, D. S., Kirsch, I., Kessler, R., & Kossowsky, J. (2017). Efficacy and safety of selective serotonin reuptake inhibitors, serotonin-norepinephrine reuptake inhibitors, and placebo for common psychiatric disorders among children and adolescents: A systematic review and meta-analysis. *JAMA Psychiatry, 74*(10), 1011–1020.

March, J. S. & Mulle, K. (1998). *OCD in children and adolescents: A cognitive-behavioral treatment manual*. New York: Guilford.

Marcks, B. A., Weisberg, R. B., Dyck, I., & Keller, M. B. (2011). Longitudinal course of obsessive-compulsive disorder in patients with anxiety disorders: A 15-year prospective follow-up study. *Comprehensive Psychiatry*, *52*(6), 670–677.

Mathes, B. M., Morabito, D. M., & Schmidt, N. B. (2019). Epidemiological and clinical gender differences in OCD. *Current Psychiatry Reports*, *21*, 1–7.

McGrath, C. A., & Abbott, M. J. (2019). Family-based psychological treatment for obsessive compulsive disorder in children and adolescents: A meta-analysis and systematic review. *Clinical Child and Family Psychology Review*, *22*(4), 478–501.

McGuire, J.F., Piacentini, J., Lewin, A.B., Brennan, E.A., Murphy, T.K., & Storch, E.A. (2015). A meta-analysis of cognitive behavior therapy and medication for child obsessive–compulsive disorder: Moderators of treatment efficacy, response, and remission. *Depression and Anxiety*, *32*, 580–593.

McKay, D., Piacentini, J., Greisberg, S., Graae, F., Jaffer, M., Miller, J., Neziroglu, F., & Yaryura-Tobias, J.A. (2003). The Children's Yale-Brown Obsessive-Compulsive Scale: Item structure in an outpatient setting. *Psychological Assessment*, *15*(4), 578–581. https://doi.org/10.1037/1040-3590.15.4.578.

Murray, K., Jassi, A., Mataix-Cols, D., Barrow, F., & Krebs, G. (2015). Outcomes of cognitive behaviour therapy for obsessive–compulsive disorder in young people with and without autism spectrum disorders: A case controlled study. *Psychiatry Research*, *228*, 8–13.

Olatunji, B.O., Davis, M.L., Powers, M.B., & Smits, J.A. (2013). Cognitive- behavioral therapy for obsessive-compulsive disorder: A meta-analysis of treatment outcome and moderators. *Journal Psychiatry Research*, *47*(1), 33–41.

Öst, L.G., Riise, E.N., Wergeland, G.J., Hansen, B., & Kvale, G. (2016). Cognitive behavioral and pharmacological treatments of OCD in children: A systematic review and meta-analysis. *Journal of Anxiety Disorders*, *43*, 58–69.

Piacentini, J., Bergman, R. L., Chang, S., Langley, A., Peris, T., Wood, J. J., & McCracken, J. (2011). Controlled comparison of family cognitive behavioral therapy and psychoeducation/relaxation training for child obsessive-compulsive disorder. *Journal of the American Academy of Child and Adolescent Psychiatry*, *50*, 1149–1161.

Piacentini, J., & Jaffer, M. (1999). *Measuring functional impairment in youngsters with OCD: Manual for the Child OCD Impact Scale (COIS)*. Los Angeles: UCLA Department of Psychiatry.

Piacentini, J., & Langley, A. K. (2004). Cognitive-behavioral therapy for children who have obsessive-compulsive disorder. *Journal of Clinical Psychology*, *60*, 1181–1194.

Piacentini, J., Peris, T. S., Bergman, R. L., Chang, S., & Jaffer, M. (2007). BRIEF REPORT: Functional impairment in childhood OCD: Development and psychometrics properties of the child obsessive-compulsive impact scale-revised (COIS-R). *Journal of Clinical Child & Adolescent Psychology*, *36*(4), 645–653. https://doi.org/10.1080/15374410701662790.

Reuman, L., Buchholz, J., & Abramowitz, J. S. (2018). Obsessive beliefs, experiential avoidance, and cognitive fusion as predictors of obsessive-compulsive disorder symptom dimensions. *Journal of Contextual Behavioral Science*, *9*, 15–20.

Riise, E.N., Kvale, G., Öst, L.G., Skjold, S.H., & Hansen, B. (2019). Does family accommodation predict outcome of concentrated exposure and response prevention for adolescents? *Child Psychiatry & Human Development*, *50*, 975–986.

Rosa-Alcázar, A.I., Iniesta-Sepúlveda, M., Storch, E.A., Rosa-Alcázar, Á., Parada-Navas, J.L., & Rodríguez, J.O. (2017). A preliminary study of cognitive-behavioral family-based treatment versus parent training for young children with obsessive-compulsive disorder. *Journal of Affective Disorders, 208*, 265–271.

Rosa-Alcázar, A.I., Rosa-Alcázar, A., & Olivares-Olivares, P. (2022). El trastorno obsesivo-compulsivo en la infancia y adolescencia. In M.A. Vallejo, & M. Fe (Eds.), *Manual de terapia de conducta en la infancia* (207–240). Dykinson.

Rosa-Alcázar, Á., Rosa-Alcázar, A.I., Olivares-Olivares, P.J., Parada-Navas, J.L., Rosa-Alcázar, E., & Sánchez-Meca, J. (2019). Family involvement and treatment for young children with obsessive-compulsive disorder: Randomized control study. *International Journal of Clinical and Health Psychology, 19*(3), 218–227.

Rosa-Alcázar, Á., Rosa-Alcázar, A.I., Parada-Navas, J.L., Olivares-Olivares, P.J., & Rosa-Alcázar, E. (2021). Predictors of parental accommodation and response treatment in young children with obsessive-compulsive disorder. *Frontiers in Psychiatry*, 737062.

Rosa-Alcázar, A., Sánchez-Meca, J., Gómez-Conesa, A., & Marín-Martínez, F. (2008). Psychological treatment of obsessive–compulsive disorder: A meta-analysis. *Clinical Psychology Review, 28*, 1310–1325.

Rosa-Alcázar, A.I., Sánchez-Meca, J., Rosa-Alcázar, Á., Iniesta- Sepúlveda, M., Olivares, J., & Parada-Navas, J.L. (2015). Psychological treatment of obsessive-compulsive disorder in children and adolescents: A meta-analysis. *The Spanish Journal of Psychology, 18*, E20.

Rudy, B.M., Lewin, A.B., Geffken, G.R., Murphy, T.K., & Storch, E.A. (2014). Predictors of treatment response to intensive cognitive-behavioral therapy for pediatric obsessive-compulsive disorder. *Psychiatry Research, 220*(1–2), 433–440.

Sánchez-Meca, J., Rosa-Alcázar, A.I., Iniesta-Sepúlveda, M., & Rosa-Alcázar, Á. (2014). Differential efficacy of cognitive-behavioral therapy and pharmacological treatments for pediatric obsessive–compulsive disorder: A meta-analysis. *Journal of Anxiety Disorders, 28*, 31–44.

Scahill, L., Riddle, M.A., McSwiggin-Hardin, M., Ort, S.I., King, R.A., Goodman, W.K., Cicchetti, D., & Leckman, J.F. (1997). Children's Yale-Brown Obsessive Compulsive Scale: Reliability and validity. *Journal of the American Academy of Child and Adolescent Psychiatry, 36*, 844–852.

Scahill L., Vitulano L.A., Brenner E.M., Lynch K.A., & King R.A. (1996). Behavioral therapy in children and adolescents with obsessive-compulsive disorder: A pilot study. *Journal of Child and Adolescent Psychopharmacology, 6*, 191–202.

Selles, R.R., Belschner, L., Negreiros, J., Lin, S., Schuberth, D., McKenney, K., Gregorowski, N., Simpson, A., Bliss, A., & Stewart, S.E. (2018). Group family-based cognitive behavioral therapy for pediatric obsessive compulsive disorder: Global outcomes and predictors of improvement. *Psychiatry Research, 260*, 116–122.

Shafran, R., Frampton, I., Herman, I., Reynolds, M., Teachman, B., & Rachman, S. (2003). The preliminary development of a new self-report measure for OCD in young people. *Journal of Adolescence, 26*, 137–42.

Sharma, E., & Math, S.B. (2019). Course and outcome of obsessive–compulsive disorder. *Indian Journal of Psychiatry, 61*(Suppl 1), S43.

Skarphedinsson, G., Weidle, B., & Ivarsson, T. (2015). Sertraline treatment of nonresponders to extended cognitive-behavior therapy in pediatric obsessive-compulsive disorder. *Journal of Child and Adolescent Psychopharmacology, 25*(7), 574–579.

Stewart, S.E., Ceranoglu, T.A., O'Hanley, T., & Geller, D.A. (2005). Performance of clinician versus self-report measures to identify obsessive-compulsive disorder in children and adolescents. *Journal of Child & Adolescent Psychopharmacology, 15*(6), 956–963.

Storch, E.A., Geffken, G.R., Merlo, L.J., Jacob, M.L., Murphy, T.K., Goodman, W.K., Larson, M.J., Fernandez, M., & Grabill, K. (2007). Family accommodation in pediatric obsessive–compulsive disorder. *Journal of Clinical Child & Adolescent Psychology, 36*(2), 207–216. https://doi.org/10.1080/15374410701277929.

Storch, E.A., Goddard, A.W., Grant, J.E., De Nadai, A.S., Goodman, W.K., Mutch, P.J., McDougle, C., & Murphy, T.K. (2013). Double-blind, placebo-controlled, pilot trial of paliperidone augmentation in serotonin reuptake inhibitor-resistant obsessive-compulsive disorder. *The Journal of Clinical Psychiatry, 74*(6), 4760.

Storch, E.A., Khanna, M., Merlo, L.J., Loew, B.A., Franklin, M., Reid, J.M., Goodman, W., & Murphy, T.K. (2009). Children's Florida obsessive compulsive inventory: Psychometric properties and feasibility of a self-report measure of obsessive–compulsive symptoms in youth. *Child Psychiatry and Human Development, 40*, 467–483.

Storch, E.A., Lewin, A.B., Geffken, G.R., Morgan, J.R., & Murphy, T.K. (2010). The role of comorbid disruptive behavior in the clinical expression of pediatric obsessive-compulsive disorder. *Behaviour Research and Therapy, 48*, 1204–1210.

Storch, E.A., McGuire, J.F., Wu, M.S., Hamblin, R., McIngvale, E., Cepeda, S.L., Scheider, S., Rufino, K., Rasmussen, S., Precio, L., & Goodman, W.K. (2019). Development and psychometric evaluation of the Children's Yale-Brown Obsessive-Compulsive Scale Second Edition. *Journal of the American Academy of Child & Adolescent Psychiatry, 58*(1), 92–98.

Storch, E.A., Murphy, T.K., Adkins, J.W., Lewin, A.B., Geffken, G.R., Johns, N.B., Jann, K.E., & Goodman, W.K. (2006). The Children's Yale-Brown Obsessive-Compulsive Scale: Psychometric properties of child- and parent-report formats. *Journal of Anxiety Disorders, 20*(8), 1055–1070. https://doi.org/10.1016/j.janxdis.2006.01.006.

Storch, E.A., Murphy, T.K., Geffken, G.R., Bagner, D.M., Soto, O., Sajid, M., Allen, P., Killiany, E., & Goodman, W.K. (2005). Factor analytic study of the Children's Yale–Brown Obsessive–Compulsive Scale. *Journal of Clinical Child and Adolescent Psychology, 34*(2), 312–319.

Storch, E.A., Park, J.M., Lewin, A.B., Morgan, J.R., Jones, A.M., & Murphy, T.K. (2011). The Leyton Obsessional Inventory – Child Version Survey Form does not demonstrate adequate psychometric properties in American youth with pediatric obsessive-compulsive disorder. *Journal of Anxiety Disorders, 25*(4), 10.1016/j.janxdis.2011.01.005. https://doi.org/10.1016/j.janxdis.2011.01.005.

Strauss, C., Hale, L., & Stobie, B. (2015). A meta-analytic review of the relationship between family accommodation and OCD symptom severity. *Journal of Anxiety Disorders, 33*, 95–102.

Sukhodolsky, D.G., Gorman, B.S., Scahill, L., Findley, D., & McGuire, J. (2013). Exposure and response prevention with or without parent management training for children with obsessive-compulsive disorder complicated by disruptive behavior: A multiple-baseline across-responses design study. *Journal of Anxiety Disorders, 27*(3), 298–305.

Tibi, L., van Oppen, P., van Balkom, A.J., Eikelenboom, M., Hendriks, G.J., & Anholt, G.E. (2020). Childhood trauma and attachment style predict the four-year course of obsessive compulsive disorder: Findings from the Netherlands obsessive compulsive disorder study. *Journal of Affective Disorders, 264*, 206–214.

Toro, J. (2006). Trastornos obsesivos en la infancia y la adolescencia. In J. Vallejo, & G.E. Berrios (Eds.), *Estados obsesivos* (pp. 433–459). Masson.

Torp, N.C., Dahl, K., Skarphedinsson, G., Compton, S., Thomsen, P.H., Weidle, B., Hybel, K., Valderhaug, R., Melin, K., Nissen, J., & Ivarsson, T. (2015). Predictors associated with improved cognitive-behavioral therapy outcome in pediatric obsessive-compulsive disorder. *Journal of the American Academy of Child & Adolescent Psychiatry, 54*(3), 200–207.

Valderhaug, R., Larsson, B., Götestam, K. G., & Piacentini, J. (2007). An open clinical trial of cognitive-behaviour therapy in children and adolescents with obsessive–compulsive disorder administered in regular outpatient clinics. *Behaviour Research and Therapy, 45*, 577–589.

Waters, T.L., Barrett, P.M., & March, J.S. (2001). Cognitive-behavioral family treatment of childhood obsessive-compulsive disorder: Preliminary findings. *American Journal of Psychotherapy, 55*, 372.

Wu, M.S., & Storch, E.A. (2016). Personalizing cognitive-behavioral treatment for pediatric obsessive-compulsive disorder. *Expert Review of Precision Medicine and Drug Development, 1*, 397–405.

10 Internet-based Cognitive Behavioral Therapy

Nicholas R. Farrell,[1] Mia C. Nuñez,[1]
Patrick B. McGrath,[1] Jamie D. Feusner,[1–5]
and Cate W. MacDonald[1,6]

[1] NOCD, Inc., Chicago, IL

[2] Department of Psychiatry, University of Toronto,
Toronto, ON

[3] Centre for Addiction and Mental Health, Toronto, ON

[4] Department of Psychiatry and Biobehavioral Sciences,
University of California Los Angeles, Los Angeles, CA

[5] Department of Women's and Children's Health, Karolinska
Institutet, Stockholm, Sweden

[6] Harvard University, Cambridge, MA

The last 10 to 15 years have witnessed burgeoning advancements and interest in the use of technology to facilitate remote delivery of mental health services for common mental health problems. The COVID-19 pandemic and associated periods of lockdown and social distancing seemingly accelerated the use of various technologies to deliver mental health services to individuals who might otherwise be without care. Of particular note is the increased availability of internet-based cognitive behavioral therapy (IB-CBT) for a range of mental health conditions in youth (Vigerland et al., 2016). Given the prevalence of obsessive-compulsive and related disorders (OCRDs) in children and adolescents and the challenges faced in accessing evidence-based treatment for anxious youths (Salloum et al., 2016), IB-CBT presents a promising option for children and families affected by these conditions.

This chapter outlines key considerations in using IB-CBT, offers a pragmatic review of its efficacy in empirical studies to date, and provides guidance for effective implementation of IB-CBT for OCRDs in youth. In this chapter, following previous descriptions of IB-CBT as a therapist guided intervention (Andersson, 2009), our scope is limited to cognitive-behavioral treatment approaches that are guided by a mental health professional and does not include strictly self-help approaches, whether internet-based or otherwise.

DOI: 10.4324/9781003386278-10

Case Description

Tak is a 16-year-old cisgender male of Chinese descent living in a Midwestern US State. He comes from a middle-class family, and his parents have an intact marriage. At age eight, Tak began to notice symptoms of what would later be diagnosed as OCD. He tried to hide the symptoms, but as he got older, they soon became apparent to his parents.

When OCD first emerged, Tak began to fear that the doors might be unlocked, and he would lay awake at night listening for sounds. For a while he would stay in his room, but eventually he would come out and ask his parents if the doors were locked, and then would even go and check them himself, though he had been assured that they were locked. Within a month, he began to sneak around the house after his family went to bed to check the locks; eventually this would happen multiple times a night.

After being caught out of bed in the middle of the night for the third time, Tak's father told him that he had to stay in his room or he would be punished, but Tak pleaded with him to install more locks on the door. Tak's mother finally learned that Tak had seen a program on TV where a house was robbed, and the entire family was assaulted. To ease Tak's fears, his parents agreed that they could get a security system, and Tak could have a monitor in his room to watch the cameras.

While this helped Tak feel better for a few weeks, he started to watch the monitor more and more, which disrupted his sleep. Eventually, the family removed the monitor from his room and took Tak to his pediatrician, who said many children worry about these things and prescribed Tak a low dose antidepressant. Tak's physician also recommended he work with a counselor in the clinic who could help him practice some relaxation techniques. Tak was able to get some relief from the antidepressants and the work with his counselor. In addition, his mother gave frequent assurance that he was safe, and his counselor told him there was nothing to worry about.

Then, in church, Tak heard the preacher talk about Hell, and he began to worry that he and his family could commit a sin and go to Hell for it. Quickly Tak stopped playing video games and began to read all the holy books and scriptures that he could get his hands on. Initially his parents were impressed that their son was no longer playing so many video games, but his mom soon realized that Tak was not sleeping again, and she became concerned. When she confronted Tak, he told her about his fears of Hell and the whole family ending up there. His mom tried to assure him that they were not going to Hell, but Tak became very distraught. Finally, his mother called the preacher who came over to their house and talked to Tak. Tak was at first consoled, but even the preacher confessed to Tak's mother that he did not know what to do and could only recommend a weekly prayer circle among their family in the home.

Tak's OCD intensified in the next year. He also began to spend more and more time in the bathroom washing his hands, especially after he had gone to the bathroom. The time Tak was spending in the bathroom began to make him late for school and his parents late for work. Tak's new behaviors only further frustrated the family in addition to the water and gas bill increasing every month due to Tak's time in the bathroom.

One day, Tak's preacher called his mother and told her that he had attended an online conference on OCD and religion, and the cases he learned about reminded him a lot of Tak. When Tak's mother started to research OCD, she was amazed to see that everything that had happened with Tak could fit under the OCD umbrella – his need to have things in his room be "just right," his fear of people breaking into the house, and his scrupulous religious concerns, in addition to his increasing time spent in the bathroom.

At first, Tak's parents struggled to find appropriate treatment for him. They lived in a rural area, and the only CBT-trained provider was over an hour away. Additionally, this provider did not accept the family's insurance, and Tak's parents could not afford to pay for treatment out of pocket. Finally, Tak's mother learned of IB-CBT and she reached out to book an appointment.

IB-CBT worked extremely well for Tak and his parents. Together, they learned more about his condition and how to "outsmart" it, primarily via confronting Tak's feared scenarios and stopping his compulsions (i.e., exposure and response prevention [ERP]). During their virtual sessions, Tak and his therapist would tour his home and practice not checking the locks or putting things in his room "just right" while living with the uncertainty over whether his feared outcomes would happen. These hands-on virtual experiences in the home were the tipping point for Tak, making significant changes in reducing the severity of his obsessions and compulsions. Tak's parents also benefited from education and coaching they received during the virtual sessions on eliminating their accommodation of his OCD (e.g., not giving him reassurance).

Clinical Rationale for Internet-Based Cognitive Behavioral Therapy

Later in this chapter, we elaborate on some of the general advantages associated with using IB-CBT to treat OCRDs in youth. In this section, we provide a rationale for our readers to understand why, in many circumstances, it may be equally or even more clinically advantageous to deliver CBT to youth with OCRDs via internet-based methods as opposed to traditional in-person settings. Whereas in-person delivery of CBT for youth has advantages over IB-CBT (e.g., perceiving patients' non-verbal cues and body language better in-person vs. videoconferencing), we assert there is a strong rationale to support the use of IB-CBT for youth with OCRDs.

For youth who struggle with OCRDs, especially those with a strong anxiety-based component such as OCD and body dysmorphic disorder (BDD), it is important that exposure therapy tasks incorporate scenarios and stimuli that commonly elicit elevated anxiety. For many youth, these scenarios and stimuli will not be present in a traditional clinical setting. This was certainly true of Tak, who needed to complete exposure tasks involving stimuli that were almost exclusively located inside his home (e.g., using his bathroom without excessive washing or cleaning). Although efforts can be made to approximate young patients' feared stimuli in traditional clinical settings, experience suggests these efforts are not always successful. Accordingly, IB-CBT can effectively bridge this gap by allowing exposure tasks to occur with the naturalistic scenarios and stimuli that consistently provoke fear for youth patients. To illustrate, Tak was able to benefit from exposure tasks with virtual support from his therapist in which he walked around his home while imagining a potential burglary without repeatedly checking locks. Of course, this type of exposure task would likely not have been feasible without an internet-based delivery method.

For many youth with OCRDs, the key problematic behaviors that are targeted in CBT may primarily manifest in either the home environment or another physical location that would be very challenging to access in a traditional in-person format. For example, an adolescent with BDD may primarily engage in excessive appearance checking and self-grooming behaviors when in a specific well-lit bathroom with a large vanity mirror in the home. As another example, a young child with persistent motor and vocal tics (i.e., Tourette's disorder) may experience the greatest degree of tic expression when in a certain physical location outside of the home, such as a family automobile or a nearby park. IB-CBT allows youth and their caregivers to receive therapeutic guidance and support in real-time in these physical locations, which is often not feasible when CBT is conducted in a traditional clinical setting. Imagine a scenario where Tak may have been encouraged by his in-person therapist to practice refraining from checking the locks when closing doors in the clinic/hospital. Although it is possible that this approach could be somewhat helpful for Tak, as he may have had concerns about being responsible for a break-in at the clinical setting, it stands to reason that this same practice would be more effective when done in Tak's home environment where his concerns about a break-in were the highest.

Finally, the rationale for the use of IB-CBT to treat OCRDs in youth is further strengthened by the seemingly ubiquitous presence of technology/internet-based platforms in the daily lives of youth. Given the familiarity that many children and adolescents have with internet-based tools, it can be assumed that this will contribute to increased levels of acceptance and cooperation by youth patients (Sweeney et al., 2019). This may be especially true when IB-CBT is supported by adjunctive technological "add-ons," such as electronically accessible education materials and internet-based communities of individuals who experience similar OCRDs (e.g., Feusner et al., 2022). Indeed, as outlined in the next section of this chapter, IB-CBT appears to be very well-accepted and consistently associated with favorable treatment outcomes for youth with OCRDs.

Empirical Support for Internet-Based Cognitive Behavioral Therapy

There is a large body of literature supporting the effectiveness of IB-CBT in the treatment of OCRDs in adults. According to meta-analyses, the benefits associated with IB-CBT are comparable to those observed in traditional face-to-face CBT in adult samples (e.g., Salazar de Pablo et al., 2023). Importantly, although there has been less study of IB-CBT in youth, one recent meta-analysis that included studies with patients of all ages found no appreciable differences in the effects of IB-CBT between adults and youth (Salazar de Pablo et al., 2023). Whereas there has been less research on the effects of IB-CBT for OCRDs in youth as compared to adult samples, the body of literature supporting the use of IB-CBT in youth has grown impressively over the past 10 to 15 years.

Do Youth With Obsessive-Compulsive Disorder Experience Benefits From Internet-Based Cognitive Behavioral Therapy?

Two recent systematic reviews of studies assessing the impact of IB-CBT for OCD in youth provide evidence for the significant benefits associated with this treatment approach (Babiano-Espinosa et al., 2019; Sampson et al., 2021). Although the number of studies supporting IB-CBT for OCRDs in youth is relatively small, the available data are promising.

Collectively, the extant studies indicate that young patients on average experience significant decreases in the severity of their OCD symptoms and associated functional impairment from pre- to post-IB-CBT (Aspvall et al., 2020; Comer et al., 2017; Hollmann et al., 2022; Lenhard et al., 2017; Storch et al., 2011), which has been primarily assessed via the Children's Yale-Brown Obsessive Compulsive Scale (Scahill et al., 1997). In the studies employing traditional randomized controlled trial methodology, IB-CBT performed superior to waitlist control conditions (Hollmann et al., 2022; Lenhard et al., 2017; Storch et al., 2011) and preliminary results were not significantly different statistically from in-person CBT (Comer et al., 2017). When available, the remission rates calculated for these studies showed that a majority of young patients experienced remission of their symptoms by the end of treatment: 60 percent (Farrell et al., 2016), 64 percent (Hollmann et al., 2022), and 56 percent (Storch et al., 2011); though definitions of remission varied across these studies. Parents were actively involved in the treatment process in all studies.

The clinical benefits of IB-CBT for treating OCD in youth do not appear to be limited to a single delivery methodology. The existing studies have used a range of approaches for implementing IB-CBT, spanning from a "pure" videoconferencing approach (e.g., Hollmann et al., 2022) to hybrid methods that integrate in-person sessions with videoconferencing sessions to varying extents (Farrell et al., 2016) as well as adjunctive psychoeducational components. Additionally, there is further methodological variance in IB-CBT based on the extent of therapist involvement, which ranges from teletherapy with a therapist guiding all of the sessions (Comer et al., 2017) to an asynchronous, self-guided IB-CBT curriculum with occasional involvement and oversight from a therapist (Lenhard et al., 2017). Although research on IB-CBT for anxiety disorders in youth has found that greater consistency of therapist contact is associated with greater likelihood of experiencing symptom reduction/remission (March et al., 2021), this has not yet been thoroughly assessed in OCD in youth.

Are Internet-Based Cognitive Behavioral Therapy Gains Well-Maintained?

Similar to traditional CBT for youth delivered in clinical settings, IB-CBT appears to produce durable benefits for youth with OCD. Of the available studies that have collected, follow-up data at one or more time points in the post-treatment period all show that patients' gains were maintained at the follow-up time points. In fact, several studies revealed that youth patients on average experienced further reductions in their OCD symptom severity in the time between the end of treatment and the follow-up time points of three months (Babiano-Espinosa et al., 2021) and six months (Aspvall et al., 2020; Babiano-Espinosa et al., 2021; Farrell et al., 2016). With regard to remission rates, it was observed that at the various follow-up time points assessed in the studies, criteria for remission were met in approximately one-half to three-fourths of patients, which provides further evidence for the durability of IB-CBT for OCD in youth.

How is Internet-Based Cognitive Behavioral Therapy Accepted by Youth and Caregivers?

Many of the studies establishing the efficacy of IB-CBT for OCD in youth have also examined treatment acceptability via collection of satisfaction ratings given by youth patients (Lenhard et al., 2017), their caregivers (Comer et al., 2017; Storch et al., 2011), or both (Hollmann et al., 2021; Hollman et al., 2022). Across these studies, IB-CBT is consistently associated with high acceptability by both youth patients and their caregivers. Of particular note, ratings of therapist alliance were high and comparable to traditional in-person CBT (Comer et al., 2017).

Additionally, when examining favorability ratings of IB-CBT as compared to traditional in-person CBT, a majority of respondents did not indicate a superiority of one over the other (Hollman et al., 2021; Lenhard et al., 2017). Finally, the low treatment dropout rates that were consistently observed across these studies lend support to the acceptability of IB-CBT in youth. The systematic review by Babiano-Espinosa and colleagues (2019) found a dropout rate of just 4.2 percent when amalgamating dropouts from all of the studies reviewed, and several of these studies did not have a single patient dropout. It is unclear what dropout rates are in real-world samples, as this has not been reported in the literature. Johnco and colleagues (2020) conducted a meta-analysis of dropout rates for in-person CBT in youth with OCD and found an estimated dropout rate of 10%.

What About Other Obsessive-Compulsive-Disorder-Related Disorders?

Although most empirical studies of IB-CBT in youth have focused on OCD specifically, there has been some research assessing the effects of IB-CBT when applied to other OCRDs in children and adolescents. Two large studies have provided empirical support for the use of IB-CBT in the treatment of chronic tics and Tourette's disorder in youth. In one study, IB-CBT yielded significant reductions in tic severity and was found to be superior to an educational control that was also delivered via the internet (Hollis et al., 2021). A similar study conducted with over 200 Swedish children reported comparable outcomes; youth who received IB-CBT experienced greater reductions in tic frequency and intensity as compared to youth who received internet-based education only in the control condition (Andrén et al., 2022). In the area of BDD, although there have not been any empirical studies using IB-CBT with youth to date, Hartmann and colleagues (2021) have developed an IB-CBT protocol based on cognitive behavioral therapy (CBT) for BDD in youth. This research holds promise to make treatment more available to youth with BDD, as similar research has shown that IB-CBT is both effective and feasible for adults with BDD (Enander et al., 2016). Unfortunately, we were unable to locate any empirical studies of IB-CBT for body-focused repetitive behaviors using youth samples. This is an important gap that future research should address.

Adaptations for Internet-Based Delivery of Cognitive Behavior Therapy

The empirical research reviewed in the prior section is encouraging in its attestation of the effectiveness of IB-CBT for youth. In these studies and in regular practice, small but meaningful adaptations to the delivery of IB-CBT can optimize the quality of the experience for youth and their families. In this section, we review important considerations for adapting IB-CBT for OCRDs for youth.

Preparing for Sessions

For the teletherapy experience to be of optimal benefit, often the patient must prepare themselves and their environment to ensure the environment is set up for success. IB-CBT providers should assist young patients (and when necessary, their caregivers) in identifying a quiet, private space in which they can participate in sessions. The patient must have access to a safe and reliable internet connection and will need to download video conferencing software and any additional applications that are to be used. To preserve session time, a caregiver can help the young patient ensure they can access treatment platforms prior to their first session.

Providers should also prepare themselves for delivering teletherapy services. One should familiarize themself with relevant guidelines delineating teletherapy best practices, such as the APA's *Guidelines for the Practice of Telepsychology* (APA, 2024). Additional preparation may include updating one's internet security measures or additional training for technological literacy.

Many providers and patients express concern that virtual treatment will lack desirable interpersonal therapy elements present in in-person sessions, especially with children under the age of 13 (Wiese et al., 2022). Relatively simple preparations could help providers feel more confident in their ability to build rapport with and engage young children. Providers should ensure that their camera angle allows for their face to be clear and visible, and they should make an effort to face the camera for the majority of the session. The providers should also inform the young patient and any caregivers present if they are going to be taking notes during the session, so the provider's attention does not seem otherwise divided. The provider may also want to allocate more time towards building rapport with the child than they would in an in-person setting, as establishing a strong therapeutic working alliance may be hindered by the absence of physical presence in the same space. As one example, orienting the child to the provider's office space and having the child do the same may also increase feelings of connectedness and familiarity for the child. In our experience, young patients seem to appreciate the opportunity to "tour" us through their home and show us their living space and bedroom.

In-Session Exercises

As discussed previously in this chapter, in-office CBT sessions may be limited to imaginal exposures or to in-vivo exposure stimuli that the patient is willing and able to bring with them to session. Virtual delivery overcomes this barrier as the provider can meet with the patient in their daily environment. As depicted in our earlier case example, Tak's therapist was able to provide live support and coaching as he completed exposures in his home environment where the fear of a home invasion was the greatest. Telehealth providers should capitalize upon this opportunity by allocating as much session time as possible to active engagement in exposure exercises as indicated in the treatment plan.

In addition to the ability to complete exposures with various stimuli in the home environment, the provider can also observe safety behaviors the young patient does in the home and intervene. The telehealth platform may even afford the provider the opportunity to schedule sessions at perhaps less-conventional times so that session time can occur when a young patient would ordinarily be completing various routines that may be affected by OCD (e.g., brushing teeth, completing schoolwork, etc.). Lastly, IB-CBT providers can also take advantage of their ability to "travel" with the young patient to places outside of the home that may be relevant for treatment (e.g., accompanying the child on a video call outside of their school). Time can be spent in session planning whether the patient should attend the subsequent session in a different location.

Web-Based Enhancements

Providers can further adapt their practice with the use of internet-based technology. Children have increasing access to mobile devices (Radesky et al., 2020), and for those who do not, the parent's device can be used with supervision. Use of appropriate applications for treatment can provide educational materials, guided exercises, and other materials that would traditionally be given as handouts in in-person therapy sessions. Internet-based technology can further be used with ERP to develop treatment materials that allow for real-time collaboration both in and outside of session and for recording of homework.

Features of the chosen web-based platform can also enhance treatment. Many platforms include shared whiteboards and screen sharing capabilities which allow all parties to view and interact with the same information/material. These features allow for shared brainstorming of, for instance, new ERP exercises, or for shared viewing of a triggering picture or article for exposure. Further, there are multiple applications available that allow the user to complete common IB-CBT tasks virtually, such as creating an exposure hierarchy, tracking completed exposure tasks, or self-monitoring urges for tics and/or BFRBs. Finally, web-based tools can also be used to increase a young patient's treatment engagement. Applications are available that allow for reward tracking, and the internet can itself be used as a reward. Providers can reward a child for engaging in a difficult exposure task with a brief web-based game or similar activity.

Safety

Active suicidality in youth is generally not considered a contraindication for telehealth treatment (Myers et al., 2017). Though providers may have reservations, evidence suggests that active suicidality in youth can be safely assessed and intervened upon via telehealth even in emergent situations (e.g., Hetrick et al., 2017). Providers should take all safety precautions they normally would take for in-person sessions (e.g., assessing suicide risk, developing safety plan as needed, etc.) with additional considerations.

Before engaging in telehealth treatment sessions, providers should plan how they intend to assess for and respond to safety concerns (Holland et al., 2021). Providers should always have a current address for the young patient's location and verify that this information is correct at the outset of each session, as this information allows the provider to know where to send emergency services if they are needed. Additionally, providers should regularly conduct safety assessments using standardized measures and ideally will conduct these assessments with a clear view of the young patient to allow for assessment of body language and other cues. Safety plans should include crisis resources in the young patient's local geographic area.

Other complications may arise as a function of not meeting with youth patients in a traditional in-person clinic setting. In the same way that caregivers may spend some in-person session time in a waiting room, it is important that parents be home with the youth patient during virtual session time even if not present in the room. Caregivers may be tempted to allow older adolescents to do their sessions at home alone, but this puts the provider in a difficult position should the adolescent leave in the middle of the session or disclose safety concerns.

Additional Considerations

The above recommendations for how CBT can be effectively adapted for youth with OCRDs using an internet-based delivery format are not exhaustive. Providers should review published guidelines carefully, especially for considerations regarding informed consent, confidentiality, security, and legal considerations (Joint Task Force for the Development of Telepsychology Guidelines for Psychologists, 2013; Lin et al., 2021). Whenever possible, we would encourage providers who plan to use IB-CBT to seek consultation from a clinician with at least some experience using IB-CBT with youth patients.

Advantages

There are many advantages of using IB-CBT to treat OCRDs in youth. First, teletherapy has brought an unprecedented level of accessibility (Wade et al., 2020). Presently, a phone or computer and an internet connection can get you access to specialists in various diagnoses and treatments in many parts of the world. Until recently, most specialists were centered around major cities and universities, therefore requiring people to travel to see them in person, sometimes at considerable time and expense. With teletherapy, those experts are accessible to anyone able to connect to them virtually. Further, teletherapy can give access to those who otherwise would not be able to attend in-person therapy sessions even if the office is located relatively nearby. To illustrate, a patient who was not able to leave the premises of their school for long enough to go to a session may be able to have a virtual session during a scheduled break. In addition, extended family or other caregivers, such as nannies or grandparents, can also join sessions relatively easily to be trained in the elimination of compulsions and other safety behaviors (e.g., avoidance) that maintain OCRDs. Or, for families who lack access to reliable transportation, teletherapy offers them a chance to have access to a service that those with reliable transportation may take for granted. Even parents or other caregiving figures who are not able to be physically present in the same physical space as the young patient may nonetheless be able to join virtual sessions if given the appropriate information and directions to do so.

Hoarding

In the case of hoarding, which often requires home visits for successful interventions (Frost & Hristova, 2011), in-person therapists would have to travel to the home to meet and assess the hoarding, which often occurs at the expense of the family (both session cost and therapist travel time). Virtual sessions for hoarding also have the advantage of allowing the therapist and child to practice sorting and discarding tasks together in the home environment where the clutter resides versus the family needing to bring many items with them into the therapy office.

Stigma

For families who are concerned about the stigma of mental health treatment, teletherapy offers a private forum to meet with a therapist. There are no drives to offices, no sitting in waiting rooms, and no potential for awkward chance meetings of people between sessions. Further, there are some states that allow children and adolescents to independently consent to their mental health treatment (Kerwin et al., 2015), and teletherapy can put access to those sessions into the hands of individuals, instead of them having to figure out transportation to an office to meet with a therapist. For some youth that are not yet ready to inform their parents of the work they are doing, this option gives them access to the care that they need when they reach the legal age of consent in their state.

Commute

Teletherapy happening in the home is convenient for the patient and therapist. The patient need not take extra time out of their day for travel as transportation issues are one of the top reported reasons for nonattendance (Long et al., 2016). Their parents or guardians need not pack up the patient and the entire family and drive them all to a possibly faraway appointment and juggle sitting in the session with supervising the other children are in the waiting room. It is not surprising that research in telepsychiatry shows that people are more likely to attend appointments if they are virtual versus in-person (Molfenter, 2013). Similar studies for teletherapy are lacking presently but are important to research for the future.

Disadvantages

"Screen Fatigue"

Today's youth are often quite adept at using technology and have a level of comfort with it that can exceed that of adults in their lives. However, children and adolescents might be tired of using their devices for educational purposes throughout their day and may want to focus more on fun activities. Increased exposure to devices such as computers and smartphones has been known to increase stress and burnout levels (Mheidly et al., 2020). If children are online for school all day and then for their tutoring and then a therapy session, they could become quite "screen fatigued" from these experiences. On the clinician side, burnout is a similar phenomenon that exists within psychotherapists who work online or face-to-face (McCormack et al., 2018). However, most articles cite emotional exhaustion as the cause of burnout, as there is less information on online therapist/therapy burnout. Related to the notion of "screen fatigue," it may be that virtual therapy sessions provide less opportunities immediately after the session for the young person and their family to review what was learned and other key takeaways from the session. To illustrate, the young person's parent may immediately join a virtual work meeting when the therapy session is complete. With this in mind, clinicians may consider guiding the young person and their parents/caregivers to review and consolidate their key learnings near the end of the therapy session.

Affordability/Accessibility

There are many people who do not have access to a computer, a smartphone, or even to an internet connection (Vogels, 2021). Without technological capabilities, teletherapy is not impossible, but it could be difficult to take advantage of all that it has to offer. It may require doing therapy in a place with privacy concerns (e.g., reserving a room at a public library) or with devices that may risk one's confidentiality (e.g., needing to borrow an electronic device from family or friends).

Online therapy may be more cost effective than in-person therapy for the client (Hollmann et al., 2021; Ruwaard et al., 2012). It is also cheaper for the provider due to substantially less cost in overheads (office space rent and utilities) and potentially a smaller time commitment (Hollmann et al., 2021), but it could still be unaffordable for some. Additionally, not all providers, in person or online, take all or any insurances, therefore pricing themselves out of being able to assist numerous individuals in need of care (Ruwaard et al., 2012).

Privacy

There are several concerns around privacy that must be considered (Lin et al., 2021). First, it is imperative to know the laws of the state(s) that you are providing care in. Each state has different laws around ages of assent and consent, and therefore a provider with multiple licenses will have to be familiar with an increasing number of laws and regulations that guide their practice. Second, it cannot be assumed that a child will be forthcoming when a parent or guardian is in the session with them. It may be crucial to convince family members that there is a time to meet together and also a time to meet individually with the child/adolescent to get a more forthcoming account of their symptoms, homework completion, self-monitoring, etc. Third, it is not possible to know what is happening off camera. Is there a device that may be recording the session, or is there someone in the room or even within earshot of the room that will know what is happening, leading the patient to potentially withhold information due to their concerns about being observed? Finally, it is never a certainty there is not someone else that is able to access the system and either watch or listen if there are not appropriate encryptions in place.

Observations

When a session is being conducted online, the therapist is not likely able to observe the whole person (Lin et al., 2021). Thus, is it possible the young patient may be engaging in a compulsion below the camera view (e.g., picking at their skin, or pulling their leg hair)? In teletherapy sessions, it may be difficult for the clinician to assess these concerns and be sure that the young patient is fully engaged in the session and is not doing any covert safety behaviors or rituals. If a patient is found to be continuously engaging in these behaviors, it may be possible to have the camera further back or at a wider angle so a fuller view of the young patient will be available for the therapist to assess what is happening in the session. Additionally, virtual sessions do not always allow for a clinician to make observations based on important sensory input that is better detected in face-to-face settings. For example, a clinician who suspects a young patient may not be engaging in appropriate hygienic routines may be able to smell this and/or have better ability to see it if the young person is in the office vs. merely being seen on a screen.

Distractions

From our personal experiences, we have noted that teletherapy sessions can naturally have more distractions (Lin et al., 2021). Many things can happen such as doorbell rings, the therapist and/or patient receives texts or phone calls in the middle of the session, or a pet interferes with the session in some way (e.g., dog barking loudly, cat walking on laptop computer keys, etc.). It could also be tempting for the patient to do the session from bed or on the floor or in low lighting. We have had to ask our patients to be in a well-lit room with the phone or laptop on a surface and not in their hands (causing a few of us a feeling of vertigo throughout the session). It is also easier for people to leave the session if they are at home vs. in an office, where certain psychological principles of demand might lead someone to stay in a session instead of escaping as a safety precaution. With appropriate precautionary measures, many of these distractions can be foreseen and minimized, but they are bound to occur at least occasionally.

Technical Difficulties

Working online is never without its complications. While children are usually skilled with applications and other online capabilities, they are not immune to technical issues. For younger children, parents may also find themselves struggling with the technology. This could lead to the therapist spending additional time troubleshooting or helping them set up the therapy for future use (Hollmann et al., 2021). To mitigate this concern, it would be worth assessing families for their technical comfort and even supplying instructions, videos, or personalized aid to help clients prior to and/or during the sessions. Even with these concerns, slow connection, lost service, and other video/audio concerns can come up that hinder the session (Lin et al., 2021).

Dissemination and Access

As noted earlier in this chapter, perhaps the most obvious advantage to using IB-CBT to treat OCRDs in youth is that evidence-based treatment is more accessible to people who otherwise may have gone without care or would have received inadequate or inappropriate care. Few people with OCD receive appropriate treatment, with about 60 percent of potential patients not receiving any care (Kohn et al., 2004), and only a small fraction of adults receiving ERP (Blanco et al., 2006). While ERP access has not been investigated as thoroughly in youth, clinical experience suggests this is also the case for children (Storch et al., 2011).

Several factors are at play in limiting the number of patients who receive ERP and other appropriate treatment for OCRDs. Some of the most prominent of these factors include availability of trained therapists, cost of treatment, the time commitment required by patients and families, and geographical limitations (e.g., O'Neill & Feusner, 2015; Pinciotti et al., 2022; Sequeira et al., 2021). Fortunately, IB-CBT can address several of these limitations. Providers are often able to maintain more flexible schedules and may be able to see more young patients due to time savings from, as one example, not having a commute to an office (Long et al., 2016). IB-CBT may also allow for virtual training of new providers, which could increase availability of skilled CBT providers. Convenience for the young patient and their family could also lead to treatment being perceived as more accessible and feasible.

However, there are unique access considerations for IB-CBT. These include access to digital platforms and devices, technological literacy concerns, and public policy barriers (Siegal et al., 2021). Unfortunately, these limitations seem to differentially affect underserved populations at a greater frequency (e.g., Falicov et al., 2020). Although many people can easily access the internet from a personal phone, computer, or other electronic device, people from disadvantaged socioeconomic backgrounds may not have access to a private space in which to attend sessions (Barney et al., 2020).

Technological literacy divides can also present barriers even if accessing the internet is not a concern. Older adults are considerably less skilled with technology than their younger counterparts, and this inequality is more pronounced for low-socioeconomic-status (SES) older adults (Hargittai et al., 2019). This can present a barrier for treatment of children when primary caregivers are grandparents or other older adults. Treatment delivered via telephone without a video component has been proposed as a solution to barriers to internet access and literacy, however, this can present cost concerns as insurances often do not reimburse for these services (Westby et al., 2021). Widespread adoption of telehealth delivery of treatment for OCRDs certainly is a step in the right direction to increase accessibility of care, but ultimately more needs to be done to increase access for underserved populations.

Summary

IB-CBT presents a viable alternative option to traditional in-person treatment for young individuals and their families in need of help for OCRDs. Given the promising effectiveness data associated with IB-CBT for OCRDs in youth and the many advantages of overcoming common barriers to accessing treatment, future work should seek to make IB-CBT available and affordable. Additionally, in following the suggestions for safe and effective delivery of IB-CBT outlined in this chapter, clinicians may consider transitioning or modifying some of their clinical practice in order to provide IB-CBT and make this treatment available to a wider audience. Though there are unique challenges inherent in doing CBT via teletherapy with young people, we contend that with appropriate preparation, the risks of these challenges are greatly outweighed by the gains associated with IB-CBT.

References

American Psychological Association. (2024, Jun). *Guidelines for the practice of telepsychology.* https://www.apa.org/practice/guidelines/telepsychology.

Andersson, G. (2009). Using the internet to provide cognitive behaviour therapy. *Behaviour Research and Therapy, 47*(3), 175–180. https://doi.org/10.1016/j.brat.2009.01.010.

Andrén, P., Holmsved, M., Ringberg, H., Wachtmeister, V., Isomura, K., Aspvall, K., Lenhard, F., Hall, C. L., Davies, E.B., Murphy, T., Hollis, C., Sampaio, F., Feldman, I., Bottai, M., Serlachius, E., Andersson, E., Fernández de la Cruz, L., & Mataix-Cols, D. (2022). Therapist-supported internet-delivered exposure and response prevention for children and adolescents with tourette syndrome: A randomized clinical trial. *JAMA Network Open, 5*(8), e2225614. https://doi.org/10.1001/jamanetworkopen.2022.25614.

Aspvall, K., Lenhard, F., Melin, K., Krebs, G., Norlin, L., Näsström, K., Jassi, A., Turner, C., Knoetze, E., Serlachius, E., Andersson, E., & Mataix-Cols, D. (2020). Implementation of internet-delivered cognitive behaviour therapy for pediatric obsessive-compulsive disorder: Lessons from clinics in Sweden, United Kingdom and Australia. *Internet Interventions, 20,* 100308. https://doi.org/10.1016/j.invent.2020.100308.

Babiano-Espinosa, L., Wolters, L.H., Weidle, B., Compton, S.N., Lydersen, S., & Skokauskas, N. (2021). Acceptability and feasibility of enhanced cognitive behavioral therapy (eCBT) for children and adolescents with obsessive–compulsive disorder. *Child and Adolescent Psychiatry and Mental Health, 15*(1), 47. https://doi.org/10.1186/s13034-021-00400-7.

Babiano-Espinosa, L., Wolters, L.H., Weidle, B., Op De Beek, V., Pedersen, S.A., Compton, S., & Skokauskas, N. (2019). Acceptability, feasibility, and efficacy of Internet cognitive behavioral therapy (iCBT) for pediatric obsessive-compulsive disorder: A systematic review. *Systematic Reviews, 8*(1), 284. https://doi.org/10.1186/s13643-019-1166-6.

Barney, A., Buckelew, S., Mesheriakova, V., & Raymond-Flesch, M. (2020). The COVID-19 pandemic and rapid implementation of adolescent and young adult telemedicine: Challenges and opportunities for innovation. *The Journal of Adolescent Health: Official Publication of the Society for Adolescent Medicine, 67*(2), 164–171. https://doi.org/10.1016/j.jadohealth.2020.05.006.

Blanco, C., Olfson, M., Stein, D.J., Simpson, H.B., Gameroff, M.J., & Narrow, W.H. (2006). Treatment of obsessive-compulsive disorder by U.S. psychiatrists. *The Journal of Clinical Psychiatry, 67*(6), 946–951. https://doi.org/10.4088/jcp.v67n0611.

Comer, J.S., Furr, J.M., Kerns, C.E., Miguel, E., Coxe, S., Elkins, R.M., Carpenter, A.L., Cornacchio, D., Cooper-Vince, C.E., DeSerisy, M., Chou, T., Sanchez, A.L., Khanna, M., Franklin, M.E., Garcia, A.M., & Freeman, J.B. (2017). Internet-delivered, family-based treatment for early-onset OCD: A pilot randomized trial. *Journal of Consulting and Clinical Psychology, 85,* 178–186. https://doi.org/10.1037/ccp0000155.

Enander, J., Andersson, E., Mataix-Cols, D., Lichtenstein, L., Alström, K., Andersson, G., Ljótsson, B., & Rück, C. (2016). Therapist guided internet based cognitive behavioural therapy for body dysmorphic disorder: Single blind randomised controlled trial. *BMJ, 352,* i241. https://doi.org/10.1136/bmj.i241.

Falicov, C., Niño, A., & D'Urso, S. (2020). Expanding possibilities: Flexibility and solidarity with under-resourced immigrant families during the COVID-19 pandemic. *Family Process, 59*(3), 865–882. https://doi.org/10.1111/famp.12578.

Farrell, L.J., Oar, E.L., Waters, A.M., McConnell, H., Tiralongo, E., Garbharran, V., & Ollendick, T. (2016). Brief intensive CBT for pediatric OCD with E-therapy maintenance. *Journal of Anxiety Disorders, 42,* 85–94. https://doi.org/10.1016/j.janxdis.2016.06.005.

Feusner, J.D., Farrell, N.R., Kreyling, J., McGrath, P.B., Rhode, A., Faneuff, T., Lonsway, S., Mohideen, R., Jurich, J.E., Trusky, L., & Smith, S.M. (2022). Online video teletherapy treatment of obsessive-compulsive disorder using exposure and response prevention: Clinical outcomes from a retrospective longitudinal observational study. *Journal of Medical Internet Research, 24*(5), e36431. https://doi.org/10.2196/36431.

Frost, R.O., & Hristova, V. (2011). Assessment of hoarding. *Journal of Clinical Psychology, 67*(5), 456–466. https://doi.org/10.1002/jclp.20790.

Hargittai, E., Piper, A.M., & Morris, M.R. (2019). From internet access to internet skills: Digital inequality among older adults. *Universal Access in the Information Society, 18*(4), 881–890. https://doi.org/10.1007/s10209-018-0617-5.

Hartmann, A.S., Schmidt, M., Staufenbiel, T., Ebert, D.D., Martin, A., & Schoenenberg, K. (2021). ImaginYouth–A therapist-guided internet-based cognitive-behavioral program for adolescents and young adults with body dysmorphic disorder: Study protocol for a two-arm randomized controlled trial. *Frontiers in psychiatry, 12,* 682965. *https://doi.org/10.3389/fpsyt.2021.682965.*

Hetrick, S.E., Yuen, H.P., Bailey, E., Cox, G.R., Templer, K., Rice, S.M., Bendall, S., & Robinson, J. (2017). Internet-based cognitive behavioural therapy for young people with suicide-related behaviour (Reframe-IT): A randomised controlled trial. *Evidence-Based Mental Health, 20*(3), 76–82. https://doi.org/10.1136/eb-2017-102719.

Holland, M., Hawks, J., Morelli, L.C., & Khan, Z. (2021). Risk assessment and crisis intervention for youth in a time of telehealth. *Contemporary School Psychology, 25*(1), 12–26. https://doi.org/10.1007/s40688-020-00341-6.

Hollis, C., Hall, C.L., Jones, R., Marston, L., Novere, M.L., Hunter, R., Brown, B.J., Sanderson, C., Andrén, P., Bennett, S.D., Chamberlain, L.R., Davies, E.B., Evans, A., Kouzoupi, N., McKenzie, C., Heyman, I., Khan, K., Kilgariff, J., Glazebrook, C., . . . Murray, E. (2021). Therapist-supported online remote behavioural intervention for tics in children and adolescents in England (ORBIT): A multicentre, parallel group, single-blind, randomised controlled trial. *The Lancet Psychiatry, 8*(10), 871–882. https://doi.org/10.1016/S2215-0366(21)00235-2.

Hollmann, K., Allgaier, K., Hohnecker, C.S., Lautenbacher, H., Bizu, V., Nickola, M., Wewetzer, G., Wewetzer, C., Ivarsson, T., Skokauskas, N., Wolters, L.H., Skarphedinsson, G., Weidle, B., de Haan, E., Torp, N.C., Compton, S.N., Calvo, R., Lera-Miguel, S., Haigis, A., . . . Conzelmann, A. (2021). Internet-based cognitive behavioral therapy in children and adolescents with obsessive compulsive disorder: A feasibility study. *Journal of Neural Transmission, 128*(9), 1445–1459. https://doi.org/10.1007/s00702-021-02409-w.

Hollmann, K., Hohnecker, C.S., Haigis, A., Alt, A.K., Kühnhausen, J., Pascher, A., Wörz, U., App, R., Lautenbacher, H., Renner, T.J., & Conzelmann, A. (2022). Internet-based cognitive behavioral therapy in children and adolescents with obsessive-compulsive disorder: A randomized controlled trial. *Frontiers in Psychiatry, 13.* https://www.frontiersin.org/articles/10.3389/fpsyt.2022.989550.

Johnco, C., McGuire, J.F., Roper, T., & Storch, E.A. (2020). A meta-analysis of dropout rates from exposure with response prevention and pharmacological treatment for youth with obsessive compulsive disorder. *Depression and Anxiety, 37,* 407–417.

Joint Task Force for the Development of Telepsychology Guidelines for Psychologists. (2013). Guidelines for the practice of telepsychology. *The American Psychologist, 68*(9), 791–800. https://doi.org/10.1037/a0035001.

Kerwin, M.E., Kirby, K.C., Speziali, D., Duggan, M., Mellitz, C., Versek, B., & McNamara, A. (2015). What can parents do? A review of state laws regarding decision making for adolescent drug abuse and mental health treatment. *Journal of Child & Adolescent Substance Abuse, 24*(3), 166–176. https://doi.org/10.108 0/1067828X.2013.777380.

Kohn, R., Saxena, S., Levav, I., & Saraceno, B. (2004). The treatment gap in mental health care. *Bulletin of the World Health Organization, 82*(11), 858–866.

Lenhard, F., Andersson, E., Mataix-Cols, D., Rück, C., Vigerland, S., Högström, J., Hillborg, M., Brander, G., Ljungström, M., Ljótsson, B., & Serlachius, E. (2017). Therapist-guided, internet-delivered cognitive-behavioral therapy for adolescents with obsessive-compulsive disorder: A randomized controlled trial. *Journal of the American Academy of Child and Adolescent Psychiatry, 56*(1), 10–19.e2. https://doi.org/10.1016/j.jaac.2016.09.515.

Lin, T., Stone, S.J., Heckman, T.G., & Anderson, T. (2021). Zoom-in to zone-out: Therapists report less therapeutic skill in telepsychology versus face-to-face therapy during the COVID-19 pandemic. *Psychotherapy*, *58*(4), 449. https://doi.org/10.1037/pst0000398.

Long, J., Sakauye, K., Chisty, K., & Upton, J. (2016). The empty chair appointment. *SAGE Open*, *6*(1), 2158244015625094. https://doi.org/10.1177/2158244015625094.

March, S., Batterham, P.J., Rowe, A., Donovan, C., Calear, A.L., & Spence, S.H. (2021). Trajectories of change in an open-access internet-based cognitive behavior program for childhood and adolescent anxiety: Open trial. *JMIR Mental Health*, *8*(6), e27981. https://doi.org/10.2196/27981.

McCormack, H.M., MacIntyre, T.E., O'Shea, D., Herring, M.P., & Campbell, M.J. (2018). The prevalence and cause(s) of burnout among applied psychologists: A systematic review. *Frontiers in Psychology*, *9*, 1897. https://doi.org/10.3389/fpsyg.2018.01897.

Mheidly, N., Fares, M.Y., & Fares, J. (2020). Coping with stress and burnout associated with telecommunication and online learning. *Frontiers in Public Health*, *8*. https://www.frontiersin.org/articles/10.3389/fpubh.2020.574969.

Molfenter, T. (2013). Reducing appointment no-shows: Going from theory to practice. *Substance Use & Misuse*, *48*(9), 743–749. https://doi.org/10.3109/10826084.2013.787098.

Myers, K., Nelson, E.-L., Rabinowitz, T., Hilty, D., Baker, D., Barnwell, S.S., Boyce, G., Bufka, L.F., Cain, S., Chui, L., Comer, J.S., Cradock, C., Goldstein, F., Johnston, B., Krupinski, E., Lo, K., Luxton, D.D., McSwain, S.D., McWilliams, J., . . . Bernard, J. (2017). American telemedicine association practice guidelines for telemental health with children and adolescents. *Telemedicine Journal and E-Health: The Official Journal of the American Telemedicine Association*, *23*(10), 779–804. https://doi.org/10.1089/tmj.2017.0177.

O'Neill, J., & Feusner, J.D. (2015). Cognitive-behavioral therapy for obsessive–compulsive disorder: Access to treatment, prediction of long-term outcome with neuroimaging. *Psychology Research and Behavior Management*, *8*, 211–223. https://doi.org/10.2147/PRBM.S75106.

Pinciotti, C.M., Bulkes, N.Z., Horvath, G., & Riemann, B.C. (2022). Efficacy of intensive CBT telehealth for obsessive-compulsive disorder during the COVID-19 pandemic. *Journal of Obsessive-Compulsive and Related Disorders*, *32*, 100705. https://doi.org/10.1016/j.jocrd.2021.100705.

Radesky, J.S., Weeks, H.M., Ball, R., Schaller, A., Yeo, S., Durnez, J., Tamayo-Rios, M., Epstein, M., Kirkorian, H., Coyne, S., & Barr, R. (2020). Young children's use of smartphones and tablets. *Pediatrics*, *146*(1), e20193518. https://doi.org/10.1542/peds.2019-3518.

Ruwaard, J., Lange, A., Schrieken, B., Dolan, C.V., & Emmelkamp, P. (2012). The effectiveness of online cognitive behavioral treatment in routine clinical practice. *PLOS ONE*, *7*(7), e40089. https://doi.org/10.1371/journal.pone.0040089.

Salazar de Pablo, G., Pascual-Sánchez, A., Panchal, U., Clark, B., & Krebs, G. (2023). Efficacy of remotely-delivered cognitive behavioural therapy for obsessive-compulsive disorder: An updated meta-analysis of randomised controlled trials. *Journal of Affective Disorders*, *322*, 289–299. https://doi.org/10.1016/j.jad.2022.11.007.

Salloum, A., Johnco, C., Lewin, A.B., McBride, N.M., & Storch, E.A. (2016). Barriers to access and participation in community mental health treatment for anxious children. *Journal of affective disorders*, *196*, 54–61. *https://doi.org/10.1016/j.jad.2016.02.026*.

Sampson, F., Tafuto, B., Jose, N., & Kim, L.P. (2021). Technology-based CBT in reducing symptoms of OCD in children: A systematic review. *Journal of Public Health Issues and Practices*, *5*(1). https://doi.org/10.33790/jphip1100177.

Scahill, L., Riddle, M.A., McSwiggin-Hardin, M., Ort, S.I., King, R.A., Goodman, W.K., Cicchetti, D., & Leckman, J.F. (1997). Children's Yale-Brown Obsessive Compulsive Scale: reliability and validity. *Journal of the American Academy of Child and Adolescent Psychiatry, 36*, 844–852.

Sequeira, A., Alozie, A., Fasteau, M., Lopez, A.K., Sy, J., Turner, K.A., Werner, C., McIngvale, E., & Björgvinsson, T. (2021). Transitioning to virtual programming amidst COVID-19 outbreak. *Counselling Psychology Quarterly, 34*(3–4), 538–553. https://doi.org/10.1080/09515070.2020.1777940.

Siegel, A., Zuo, Y., Moghaddamcharkari, N., McIntyre, R.S., & Rosenblat, J.D. (2021). Barriers, benefits and interventions for improving the delivery of telemental health services during the coronavirus disease 2019 pandemic: A systematic review. *Current Opinion in Psychiatry, 34*(4), 434–443. https://doi.org/10.1097/YCO.0000000000000714.

Storch, E.A., Caporino, N.E., Morgan, J.R., Lewin, A.B., Rojas, A., Brauer, L., Larson, M.J., & Murphy, T. K. (2011). Preliminary investigation of web-camera delivered cognitive-behavioral therapy for youth with obsessive-compulsive disorder. *Psychiatry Research, 189*(3), 407–412. https://doi.org/10.1016/j.psychres.2011.05.047.

Sweeney, G.M., Donovan, C.L., March, S., & Forbes, Y. (2019). Logging into therapy: Adolescent perceptions of online therapies for mental health problems. *Internet Interventions, 15*, 93–99. https://doi.org/10.1016/j.invent.2016.12.001.

Vigerland, S., Lenhard, F., Bonnert, M., Lalouni, M., Hedman, E., Ahlen, J., Olén, O., Serlachius, E., & Ljótsson, B. (2016). Internet-delivered cognitive behavior therapy for children and adolescents: A systematic review and meta-analysis. *Clinical Psychology Review, 50*, 1–10. https://doi.org/10.1016/j.cpr.2016.09.005.

Vogels, E.A. (2021, June 22). Digital divide persists even as Americans with lower incomes make gains in tech adoption. *Pew Research Center*. https://www.pewresearch.org/fact-tank/2021/06/22/digital-divide-persists-even-as-americans-with-lower-incomes-make-gains-in-tech-adoption/.

Wade, S.L., Gies, L.M., Fisher, A.P., Moscato, E.L., Adlam, A.R., Bardoni, A., Corti, C., Limond, J., Modi, A.C., & Williams, T. (2020). Telepsychotherapy with children and families: Lessons gleaned from two decades of translational research. *Journal of Psychotherapy Integration, 30*, 332–347. https://doi.org/10.1037/int0000215.

Westby, A., Nissly, T., Gieseker, R., Timmins, K., & Justesen, K. (2021). Achieving equity in telehealth: "Centering at the margins" in access, provision, and reimbursement. *Journal of the American Board of Family Medicine: JABFM, 34*(Suppl), S29–S32. https://doi.org/10.3122/jabfm.2021.S1.200280.

Wiese, A.D., Drummond, K.N., Fuselier, M.N., Sheu, J.C., Liu, G., Guzick, A.G., Goodman, W.K., & Storch, E.A. (2022). Provider perceptions of telehealth and in-person exposure and response prevention for obsessive-compulsive disorder. *Psychiatry Research, 313*, 114610.

11 Psychopharmacology of Obsessive-Compulsive Disorder in Children and Adolescents

Aarya Krishnan Rajalakshmi,[1,2] *Aditya Kumar Singh Pawar*[1,2] *and Daniel A. Geller*[3,4]

[1] *Kennedy Krieger Institute, Baltimore, MD*

[2] *Johns Hopkins University School of Medicine, Baltimore, MD*

[3] *Massachusetts General Hospital, Boston, MA*

[4] *Harvard Medical School, Boston, MA*

Introduction

Pediatric obsessive-compulsive disorder (OCD) is a common and debilitating mental health condition that affects approximately 1–3 percent of children and adolescents worldwide. While cognitive-behavioral therapy (CBT) has been seen to be consistently effective in the treatment of pediatric OCD, it may not be sufficient for all cases. Medication is a valuable adjunctive treatment option for OCD in children and adolescents. This chapter provides an evidence-based overview of the current state of psychopharmacology for pediatric OCD.

When Should Medication Be Introduced for Obsessive-Compulsive Disorder in Children and Adolescents?

Evidence-based first-line treatments for pediatric OCD include CBT and medication.

CBT is recommended as the initial treatment approach for children and adolescents presenting with mild to moderate OCD. However, certain factors support early introduction of medication including patient factors, therapy factors, and illness factors (Geller, March, & AACP Committee on Quality Issues, 2012).

1. Patient factors: An unwillingness to participate in CBT or an inability to tolerate the distress that is key to exposure and response prevention (ERP) based approaches.

DOI: 10.4324/9781003386278-11

2. Therapy factors: Unavailability of or delays in access to therapists who have the necessary skill and expertise required to deliver ERP or lack of progress despite adequate ERP.
3. Illness factors: Moderate to severe illness as reflected by a score on the Children's Yale-Brown Obsessive-Compulsive Scale (CY-BOCS) over 23, significant impairment or pronounced distress from the illness, poor insight into the pathological nature of symptoms and the need for change, comorbid illnesses – including but not limited to depression, anxiety, or disruptive behavioral disorders – that can impact motivation, and challenging engagement with or diminished response to standard CBT for OCD.

In clinical settings, it is not uncommon to encounter one or more of these circumstances in the treatment-seeking population. This in turn necessitates the early introduction of medication in conjunction with, or at times even ahead of, CBT, with the goal of relieving distress, ameliorating symptoms until CBT can be accessed, or enabling meaningful participation in CBT.

Pharmacological Interventions for Pediatric Obsessive-Compulsive Disorder

Medications that are approved for the treatment of pediatric OCD belong to the broad class of serotonin uptake inhibitors which includes clomipramine (CMI) and selective serotonin reuptake inhibitors (SSRIs).

Clomipramine was the first drug to gain approval for the treatment of OCD in the pediatric age group. Clomipramine belongs to the class of tricyclic antidepressants (TCAs) and is a tertiary amine. In 1989 the United States Food and Drug Administration (FDA) first approved clomipramine for the treatment of OCD in those aged ten years and older. Clomipramine has a specific and distinguishing effect regarding inhibiting serotonin reuptake and it is believed that its role within the serotoninergic system may confer its therapeutic effect for OCD.

As with other TCAs, clomipramine is known to have actions on multiple receptors including the cholinergic, histaminergic, and adrenergic systems. The effect on these neurotransmitters is associated with side effects such as blurred vision, dryness of mouth, nausea, constipation, tachycardia, dizziness, postural hypotension sedation, increased appetite, and weight gain. More troublesome adverse effects include elevated arrhythmogenic potential via prolongation of the QTc interval, the risk of lowering seizure threshold especially at higher doses, and the risk of fatal overdose. This side effect profile led to a decline in the popularity of TCAs, especially for use with children, and careful lab monitoring of patients including monitoring of metabolic parameters, monitoring of plasma drug levels (especially at higher doses), and use of electrocardiograms (EKGs; Biederman, 1991; Flament et al., 1985). While subsequent studies continued to observe similar benefits with the use of clomipramine, the tolerability profile and the need for close lab monitoring limited its use, especially in youth.

The years that followed witnessed the subsequent approval and increasing use of SSRIs which gained popularity as effective medications for OCD, especially in the younger population, owing to their more favorable tolerability profiles and relative safety. Sertraline, fluoxetine and fluvoxamine have FDA approval in the US for the treatment of pediatric OCD in children aged six, seven, and eight and above, respectively, on the basis of data from randomized controlled trials that established their superiority over placebo (March et al., 1998; Geller et al., 2001; Riddle et al., 2001).

All SSRIs seem to show comparable benefit, as there is no data that supports relative superiority of one SSRI over the others (Geller et al., 2003b; Varigonda, Jakubovski, & Bloch, 2016). The choice of medication is guided by factors that include an individual history of response, a family history of response, and pharmacokinetic factors (for instance, the long half-life of fluoxetine could be advantageous in the situation of anticipated inadequate compliance). It is appropriate to have a discussion with parents about the above factors. It would be acceptable to start any of these approved SSRI medications.

Dosing and Duration of Treatment

The recommended approach for the use of medication in children involves starting medication at the lower end of the suggested optimal dose range and titrating upwards every two to three weeks until the maximal tolerated dose is reached while monitoring for symptom improvement. The FDA-recommended dose ranges utilized in pediatric OCD are as follows:

- Fluoxetine: 20–60mg
- Fluvoxamine: 100–300mg
- Sertraline: 100–200mg
- Clomipramine: 25–150mg.

Studies of medication treatment for adult OCD have identified a dose-response relationship with SSRI medication but similar data does not exist for the pediatric age group (Bloch et al., 2010). Most of the existing data on the use of these medications in children and adolescents comes from studies that have used medication at or close to the FDA-recommended maximal doses. Hence it is difficult to assess whether higher doses clearly confer incremental benefit in this population. A meta-analysis that looked at dose-response relationships in adult OCD noted an increased rate of discontinuation due to side effects though not a significant increase in all-cause discontinuation (Bloch et al., 2010). The authors concluded that, in general, the benefits of medication treatment outweighed concerns related to side effects in adults with OCD; however, this dose-response relationship may be important to consider when treating children for whom tolerability and safety is paramount. Further, there are distinct concerns about the tolerability of SSRIs in children, particularly regarding the risks of behavioral activation, mania, and suicidal ideation. It is thus prudent to utilize an approach that involves gradual titration while closely monitoring tolerability as opposed to a brisk up-titration to the highest effective dose point (Geller et al., 2012).

Guidelines suggest that to constitute an optimal trial of effectiveness, medication for OCD needs to be continued for a period of at least ten to twelve weeks at the maximum recommended or maximum tolerated dose. Continuing an effective medication regime for at least six to twelve months following symptom remission is encouraged. In adult OCD treatment studies, it has been observed that adults who were randomly assigned to discontinue SSRI medication were twice as likely to relapse compared to those who remained on medication (Fineberg et al., 2007). There are no such prospective trials of medication discontinuation for pediatric OCD that could serve as an evidence base for treatment duration or discontinuation decisions in this age group, though a study of this nature is underway (Leuchter et al., 2023). Moreover, there are data to suggest that natural remission of OCD may not be infrequent in adolescence (Bloch & Storch, 2015). The general approach in children remains one of ensuring that medication is continued for at least six months to one year of stability and then weighing the pros and cons of drug discontinuation. If a decision is made to withdraw medication, it would be most appropriate to initiate a gradual taper at a time of minimum stress and demands and provide evidence-based psychosocial support so that the impact of a relapse is minimized if it were to occur. Educating parents on the significance of early identification of signs of worsening symptoms and the importance of seeking care without delay cannot be over emphasized. In situations in which CBT was a part of the effective treatment regime for the child, booster sessions may provide useful support when medication taper is initiated and ongoing.

Safety and Tolerability

In situations where medication is recommended for the treatment of OCD in a child or adolescent, a detailed discussion with parents about what is known of the safety and tolerability profiles of these agents is a vital step in the treatment process. Understandably, parents are keen to understand what is to be expected short-term and long-term with these medications. In general, SSRI medications are seen to be relatively safe and well-tolerated across age groups and this is a useful message with which to start the discussion. At the same time, it is also important to discuss the limits of our knowledge when it comes to long-term treatment with SSRIs. Changes in sleep, headache, symptoms of gastrointestinal distress (including nausea, abdominal discomfort, and diarrhea), weight changes, behavioral activation, and sexual dysfunction are all known side effects associated with SSRIS (Mills & Strawn, 2020; Solmi et al., 2020). Particularly significant aspects that deserve discussion prior to starting an SSRI in youth pertains to behavioral activation, the FDA "black box" warning for suicidality, and the risk of switch to mania.

Behavioral activation is a presentation described as a state of heightened activity, restlessness, and disinhibition without the euphoria or grandiosity that defines manic states (Reinblatt et al., 2009). Treatment-induced activation is estimated to occur in between 10–50 percent of individuals across pediatric treatment studies and has been noted to contribute significantly to discontinuation of SSRIs, particularly in younger children (Safer & Zito, 2006). Activation has been observed to negatively impact response to treatment for pediatric OCD and hence deserves attention and intervention (Reid et al., 2015). Our current understanding suggests that the risk of behavioral activation is higher with younger children, rapid dose titration, and higher plasma drug levels, which in turn is possibly linked to individual differences in metabolism of these drugs (Reinblatt et al., 2009; Riddle et al., 1991; Safer & Zito, 2006; Walkup et al., 2008). Dose reduction serves as a useful strategy to manage activation-related adverse effects (Riddle et al., 1991). These observations further highlight the importance of a conservative approach while using medication in treating children; an approach that involves starting low and a measured rate of up titration so as to promote tolerability, limit the probability of adverse effects and lessen the chances of treatment discontinuation.

Children who receive antidepressant treatment are at a relatively higher risk for a switch to mania compared to adolescents and adults. Administering an antidepressant agent to as few as 10 children in the 10 to 14 age group may potentially lead to at least one occurrence of manic conversion (Martin et al., 2004). Other risk markers, such as a family history of bipolar disorder, elevate vulnerability for switch to mania, necessitating close monitoring of this group.

The FDA black box warning for suicide often arises as an understandable source of worry that fuels reluctance in parents when SSRI treatment is recommended. It is useful to clarify that there have been no suicides reported in any pediatric OCD medication trials. In the context of OCD treatment, there is no data to suggest a clear increase in the risk of suicidal thinking or behaviors associated with SSRI medication (Bridge et al., 2007; Mills & Strawn, 2020). It is helpful to present measures that demonstrate the clear risk/benefit advantage of using SSRIs in the treatment of pediatric OCD. Data from a large meta-analysis examining concerns related to suicidality in SSRI-treated youth arrived at a "number needed to treat" (NNT) of six based on response to SSRIs for OCD versus placebo and a "number needed to harm" (NNH) of 200 relating to the absolute risk of suicidal thinking or behavior in those receiving SSRI treatment (Bridge et al., 2007). These numbers attest to how treatment effects and gains far outweigh risks.

Defining Outcomes

After initiation of medication, it is important to monitor response to treatment. The CY-BOCS and the second edition of the CY-BOCS (CY-BOCS-II) are the gold standard clinician-administered tools that helps establish baseline OCD severity and gauge change throughout treatment (Scahill, 1997; Storch, 2019). In the context of OCD treatment, "response" is understood as >/=35 percent reduction in CY-BOCS severity scores as well as a Clinical Global Impression – Improvement (CGI-I) score of one or two (much or very much improved) for a period of at least one week. Partial response is considered between 25–35 percent reduction in scores along with a CGI-I score of at least three (minimally improved) for a period of at least one week. Remission is when the OCD diagnostic criteria are no longer met or when a CY-BOCS score of </=12 along with a CGI-I score of one or two for at least one week is achieved (Mataix-Cols et al., 2016).

Treatment Resistance

When initiation of an SSRI is not met with adequate improvement to qualify for response parameters as described above, the initial approach would be to increase the medication dose so long as it is tolerated well. It is advised to continue dose titration every three weeks until the maximum recommended dose or maximum tolerated dose is reached while assessing for trends towards improvement. It is appropriate to ensure that treatment has continued for at least ten weeks, if not twelve weeks, at the highest approved dose within the limits of tolerability.

About a quarter to one third of pediatric patients do not show response to first line treatment for OCD as gathered by the Pediatric OCD Treatment Study (The Pediatric OCD Treatment Study (POTS) Team, 2004). Treatment refractory OCD is understood as the lack of adequate symptom improvement after treatment with at least two serotonin reuptake inhibitors (SSRIs or clomipramine) at maximum recommended or maximum tolerated doses for a period of at least ten to twelve weeks and adequate CBT which is constituted by at least eight to ten sessions.

The first step of management when met with treatment resistance is to re-examine more closely each component to satisfactorily ascertain the accuracy of the OCD diagnosis as well as the adequacy of treatment, inclusive of medication trials as well as CBT.

OCD in children is not always straightforward to diagnose. Comorbidity is the rule that further impacts the ease of discerning OCD symptoms in a child who may also have other symptoms that may impact presentation. Other clinical conditions including complex tics, ruminations of major depression, worries of generalized anxiety disorder, emerging psychosis, repetitive behaviors of autism spectrum disorder, and ego syntonic traits of perfectionism may mimic OCD and may be harder to tell apart in children who are unable to clearly articulate internal experiences (Bloch & Storch, 2015). Misdiagnosis of any of these conditions as OCD may not be followed by the expected pattern of response to standard OCD combination treatment of SSRI medication and ERP. Thus, in situations where standard approaches to treatment are met with an inadequate response, it may be prudent to reassess the diagnosis before proceeding with additional interventions.

Similarly, ensuring adherence to medication, re-affirming that medication treatment met consensus definitions of an adequate medication trial, and confirming the nature of received CBT to ensure that the vital ingredients of exposure and response prevention were practiced in a graded manner with parental involvement replete with homework assignments, is a part of ascertaining that standard treatments were indeed employed in the recommended fashion.

If improvement continues to be lacking at this point, it is useful to assess for moderators that are known to impact response to treatment for pediatric OCD, which include but are not limited to the following.

1) Comorbid tic disorders: Tics are known to be highly comorbid with OCD with about one third of those with Tourette's disorder developing OCD. OCD with tics has been seen to have certain distinct clinical features that have been repeatedly observed when these conditions are comorbid (Hanna et al., 2002; Leckman et al., 2010; Leckman et al., 1994; Zohar et al., 1997).There has been some concern for a lower response to SSRIs when used in the treatment of OCD with tics (Geller et al., 2003a; March et al., 2007)

2) Hoarding: Symptoms of hoarding have been seen to portend a poorer response to treatment with SRIs among youth (Masi et al., 2005; Bloch et al. 2014) with specifically tailored CBT approaches being recommended as the mainstay of treatment (McKay, 2016; Tolin et al., 2015).

3) Insight: About one third of children and adolescents with OCD present with limited insight into the excessive or meaningless nature of their obsessions or compulsive rituals. This can understandably affect their motivation to engage in treatment, especially when CBT involves endurance of distress. Poor insight has been associated with attenuated

response to treatment (Garcia et al., 2010; Storch et al., 2014; Storch et al., 2008).

4) Family accommodations: These include actions taken by the family to tolerate and accommodate the child's rituals, offer reassurance, complete tasks on the child's behalf, or other actions with the intention of relieving distress but which can inadvertently reinforce symptoms. Family accommodation occurs frequently in the families of youth with OCD and there is concern that these actions can impede response. As a result, family involvement in treatment is necessary to address and limit these accommodations effectively (Bipeta et al., 2013; Lebowitz et al., 2013; Merlo et al., 2009).

Once there has been devoted effort to assess these factors and tailor approaches to treatment to address the impact of these influences to the greatest extent possible, it is prudent to consider the role of adjunctive treatments. Approaches for treatment-resistant OCD might include augmentation with the below classes of medication.

Clomipramine

If the initial two SRI trials did not include clomipramine, it could be useful to introduce clomipramine to augment response to an SSRI. Meta-analyses of randomized controlled trial data of medication in pediatric OCD have noted superiority over SSRIs (Geller et al., 2003b; Varigonda et al., 2016) while also raising questions pertaining to confounding factors such as the year of publication, nature of the studies, or the participants included. Despite such an edge, tolerability concerns have been the biggest limiting factor with the use of clomipramine; as a result, it is not conventionally employed as the initial medication choice. But in situations that involve treatment resistance to the use of SSRIs, clomipramine may be a useful addition to the treatment regime.

There is a unique pharmacokinetic benefit to the combination of fluvoxamine and clomipramine. Through its inhibition of CYP1A2 and 2 C19, and moderate inhibition of CYP 2D6, fluvoxamine inhibits the enzymatic conversion of CMI to desmethylclomipramine (dCMI), which is thought to have more adrenergic receptor action. By tilting the balance towards more of clomipramine than desmethylclomipramine, it promotes more of the needed serotoninergic activity while limiting unwanted adrenergic effects that are responsible for arrhythmogenic potential. When a non-fluvoxamine SSRI like fluoxetine or sertraline is augmented with clomipramine, there is some theoretical concern that the CYP 2D6 inhibition by these agents may work towards inhibiting the enzymatic breakdown of desmethylclomipramine, thus increasing serum levels of this metabolite and in turn elevating the risk of cardiac rhythm disturbances. Even while this has not been clearly substantiated in clinical settings, some caution is advised when clomipramine is used to augment fluoxetine or sertraline.

This combination of fluvoxamine and clomipramine was well tolerated when the dCMI:CMI concentration was <0.3 as seen in an adult case series of 22 patients with OCD and depression (Szegedi et al., 1996). In a retrospective chart review conducted by Fung et al. (2021), the safety of this medication combination in pediatric OCD patients was examined and found to be well tolerated. Neither of these studies provided efficacy data. Hence while there is some preliminary data to indicate that the combination may have a favorable tolerability profile, it is unclear if there is an advantage from an effectiveness standpoint.

Antipsychotics

Neuroleptic medications are one of the top choices for augmenting SSRI responses in OCD owing to observed benefits with OCD symptoms as well as their beneficial role in the treatment of frequent comorbid illnesses inclusive of tic disorders, other externalizing disorders, and mood disorders. However, no antipsychotics are FDA approved for pediatric OCD so their use is "off label." Meta-analytic data in adults confirms the benefit of adding antipsychotics to the medication regime for OCD. Aripiprazole, haloperidol, and risperidone have demonstrated convincing benefit while olanzapine, paliperidone, and quetiapine failed to demonstrate an advantage over placebo per evidence from existing controlled trials in the adult population (Dold et al., 2015).

Controlled data assessing the outcome of antipsychotic augmentation in the pediatric population is lacking. Further, significant concerns related to metabolic side effects, weight gain, and potential for movement disorders discourage early introduction of these agents into the treatment regime. Published data in children and adolescents with OCD is in the form of case reports, case series, chart reviews, and naturalistic or open-label studies. The preponderance of literature examining response to antipsychotic augmentation in pediatric OCD pertains to reports on the use of aripiprazole and risperidone.

One of the largest published data sets on the use of antipsychotics in children is the report by Masi, Pfanner, & Brovedani, (2013) on the open label use of risperidone (mean doses of 1.7±0.8 mg) and aripiprazole (8.9±3.1 mg) in a cohort of 69 children with tic-related OCD who did not respond to at least 12 weeks of SSRI monotherapy. Overall, 56.5 percent showed response (CGI-I score one or two, CGI-S score three or less, and C-GAS score 50 or more during three consecutive months after a 12-week treatment). There were no differences between response patterns for risperidone and aripiprazole and there were no instances of medication discontinuation due to side effects. Weight gain and sedation were reported in the risperidone subset while aripiprazole was associated with mild to moderate agitation. This report suggests that about half of pediatric patients with tic-related OCD respond to antipsychotic augmentation that seems well tolerated.

The same authors (Masi et al., 2010) also described a consecutive series of 39 adolescents with OCD non-responsive to two SSRI trials who were treated with aripiprazole (12.2±3.4 mg), of which 59 percent demonstrated response as defined by CGI-I scores of one or two and CGI-S scores of three or below. Mild agitation and sleep disturbances were reported in about ten percent of this cohort.

A retrospective chart review (Akyol Ardic et al., 2017) discusses response to aripiprazole (3.4±2.2 mg) augmentation in 48 children and adolescents with OCD who met accepted definitions for treatment resistance. Improvement in OCD, as measured using YBOCS, CGI-I, and CGI-S, reached statistical significance with scores dropping to subthreshold levels at the final point of observation. Statistically significant weight gain was an observation that was noted as a source of concern and is consistent with reservations that pertain to utilizing antipsychotics in the psychopharmacological treatment of pediatric OCD.

Ziprasidone is another antipsychotic with a touted relative advantage in terms of propensity for less weight gain and metabolic side effects. An open label study by Yeghiyan et al. (2008) in 14 youth with OCD and Tourette's disorder reported benefits with ziprasidone treatment (dose range of 60 to 120 mg) in at least 6 patients showing a 28 percent decrease in CY-BOCS severity measures. Though data is lacking, medication like ziprasidone and lurasidone that are associated with a relatively better tolerability profile regarding metabolic parameters may present potential benefits in situations wherein other better studied agents are associated with adverse events or minimal response.

Glutamate Modulators

Medications that affect the serotoninergic system have been the mainstay of OCD treatment followed by adjunctive benefits noted with dopaminergic modulators. The presence of a subgroup of patients who do not improve with these medications has fueled the search for medications that may affect other pathways involved in the pathogenesis of OCD. The role of the glutamatergic system has been the more recent subject of interest supported by evidence from genetic associations and neuroimaging-based findings (Grant et al., 2013). Medications that are understood to be glutamate modulators have been investigated for their role in OCD management. Those include the following.

Riluzole

Benefits associated with riluzole treatment observed in a small open-label pilot trial in six children with OCD were not replicated in a larger 12-week randomized controlled trial (RCT) that recruited 60 children (Grant et al., 2007; Grant et al., 2013). Comparisons of treatment with riluzole (up to doses of 100 mg) with placebo as an add on to pre-existing medication treatment revealed no differences in terms of OCD severity measures tracked on the CYBOCS as well as CGI scores. No statistical differences in the rate of adverse effects were reported between groups though there were five subjects who had to discontinue riluzole due to an asymptomatic elevation in transaminases, which did normalize soon after stopping the medication. There was one child in the riluzole group who was on three other medications who developed pancreatitis that improved without any sequalae.

D-Cycloserine

D-cycloserine (DCS) is an N-methyl-D-aspartate (NMDA) partial agonist and its augmentation of CBT is thought to promote the extinction of learned fear. Initial data from a small RCT showed benefits, whilst a subsequent RCT with a larger sample size of 142 youth failed to demonstrate differences between groups with CBT with or without DCS augmentation (Storch et al., 2010; Storch et al., 2016). Confounding factors like the ceiling effect of adequately delivered CBT have been speculated to impact the result. Other smaller trials have demonstrated variable findings. The group lead by Farrell et al. (2013) recorded clear benefit regarding OCD severity measures when CBT was augmented with DCS versus placebo at one month follow up. Post-session augmentation of CBT with DCS was not associated with efficacy over placebo in a small study conducted by Mataix-Cols et al. (2014).

At present, we lack compelling data suggesting an advantage of DCS augmentation of CBT for the treatment of pediatric OCD.

Memantine

Case reports have suggested benefit from memantine in the treatment of pediatric OCD but this has not been substantiated adequately through controlled trials (Hezel, Beattie, & Stewart, 2009; Pekrul & Fitzgerald, 2015). A randomized placebo-controlled trial that compared memantine and placebo, reported data from a small group of seven children with ASD and/or OCD and noted encouraging results in terms of decrease in YBOCS scores and CGI scores in the memantine group. The small sample size precluded statistical comparisons to establish superiority (Niemeyer et al., 2022).

N-Acetyl Cysteine

N-acetyl Cysteine (NAC) is an amino acid derivative that has been used in the treatment of OCD owing to postulated mechanisms involved in modulating glutamate function and serving to decrease oxidative stress (Parli et al., 2022). Case reports suggest that NAC may play a beneficial role. Two randomized controlled trials provide evidence that supports the role of NAC in pediatric OCD treatment. Ghanizadeh et al. (2017) conducted a multisite ten-week RCT wherein 34 patients aged ten to twenty-one years who failed to respond to at least one SSRI were enrolled and randomized into NAC with citalopram versus placebo with citalopram groups and followed up on CYBOCS severity as well as Pediatric Quality of Life measures. Citalopram was used in doses between 20 to 40 mg and the NAC dose at completion ranged between 1,200–2,400 mg/day. At the end of the trial there was a statistically significant improvement in OCD symptom severity as well as the Quality of Life scores in the NAC group which was not observed in the placebo group. The mean CYBOCS scores of those in the NAC group showed a substantial decline from an average of 21.0 (8.2) to 11.3 (5.7) over the ten-week period. The rate of side effects did not differ between the groups and the most commonly reported side effects in the NAC group included fatigue, dizziness, blurred vision, tremors, insomnia, and sweating.

Li et al. (2020) conducted an RCT wherein 11 children and adolescents with OCD who were on stable treatment (medication and therapy) for OCD were randomized to receive NAC (up to 2,700 mg/day) or placebo and their CYBOCS scores were monitored. NAC outperformed placebo and the difference was statistically significant. It is important to note that this trial was underpowered and represents data from a small sample that can only serve as preliminary evidence suggesting benefit.

Others

Case studies have reported benefits with other medication inclusive of stimulants, benzodiazepines, lamotrigine, vortioxetine, and sumatriptan in the treatment of pediatric OCD. However, the anecdotal nature of these reports limit conclusions and are insufficient to guide treatment at this stage until these findings can be substantiated by larger, controlled trials.

Effectiveness of Medications in Pediatric Obsessive-Compulsive Disorder

Multisite randomized placebo-controlled trials have convincingly demonstrated the superiority of individual SSRI medication and clomipramine over placebo for the treatment of pediatric OCD (DeVeaugh-Geiss et al., 1992; Geller et al., 2001; March et al., 1998; Riddle et al., 2001).

The Pediatric OCD Treatment Study (POTS) stands out as a landmark multi-site RCT that examined four arms of treatment for 12 weeks, namely: CBT, Sertraline, Placebo and CBT + Sertraline in 112 children aged seven to seventeen with OCD (The Pediatric OCD Treatment Study (POTS) Team, 2004). Each of these modalities of treatment, be it alone or in combination, outperformed placebo. The rate of clinical remission was highest for combined treatment: 53.6 percent (95 percent confidence interval [CI], 36 percent–70 percent) followed by CBT alone, 39.3 percent (95 percent CI, 24 percent–58 percent), sertraline alone, 21.4 percent (95 percent CI, 10 percent–40 percent); and placebo, 3.6 percent (95 percent CI, 0 percent–19 percent). The differences in remission rates between combined treatment and CBT were not statistically significant (p=0.42) though proved superior to medication and placebo. Additionally, though the average rates of remission from CBT were higher than that of sertraline, the differences were not statistically significant.

All treatments administered were tolerated well without notable concerns for adverse effects. The study findings laid the groundwork for treatment choices in pediatric OCD and supported the use of CBT alone or CBT along with pharmacological treatment as the first approach for a child or adolescent presenting with OCD. Medication when used in combination with CBT was thought to offset possible site-specific differences in the quality of CBT that was delivered. This observation of the advantage of combining pharmacological and cognitive behavioral treatments holds definite value in real world settings wherein significant variability in the quality of CBT can be expected to be the norm.

In the past two decades, meta-analyses have proved to be a useful tool in statistically combining results from RCT and have served to ascertain the superiority of medication-based treatment to placebo. Geller et al. (2003b) conducted one of the earliest meta-analyses of published randomized, controlled medication trials in children and adolescents with OCD to assess evidence for differential efficacy. Included data pertained to 1,044 pediatric participants with OCD from 12 studies. Cumulatively the difference that emerged in the comparison of medication with placebo was highly significant, hence rendering compelling support for the role of pharmacotherapy. The pooled effect size of 0.46 translated to a difference of about four points on the CYBOCS scale between medication and placebo which suggests that although medications are beneficial, the effects are modest. Clomipramine was significantly superior to each of the SSRIs while the SSRIs were comparably effective with no individual differences demonstrated within this group. Despite the noted superiority of clomipramine, SSRIS were still recommended as the initial choice in light of their relatively favorable tolerability profile.

A meta-analysis by Sánchez-Meca et al. (2014) included additional studies completed in the intervening years and examined the differential efficacy of CBT, pharmacological and combined treatment for pediatric OCD. The located studies yielded data on ten comparisons between pharmacological and a control group and three comparisons of combined treatment versus control. An effect size for pharmacological treatments was d=0.745 and for combined treatment was d=1.704, providing further evidence backing the role of medication alone or in combination in the treatment of OCD in youth. Within pharmacological treatments, clomipramine (d=1.305) was more efficacious than SSRIs (d=0.644), with authors recommending clomipramine as a second line choice owing to its adverse effect profile, in keeping with previous guidelines.

Ivarsson's systematic review and meta-analysis (2015), which included 14 trials, lent consistency to previous findings on the efficacy of pharmacological interventions for pediatric OCD. The calculated effect size (Hedge's g=0.48) for pharmacological treatment amounted to a 3.9-point decrease in CYBOCS severity scores. They also found no evidence supporting difference in efficacy between the individual SSRIs.

A meta-analysis published by Varigonda et al. (2016) sought to extend findings from the initial meta-analysis published by Geller et al. (2003b) using longitudinal data from each trial. Specific questions that this effort strived to answer included the time course of response to medication and the relationship between dose and response. Nine trials involving 801 children with OCD were included in this meta-analysis. For the SSRIs, seven trials with a total of 725 participants (placebo: n=351, SSRI: n=374) provided data for analysis across multiple weekly points. A significant benefit of SSRI compared to placebo was observed as early as two weeks after the initiation of treatment in pediatric OCD. Over 85 percent of the improvement observed on SSRI compared to placebo in pediatric OCD trials was observed by week two. For clomipramine only two trials with a total of 76 participants (placebo n=37, clomipramine n=39) provided data for analysis across multiple weekly points to assess OCD symptom improvement. Over 75 percent of the improvement in OCD symptoms observed with clomipramine compared to placebo in pediatric OCD trials was evident within two weeks.

These results suggest that the greatest incremental treatment gains in pediatric OCD occur early in SSRI treatment. This finding is of significance considering that existing guidelines across age groups suggest that for medication trials to be considered optimal and adequate at least eight to twelve weeks of treatment is in order. As benefits do tend to accrue over time, an adequate duration of treatment remains pertinent until there is more longitudinal data that can provide more insights into the time pattern of response.

There was no evidence for a relationship between SSRI dosing and treatment effect, although data was limited. Studies on adults with OCD have supported a strong dose response relationship. Pediatric studies performed so far do not employ fixed dose designs to do justice to this question. Most studies that were included in this meta-analysis used maximal tolerated doses and hence did not permit examination of response across different doses.

Similar to previous studies on the subject, the authors yet again established that there were no significant differences in magnitude of response to serotonergic medications between children and adults with OCD, there were no significant differences in treatment responses between SSRI agents, and that clomipramine demonstrated a significantly greater response when compared to placebo than SSRIs.

The most recent statistical synthesis of RCT data on the efficacy and acceptability of SRI medication and different formats of CBT in the treatment of pediatric OCD derives from a network meta-analysis by Cervin et al. (Unpublished). Of the 30 included RCTs, 13 included comparisons of SRIs and demonstrated a five-to-nine-point difference in the post treatment CYBOCS scores with pharmacotherapy. In a relative context this compares with a seven-to-twelve-point difference with in-person CBT and the most substantial difference amounting to 9 to 13 points with a combination of these treatments. Each of these interventions surpassed the accepted threshold of a four-point difference in scores to translate to a meaningful difference. The noted two-to-three-point difference in YBOCS scores between medication and in-person CBT raises questions pertaining to the actual clinical relevance of ranking these treatment modalities strictly based on these treatment metrics. The authors suggest that there may be other understudied but more practically relevant aspects such as patient preference and acceptability that may have a bigger role to play in determining choice and adjudging the relative utility of these treatments.

Conclusion

Psychopharmacology is an important treatment option for pediatric OCD. While CBT remains the initial treatment approach, pharmacological interventions are necessary in many cases. Available evidence suggests that clomipramine and SSRIs are the most effective pharmacological agents for the treatment of pediatric OCD, with favorable outcomes in terms of reducing symptoms and improving functioning. Tolerability profiles support use of SSRIs as the primary pharmacological agents. In circumstances of partial or no response to these medications, anti-psychotics are commonly used off label as augmenting agents, though newer agents such as glutaminergic compounds are also being examined for potential benefit Continued research in this area is needed to identify novel treatment strategies, inclusive of exploring the role of neuromodulatory approaches that can be utilized in the management of OCD in children and adolescents.

References

Akyol Ardic, U., Ercan, E.S., Kutlu, A., Yuce, D., Ipci, M., & Inci, S.B. (2017). Successful treatment response with aripiprazole augmentation of SSRIs in refractory obsessive-compulsive disorder in childhood. *Child Psychiatry & Human Development*, 48(5), 699–704. https://doi.org/10.1007/s10578-016-0694-8.

Biederman, J. (1991). Sudden death in children treated with a tricyclic antidepressant: A commentary. *Journal of the American Academy of Child & Adolescent Psychiatry*, 30(3), 495–498. https://doi.org/10.1097/00004583-199105000-00023.

Bipeta, R., Yerramilli, S.S., Pingali, S., Karredla, A.R., & Ali, M.O. (2013). A cross-sectional study of insight and family accommodation in pediatric obsessive-compulsive disorder. *Child and Adolescent Psychiatry and Mental Health*, 7(1), 20. https://doi.org/10.1186/1753-2000-7-20.

Bloch, M.H., Bartley, C.A., Zipperer, L., Jakubovski, E., Landeros-Weisenberger, A., Pittenger, C., & Leckman, J.F. (2014). Meta-analysis: Hoarding symptoms associated with poor treatment outcome in obsessive-compulsive disorder. *Molecular Psychiatry*, 19(9), 1025–1030. https://doi.org/10.1038/mp.2014.50.

Bloch, M.H., McGuire, J., Landeros-Weisenberger, A., Leckman, J.F., & Pittenger, C. (2010). Meta-analysis of the dose-response relationship of SSRI in obsessive-compulsive disorder. *Molecular Psychiatry*, 15(8), 850–855. https://doi.org/10.1038/mp.2009.50.

Bloch, M.H., & Storch, E.A. (2015). Assessment and management of treatment-refractory obsessive-compulsive disorder in children. *Journal of the American Academy of Child & Adolescent Psychiatry*, 54(4), 251–262. https://doi.org/10.1016/j.jaac.2015.01.011.

Bridge, J., Iyengar, S., Salary, C.B., Barbe, R.P., Birmaher, B., Pincus, H.A., Ren, L., & Brent, D.A. (2007). Clinical response and risk for reported suicidal ideation and suicide attempts in pediatric antidepressant treatment: A meta-analysis of randomized controlled trials. *Journal of the American Medical Association*, 297(15), 1683–1696. https://doi.org/10.1001/jama.297.15.1683.

Cervin, M., McGuire, J.F., D'Souza, J.M., De Nadai, A.S., Aspvall, K., Goodman, W.K., Andrén, P., Schneider, S.C., Geller, D.A., Mataix-Cols, D., & Storch, E.A. (Unpublished). Efficacy and acceptability of serotonin reuptake inhibitors and cognitive-behavioral therapy for pediatric obsessive-compulsive disorder: A network meta-analysis.

DeVeaugh-Geiss, J., Moroz, G., Biederman, J.B., Cantwell, D., Fontaine, R., Greist, J., Reichler, R., Katz, R., & Landau, P. (1992). Clomipramine hydrochloride in childhood and adolescent obsessive-compulsive disorder: A multicenter trial. *Journal of the American Academy of Child and Adolescent Psychiatry, 31*(1), 45–49. https://doi.org/10.1097/00004583-199201000-00008.

Dold, M., Aigner, M., Lanzenberger, R., & Kasper, S. (2015). Antipsychotic augmentation of serotonin reuptake inhibitors in treatment-resistant obsessive-compulsive disorder: An update meta-analysis of double-blind, randomized, placebo-controlled trials. *International Journal of Neuropsychopharmacology, 18*(9). https://doi.org/10.1093/ijnp/pyv047.

Farrell, L.J., Waters, A.M., Boschen, M.J., Hattingh, L., McConnell, H., Milliner, E.L., Collings, N., Zimmer-Gembeck, M., Shelton, D., Ollendick, T.H., Testa, C., & Storch, E.A. (2013). Difficult-to-treat pediatric obsessive-compulsive disorder: Feasibility and preliminary results of a randomized pilot trial of D-cycloserine-augmented behavior therapy. *Depression and Anxiety, 30*(8), 723–731. https://doi.org/10.1002/da.22132.

Fineberg, N.A., Pampaloni, I., Pallanti, S., Ipser, J., & Stein, D.J. (2007). Sustained response versus relapse: The pharmacotherapeutic goal for obsessive-compulsive disorder. *International Clinical Psychopharmacology, 22*(6), 313–322. https://doi.org/10.1097/YIC.0b013e32825ea312.

Flament, M.F., Rapoport, J.L., Berg, C.J., Sceery, W., Kilts, C., Mellstrom, B., & Linnoila, M. (1985). Clomipramine treatment of childhood obsessive-compulsive disorder: A double-blind controlled study. *Archives of General Psychiatry, 42*(10), 977–983. https://doi.org/10.1001/archpsyc.1985.01790330057007.

Fung, R., Elbe, D., & Stewart, S.E. (2021). Retrospective review of fluvoxamine-clomipramine combination therapy in obsessive-compulsive disorder in children and adolescents. *Journal of the Canadian Academy of Child and Adolescent Psychiatry, 30*(3), 150–155.

Garcia, A.M., Sapyta, J.J., Moore, P.S., Freeman, J.B., Franklin, M.E., March, J.S., & Foa, E.B. (2010). Predictors and moderators of treatment outcome in the Pediatric Obsessive Compulsive Treatment Study (POTS I). *Journal of the American Academy of Child & Adolescent Psychiatry, 49*(10), 1024–1033. https://doi.org/10.1016/j.jaac.2010.06.013.

Geller, D.A., Biederman, J., Stewart, S.E., Mullin, B., Farrell, C., Wagner, K.D., Emslie, G., & Carpenter, D. (2003a). Impact of comorbidity on treatment response in pediatric obsessive-compulsive disorder: Is the use of exclusion criteria empirically supported in randomized clinical trials? *Journal of Child & Adolescent Psychopharmacology, 13*, S19–29. https://doi.org/10.1089/104454603322126313.

Geller, D.A., Biederman, J., Stewart, S.E., Mullin, B., Martin, A., Spencer, T., & Faraone, S.V. (2003b). Which SSRI? A meta-analysis of pharmacotherapy trials in pediatric obsessive-compulsive disorder. *American Journal of Psychiatry, 160*(11), 1919–1928. https://doi.org/10.1176/appi.ajp.160.11.1919.

Geller, D.A., Hoog, S.L., Heiligenstein, J.H., Ricardi, R.K., Tamura, R., Kluszynski, S., & Jacobson, J.G. (2001). Fluoxetine treatment for obsessive-compulsive disorder in children and adolescents: A placebo-controlled clinical trial. *Journal of the American Academy of Child & Adolescent Psychiatry, 40*(7), 773–779. https://doi.org/10.1097/00004583-200107000-00011.

Geller, D.A., March, J., & AACAP Committee on Quality Issues. (2012). Practice parameter for the assessment and treatment of children and adolescents with obsessive-compulsive disorder. *Journal of the American Academy of Child & Adolescent Psychiatry, 51*(1), 98–113. https://doi.org/https://doi.org/10.1016/j.jaac.2011.09.019.

Ghanizadeh, A., Mohammadi, M.R., Bahraini, S., Keshavarzi, Z., Firoozabadi, A., & Alavi Shoshtari, A. (2017). Efficacy of n-acetylcysteine augmentation on obsessive compulsive disorder: A multicenter randomized double blind placebo controlled clinical trial. *Iranian Journal of Psychiatry*, 12(2), 134–141.

Grant, P., Lougee, L., Hirschtritt, M., & Swedo, S.E. (2007). An open-label trial of riluzole, a glutamate antagonist, in children with treatment-resistant obsessive-compulsive disorder. *Journal of Child & Adolescent Psychopharmacology*, 17(6), 761–767. https://doi.org/10.1089/cap.2007.0021.

Grant, P.J., Joseph, L.A., Farmer, C.A., Luckenbaugh, D.A., Lougee, L.C., Zarate Jr., C.A., & Swedo, S.E. (2013). 12-week placebo-controlled trial of add-on riluzole in the treatment of childhood-onset obsessive compulsive disorder. *Neuropsychopharmacology*, 39(6), 1453–1459. https://doi.org/10.1038/npp.2013.343.

Hanna, G.L., Piacentini, J., Cantwell, D.P., Fischer, D.J., Himle, J.A., & Van Etten, M. (2002). Obsessive-compulsive disorder with and without tics in a clinical sample of children and adolescents. *Depression and anxiety*, 16(2), 59–63. https://doi.org/10.1002/da.10058.

Hezel, D.M., Beattie, K., & Stewart, S.E. (2009). Memantine as an augmenting agent for severe pediatric OCD. *American Journal of Psychiatry*, 166(2), 237. https://doi.org/10.1176/appi.ajp.2008.08091427.

Ivarsson, T., Skarphedinsson, G., Kornør, H., Axelsdottir, B., Biedilæ, S., Heyman, I., Asbahr, F., Thomsen, P.H., Fineberg, N., & March, J. (2015). The place of and evidence for serotonin reuptake inhibitors (SRIs) for obsessive compulsive disorder (OCD) in children and adolescents: Views based on a systematic review and meta-analysis. *Psychiatry Research*, 227(1), 93–103. https://doi.org/10.1016/j.psychres.2015.01.015.

Lebowitz, E.R., Woolston, J., Bar-Haim, Y., Calvocoressi, L., Dauser, C., Warnick, E., Scahill, L., Chakir, A.R., Shechner, T., Hermes, H., Vitulano, L.A., King, R.A., & Leckman, J.F. (2013). Family accommodation in pediatric anxiety disorders. *Depression and Anxiety*, 30(1), 47–54. https://doi.org/10.1002/da.21998.

Leckman, J.F., Denys, D., Simpson, H.B., Mataix-Cols, D., Hollander, E., Saxena, S., Miguel, E.C., Rauch, S.L., Goodman, W.K., Phillips, K.A., & Stein, D.J. (2010). Obsessive-compulsive disorder: A review of the diagnostic criteria and possible subtypes and dimensional specifiers for DSM-V. *Depression and anxiety*, 27(6), 507–527. https://doi.org/10.1002/da.20669.

Leckman, J.F., Grice, D.E., Barr, L.C., de Vries, A.L., Martin, C., Cohen, D.J., McDougle, C.J., Goodman, W.K., & Rasmussen, S.A. (1994). Tic-related vs. non-tic-related obsessive compulsive disorder. *Anxiety*, 1(5), 208–215.

Leuchter, J.D., Kook, M., Geller, D.A., Hertz, A.G., Garcia, J., Trent, E.S., Dibbs, T., Onyeka, O., Goodman, W.K., Guzick, A.G., Wiese, A.D., Palo, A.D., Small, B.J., Simpson, H.B., Havel, L.K., Nibras, S.A., Saxena, K., & Storch, E.A. (2023). Promoting OCD WEllness and Resilience (POWER) study: Rationale, design, and methods. *Psychiatry Research Communications*, 3(2), 100111. https://doi.org/10.1016/j.psycom.2023.100111.

Li, F., Welling, M.C., Johnson, J.A., Coughlin, C., Mulqueen, J., Jakubovski, E., Coury, S., Landeros-Weisenberger, A., & Bloch, M.H. (2020). N-acetylcysteine for pediatric obsessive-compulsive disorder: A small pilot study. *Journal of Child & Adolescent Psychopharmacology*, 30(1), 32–37. https://doi.org/10.1089/cap.2019.0041.

March, J.S., Biederman, J., Wolkow, R., Safferman, A., Mardekian, J., Cook, E.H., Cutler, N.R., Dominguez, R., Ferguson, J., Muller, B., Riesenberg, R., Rosenthal, M.,

Sallee, F.R., Wagner, K.D., & Steiner, H. (1998). Sertraline in children and adolescents with obsessive-compulsive disorder: A multicenter randomized controlled trial. *Journal of the American Medical Association, 280*(20), 1752–1756. https:// doi.org/10.1001/jama.280.20.1752.

March, J.S., Franklin, M.E., Leonard, H., Garcia, A., Moore, P., Freeman, J., & Foa, E. (2007). Tics moderate treatment outcome with sertraline but not cognitive-behavior therapy in pediatric obsessive-compulsive disorder. *Biological Psychiatry, 61*(3), 344–347. https://doi.org/10.1016/j.biopsych.2006.09.035.

Martin, A., Young, C., Leckman, J.F., Mukonoweshuro, C., Rosenheck, R., & Leslie, D. (2004). Age effects on antidepressant-induced manic conversion. *Archives of Pediatrics & Adolescent Medicine, 158*(8), 773–780. https://doi.org/10.1001/ archpedi.158.8.773.

Masi, G., Millepiedi, S., Mucci, M., Bertini, N., Milantoni, L., & Arcangeli, F. (2005). A naturalistic study of referred children and adolescents with obsessive-compulsive disorder. *Journal of the American Academy of Child and Adolescent Psychiatry, 44*(7), 673–681. https://doi.org/10.1097/01.chi.000016 1648.82775.ee.

Masi, G., Pfanner, C., & Brovedani, P. (2013). Antipsychotic augmentation of selective serotonin reuptake inhibitors in resistant tic-related obsessive-compulsive disorder in children and adolescents: A naturalistic comparative study. *Journal of Psychiatric Research, 47*(8), 1007–1012. https://doi.org/10.1016/j. jpsychires.2013.04.003.

Masi, G., Pfanner, C., Millepiedi, S., & Berloffa, S. (2010). Aripiprazole augmentation in 39 adolescents with medication-resistant obsessive-compulsive disorder. *Journal of Clinical Psychopharmacology, 30*(6), 688–693. https://doi.org/ 10.1097/jcp.0b013e3181fab7b1.

Mataix-Cols, D., Fernández de la Cruz, L., Nordsletten, A.E., Lenhard, F., Isomura, K., & Simpson, H.B. (2016). Towards an international expert consensus for defining treatment response, remission, recovery and relapse in obsessive-compulsive disorder. *World Psychiatry, 15*(1), 80–81. https://doi.org/10.1002/wps.20299.

Mataix-Cols, D., Turner, C., Monzani, B., Isomura, K., Murphy, C., Krebs, G., & Heyman, I. (2014). Cognitive-behavioural therapy with post-session D-cycloserine augmentation for paediatric obsessive-compulsive disorder: Pilot randomised controlled trial. *The British Journal of Psychiatry, 204*(1), 77–78. https://doi. org/10.1192/bjp.bp.113.126284.

McKay, D. (2016). Cognitive-behavioral treatment of hoarding in youth: A case illustration. *Journal of Clinical Psychology, 72*(11), 1209–1218. https://doi. org/10.1002/jclp.22400.

Merlo, L.J., Lehmkuhl, H.D., Geffken, G.R., & Storch, E.A. (2009). Decreased family accommodation associated with improved therapy outcome in pediatric obsessive-compulsive disorder. *Journal of Consulting and Clinical Psychology, 77*(2), 355–360. https://doi.org/10.1037/a0012652.

Mills, J.A., & Strawn, J.R. (2020). Antidepressant tolerability in pediatric anxiety and obsessive-compulsive disorders: A Bayesian hierarchical modeling meta-analysis. *Journal of the American Academy of Child & Adolescent Psychiatry, 59*(11), 1240–1251. https://doi.org/10.1016/j.jaac.2019.10.013.

Niemeyer, L., Mechler, K., Dittmann, R.W., Banaschewski, T., Buitelaar, J., Durston, S., & Häge, A. (2022). Memantine as treatment for compulsivity in child and adolescent psychiatry: Descriptive findings from an incompleted randomized, double-blind, placebo-controlled trial. *Contemporary Clinical Trials Communications, 29*, 100982. https://doi.org/10.1016/j.conctc.2022.100982.

Parli, G.M., Gales, M.A., & Gales, B.J. (2022). N-acetylcysteine for obsessive-compulsive and related disorders in children and adolescents: A review. *Annals of Pharmacotherapy*, Advance online publication. https://doi.org/10.1177/10600280221138092.

The Pediatric OCD Treatment Study (POTS) Team. (2004). Cognitive-behavior therapy, sertraline, and their combination for children and adolescents with obsessive-compulsive disorder: The pediatric OCD treatment study (POTS) randomized controlled trial. *Journal of the American Medical Association Psychiatry*, 292(16), 1969–1976. https://doi.org/10.1001/jama.292.16.1969.

Pekrul, S.R., & Fitzgerald, K.D. (2015). Memantine Augmentation in a Down's Syndrome Adolescent with Treatment-Resistant Obsessive-Compulsive Disorder. *J Child Adolesc Psychopharmacol*, 25(7), 593–595. https://doi.org/10.1089/cap.2015.0073.

Reid, A.M., McNamara, J.P., Murphy, T.K., Guzick, A.G., Storch, E.A., Goodman, W.K., Geffken, G.R., & Bussing, R. (2015). Side-effects of SSRIs disrupt multimodal treatment for pediatric OCD in a randomized-controlled trial. *Journal of Psychiatric Research*, 71, 140–147. https://doi.org/10.1016/j.jpsychires.2015.10.006.

Reinblatt, S.P., DosReis, S., Walkup, J.T., & Riddle, M.A. (2009). Activation adverse events induced by the selective serotonin reuptake inhibitor fluvoxamine in children and adolescents. *Journal of Child & Adolescent Psychopharmacology*, 19(2), 119–126. https://doi.org/10.1089/cap.2008.040.

Riddle, M., King, R., Hardin, M., Scahill, L., Ort, S., Chappell, P., Rasmusson, A., & Leckman, J. (1991). Behavioral side effects of fluoxetine in children and adolescents. *Journal of Child and Adolescent Psychopharmacology*, 1(3), 193–198. https://doi.org/https://doi.org/10.1089/cap.1990.1.193.

Riddle, M.A., Reeve, E.A., Yaryura-Tobias, J.A., Yang, H.M., Claghorn, J.L., Gaffney, G., Greist, J.H., Holland, D., McConville, B.J., Pigott, T., & Walkup, J.T. (2001). Fluvoxamine for children and adolescents with obsessive-compulsive disorder: A randomized, controlled, multicenter trial. *Journal of the American Academy of Child and Adolescent Psychiatry*, 40(2), 222–229. https://doi.org/10.1097/00004583-200102000-00017.

Safer, D.J., & Zito, J.M. (2006). Treatment-emergent adverse events from selective serotonin reuptake inhibitors by age group: Children versus adolescents. *Journal of Child and Adolescent Psychopharmacology*, 16(1–2), 159–169. https://doi.org/10.1089/cap.2006.16.159.

Sánchez-Meca, J., Rosa-Alcázar, A.I., Iniesta-Sepúlveda, M., & Rosa-Alcázar, A. (2014). Differential efficacy of cognitive-behavioral therapy and pharmacological treatments for pediatric obsessive-compulsive disorder: A meta-analysis. *Journal of Anxiety Disorders*, 28(1), 31–44. https://doi.org/10.1016/j.janxdis.2013.10.007.

Scahill,L.,Riddle,M.A.,McSwiggin-Hardin,M.,Ort,S.I.,King,R.A.,Goodman,W.K., Cicchetti, D. & Leckman, J.F. (1997). Children's Yale-Brown obsessive compulsive scale: Reliability and validity. *Journal of the American Academy of Child & Adolescent Psychiatry*, 36(6), 844–852. https://doi.org/10.1097/00004583-19970 6000-00023.

Solmi, M., Fornaro, M., Ostinelli, E.G., Zangani, C., Croatto, G., Monaco, F., Krinitski, D., Fusar-Poli, P., & Correll, C.U. (2020). Safety of 80 antidepressants, antipsychotics, anti-attention-deficit/hyperactivity medications and mood stabilizers in children and adolescents with psychiatric disorders: A large scale systematic meta-review of 78 adverse effects. *World Psychiatry*, 19(2), 214–232. https://doi.org/10.1002/wps.20765.

Storch, E.A., McGuire, J.F., Wu, M.S., Hamblin, R., McIngvale, E., Cepeda, S.L., Schneider, S.C., Rufino, K.A., Rasmussen, S.A., Price, L.H., & Goodman, W.K. (2019). Development and psychometric evaluation of the children's Yale-Brown obsessive-compulsive scale second edition. *Journal of the American Academy of Child & Adolescent Psychiatry*, 58(1), 92–98.

Storch, E.A., De Nadai, A.S., Jacob, M.L., Lewin, A.B., Muroff, J., Eisen, J., Abramowitz, J.S., Geller, D.A., & Murphy, T.K. (2014). Phenomenology and correlates of insight in pediatric obsessive-compulsive disorder. *Compr Psychiatry*, 55(3), 613–620. https://doi.org/10.1016/j.comppsych.2013.09.014.

Storch, E.A., Milsom, V.A., Merlo, L.J., Larson, M., Geffken, G.R., Jacob, M.L., Murphy, T.K., & Goodman, W.K. (2008). Insight in pediatric obsessive-compulsive disorder: Associations with clinical presentation. *Psychiatry Research*, 160(2), 212–220. https://doi.org/10.1016/j.psychres.2007.07.005.

Storch, E.A., Murphy, T.K., Goodman, W.K., Geffken, G.R., Lewin, A.B., Henin, A., Micco, J.A., Sprich, S., Wilhelm, S., Bengtson, M., & Geller, D.A. (2010). A preliminary study of D-cycloserine augmentation of cognitive-behavioral therapy in pediatric obsessive-compulsive disorder. *Biological Psychiatry*, 68(11), 1073–1076. https://doi.org/10.1016/j.biopsych.2010.07.015.

Storch, E.A., Wilhelm, S., Sprich, S., Henin, A., Micco, J., Small, B.J., McGuire, J., Mutch, P.J., Lewin, A.B., Murphy, T.K., & Geller, D.A. (2016). Efficacy of augmentation of cognitive behavior therapy with weight-adjusted D-cycloserine vs. placebo in pediatric obsessive-compulsive disorder: A randomized clinical trial. *Journal of the American Medical Association Psychiatry*, 73(8), 779–788. https://doi.org/10.1001/jamapsychiatry.2016.1128.

Szegedi, A., Wetzel, H., Leal, M., Härtter, S., & Hiemke, C. (1996). Combination treatment with clomipramine and fluvoxamine: Drug monitoring, safety, and tolerability data. *Journal of Clinical Psychiatry*, 57(6), 257–264.

Tolin, D.F., Frost, R.O., Steketee, G., & Muroff, J. (2015). Cognitive behavioral therapy for hoarding disorder: A meta-analysis. *Depression and anxiety*, 32(3), 158–166. https://doi.org/10.1002/da.22327

Varigonda, A., Jakubovski, E., & Bloch, M. (2016). Systematic review and meta-analysis: Early treatment responses of selective serotonin reuptake inhibitors and clomipramine in pediatric obsessive-compulsive disorder. *Journal of the American Academy of Child and Adolescent Psychiatry*, 55(10), 851–859. https://doi.org/10.1016/j.jaac.2016.07.768.

Walkup, J.T., Albano, A.M., Piacentini, J., Birmaher, B., Compton, S.N., Sherrill, J.T., Ginsburg, G.S., Rynn, M.A., McCracken, J., Waslick, B., Iyengar, S., March, J.S., & Kendall, P.C. (2008). Cognitive behavioral therapy, sertraline, or a combination in childhood anxiety. *New England Journal of Medicine*, 359(26), 2753–2766. https://doi.org/10.1056/NEJMoa0804633.

Yeghiyan, M., Israelyan, N., & Tosalakyn, M. (2008). Ziprasidone among adolescents with overlapping OCD and Tourette's syndrome (Pilot study). *Annals of General Psychiatry*, 7, S307. https://doi.org/https://doi.org/10.1186/1744-859X-7-S1-S307.

Zohar, A.H., Pauls, D.L., Ratzoni, G., Apter, A., Dycian, A., Binder, M., King, R., Leckman, J.F., Kron, S., & Cohen, D.J. (1997). Obsessive-compulsive disorder with and without tics in an epidemiological sample of adolescents. *American Journal of Psychiatry*, 154(2), 274–276. https://doi.org/10.1176/ajp.154.2.274.

12 Psychopharmacology of Obsessive-Compulsive Related Disorders and Comorbid Disorders in Children and Adolescents

Aarya Krishnan Rajalakshmi,[1,2] *Aditya Kumar Singh Pawar*[1,2] *and Daniel A. Geller*[3,4]

[1] *Kennedy Krieger Institute, Baltimore, MD*

[2] *Johns Hopkins University School of Medicine, Baltimore, MD*

[3] *Massachusetts General Hospital, Boston, MA*

[4] *Harvard Medical School, Boston, MA*

Comorbidity in Pediatric Obsessive-Compulsive Disorder and approaches to treatment

Obsessive-compulsive disorder (OCD) in children and adolescents is frequently comorbid with other conditions. Comorbidity has been found to decrease the response to pharmacologic treatment and increase the risk of relapse in pediatric OCD (Geller et al., 2003). A thorough assessment intended to evaluate for the presence and extent of comorbidity as well as a determination of the most impairing of these illnesses becomes crucial in ensuring the appropriate choice and sequence of treatment. Common comorbidity that influences treatment decisions are discussed below.

Obsessive-Compulsive Disorder and Tic Disorders

The *Diagnostic and Statistical Manual of Mental Disorders* (DSM-5) includes a "tic related" specifier for OCD to refer to those with the illness who also have a history of tics, current or past. Tic disorders are thought to occur in 10–40 percent of children and adolescents with OCD (Leckman et al., 2010). Tic-related OCD is thought to have an earlier onset, a male predominance, and a higher proportion of symmetry-related, "just right" obsessions, aggressive content, and counting and ordering compulsions as a part of their symptomatology (Hanna et al., 2002; Leckman et al., 2010; Leckman et al., 1994; Zohar et al., 1997). Tic disorders are known to wane through adolescence

DOI: 10.4324/9781003386278-12

and there was reason to expect a similar favorable prognosis when OCD occurred with tics in childhood, though evidence from adults with OCD suggested a poorer prognosis when OCD was comorbid with tics.

Cognitive-behavioral therapy (CBT) is believed to be highly effective in OCD comorbid with tics and is recommended as the first-line treatment in children and adolescents who present with both these conditions (McGuire et al., 2015). Response to selective serotonin reuptake inhibitors (SSRIs) has been seen to be lower in those with both OCD and tics (Geller et al., 2003; March et al., 2007). In adults with OCD, tics-controlled trials have established the benefits of using antipsychotic medications (Bloch et al., 2006). Controlled data of this nature is lacking in children. A naturalistic study showed that risperidone and aripiprazole were well tolerated and effective in the treatment of tic-related pediatric OCD (Masi, Pfanner, & Brovedani, 2013).

In the absence of a robust evidence base supported by controlled trial data and concerns related to metabolic side effects, it is appropriate to follow an approach that involves ensuring CBT either in combination with or followed by SSRIs medication for OCD with tics in children. If there is no improvement, addition of low-dose antipsychotic medication may present a reasonable option.

Obsessive-Compulsive Disorder and Attention Deficit Hyperactivity Disorder

Attention deficit hyperactivity disorder (ADHD) is seen to co-occur in 25.5 percent of children and adolescents with OCD (Masi et al., 2010). Response to standard treatments for OCD was lower in children with comorbid ADHD but with higher rates of relapse following treatment (Geller et al., 2003). Treatment of both conditions is meaningful to support restored functioning and it may be prudent to start with the treatment of whichever is the most distressing and or impairing of the illnesses.

Stimulants are deemed to be the most effective class of medication in the treatment of ADHD in children. Concerns pertaining to stimulants exacerbating obsessive-compulsive symptomatology are not adequately substantiated. The addition of extended-release methylphenidate to treatment with fluvoxamine for OCD has been seen to be associated with favorable response and good tolerability surpassing placebo treatment in a randomized controlled trial (RCT) in adults (Zheng et al., 2019). Data from case studies illustrate the safety and utility of augmenting with methylphenidate and amphetamine salts in the treatment of children and young adults with OCD and comorbid ADHD (King et al., 2017; Owley et al., 2002). In the event of poor tolerability or limited benefit with stimulants, atomoxetine or alpha agonists represent suitable alternatives, the latter especially in the event of co-occurrence of tics.

Obsessive-Compulsive Disorder and Autism Spectrum Disorder

25% of youth with OCD have autism spectrum disorder (ASD; Martin et al., 2020). Establishing the diagnosis of OCD in those with ASD can pose challenges, especially in those children with limited verbal abilities. Rigidity, insistence on sameness/routine, and a strict adherence to rituals that are known to occur in ASD can bear similarities to symptoms of OCD. Establishing the ego-dystonic nature of thoughts and actions and attendant distress would be important for characterizing symptoms as OCD, a task that may not often be straightforward in clinical settings.

The accepted treatment approaches of CBT and SSRI medication, as appropriate, would be the standard of care for pediatric OCD when it co-occurs with ASD. There is a dearth of medication trials that have attempted to assess efficacy and tolerability in this subset of youth. An RCT that compared fluoxetine and placebo in the treatment of obsessive-compulsive behaviors in those children and adolescents with ASD failed to demonstrate convincingly statistically significant benefits of the medication over placebo after analyzing for confounding factors (Reddihough et al., 2019).

Obsessive-Compulsive Disorder and Depression

Distress from unremitting OCD can be associated with demoralization and it becomes important to distinguish this from clinical depression. 13 to 73 percent of children with OCD have comorbid depressive disorders. Such comorbidity has been linked to a more severe presentation with diminished response to CBT as well as pharmacological treatment (Storch et al., 2012). Severity of depressive symptoms was thought to positively correlate with suicide attempts in those with OCD. At least one out of ten patients with OCD attempted suicide over their lifetime with nearly 50 percent having suicidal ideation (Pellegrini et al., 2020).

Comorbid depression can present as an indication to consider introduction of SSRIs for the treatment of OCD in children. This is especially relevant in situations wherein depressive symptoms of poor motivation and diminished hope negatively impact engagement in CBT.

Obsessive-Compulsive Disorder and Bipolar Disorder

Overall, 15 percent of youth with OCD have comorbid bipolar disorder (BD), with an attendant increase in the likelihood of presenting with hoarding symptoms, poorer functioning, greater comorbidity (especially with anxiety disorders), and a higher rate of hospitalizations (Joshi et al., 2010). This comorbidity can pose significant challenges with treatment. While the primary pharmacological approach for OCD utilizes SSRIs, the use of SSRIs are discouraged in those with bipolar disorder as these agents could further destabilize mood.

Prioritizing the goal of mood stabilization over the treatment of OCD is recommended. A review of pediatric studies pertaining to youth with OCD and bipolar disorder suggested that the majority received mood stabilizers which is consistent with the accepted dictum of first ensuring mood stabilization (Amerio et al., 2016).

A systematic review pertaining to the treatment of the BD-OCD comorbidity in adults showed that the use of mood stabilizers alone or with second generation antipsychotics was reported in all studies. A combination of lithium and aripiprazole was seen to be effective in treating obsessive symptoms during a manic episode. The use of SSRIs was associated with a manic switch in multiple reports (Amerio et al., 2019).

Hence in pediatric patients who present with this comorbidity, it may be reasonable to consider the use of aripiprazole with or without a conventional mood stabilizing medication, considering the established benefit of aripiprazole in mood stabilization as well as emerging data on the beneficial role of this medication in treatment refractory OCD.

Obsessive-Compulsive-Related Disorders

Body Dysmorphic Disorder

Body dysmorphic disorder (BDD) is characterized by a preoccupation with perceived flaws in physical appearance that may appear either slight or absent to others, leads to repetitive behavior (checking mirrors, camouflaging rituals, etc.) and/or avoidance, and is associated with significant distress and impairment (American Psychiatric Association, 2013). It emerges in adolescence with the age of onset ranging between 4 to 17 years (Albertini & Phillips, 1999; Bjornsson et al., 2013; Rautio et al., 2022). Comorbidity is the norm and the most commonly co-occurring illnesses include depression, anxiety disorders, OCD, and substance use disorders (Mufaddel et al., 2013). High rates of suicidal ideation and attempts have been seen in those with BDD (Angelakis, Gooding, & Panagioti, 2016).

The accepted treatment approaches to BDD include a combination of SSRIs and CBT (Hong et al., 2019; Phillips, 2009). Controlled trials in adult populations with BDD established the superiority of fluoxetine to placebo and clomipramine over desipramine, indicating that modulating the serotoninergic system may have a beneficial role to play in treatment (Ipser et al., 2009). There is no controlled trial data on the pharmacotherapy of BDD in the pediatric age group. Initial case reports described benefits of treating BDD in children and adolescents with clomipramine and doxepine (Sobanski & Schmidt, 2000). Multiple subsequent case reports illustrated gains from SSRI treatment in youth. The largest published pediatric cohort was of 33 consecutive children with BDD. Ten of nineteen (53 percent) subjects treated with an SSRI had much or very much improvement in BDD symptoms. Favorable SSRI response was seen regardless of comorbid depression and OCD. Mean duration of treatment was 8±3 weeks (Albertini & Phillips, 1999).

In the absence of high-quality, controlled pediatric studies, available evidence from adult trials as well as case series in children serve as the basis for choosing SSRIs as first-line medication in the treatment of pediatric BDD. SSRIs are useful in addressing primary symptoms of BDD as well as comorbid depressive and anxiety disorders. The tolerability profile of SSRIs supports choosing this class of medication over clomipramine. It may be appropriate to introduce clomipramine after failed trials with one or two SSRI medication. Insight often tends to be limited in those with BDD (Hartmann et al., 2013; Phillips et al., 2014). It is noteworthy that evidence from adult pharmacotherapy trials suggests benefits from SSRI medication regardless of the degree of insight (Ipser et al., 2009).

Antipsychotics have been tried in BDD with mixed results (Rashid, Khan, & Fineberg, 2015) and there is no data on the use of antipsychotic medication as a standalone or augmentative approach in children and adolescents. In the event of an absence of response from trials of SSRIs and clomipramine for pediatric BDD in conjunction with CBT, augmentation with antipsychotics may be considered after weighing risks and benefits.

A four year follow up of adults and adolescents with BDD suggested that the illness often tended to run a chronic course with a higher likelihood of relapse. This gives reason to support maintenance treatment. Longitudinal follow up data from a RCT of CBT in youth with BDD demonstrated significant gains from CBT that were also maintained over time, although it emerged that a considerable proportion remained symptomatic and vulnerable to negative events at a 12-month point (Krebs et al., 2017).

Body-Focused Repetitive Behaviors

Body-focused repetitive behaviors are classified as obsessive-compulsive and related disorders (OCRDs) in the DSM-5 and are described as repetitive behavior focused on various body sites (skin picking, hair pulling, nail biting, etc.) associated with repeated attempts to stop difficulties in controlling these behaviors, attendant distress, and functional impairment. The best characterized of these include trichotillomania and excoriation disorder.

Trichotillomania (Hair Pulling Disorder)

Trichotillomania (TTM) is described as repetitive pulling out of one's hair resulting in hair loss that is accompanied by repeated attempts to decrease or stop hair pulling. This behavior causes clinically significant distress or impairment. Onset is most commonly in adolescence although onset in the younger years has also been described (Walther et al., 2014) Comorbidity is frequent with other body-focused repetitive behavior disorders, OCD, depression, and anxiety disorders (Duke et al., 2010; Panza et al., 2013). Recommended first-line treatment is behavior therapy with specific reference to habit reversal training (HRT) (Bloch et al., 2007; Flessner et al., 2010; McGuire et al., 2014).

When it comes to pharmacological treatment, SSRIs and clomipramine are frequently used, and RCTs have shown benefit, though with some variability across studies. These studies however mostly included adult participants if not a mix of different age groups (McGuire et al., 2014). Individual controlled trials have shown superiority of olanzapine over placebo as well as N-acetylcysteine (NAC) over placebo when used in adults for the treatment of TTM (Grant et al., 2009; Van Ameringen et al., 2010).

A recent well-powered double-blind placebo controlled RCT by Grant et al. (2023) randomized 100 adults with body-focused repetitive behavior (trichotillomania and skin picking disorder [SPD]) to memantine (up to 20 mg/day) and placebo and demonstrated convincing evidence for the superiority of memantine with no difference in discontinuation rates between treatments. Per the NIHM Trichotillomania Symptoms Severity Scale (NIHM-SSS), the memantine group showed a 56 percent reduction in severity compared to 9 percent in the control group, with statistically significant differences emerging at week four. The memantine group also reported a 33 percent reduction on the self-reported Massachusetts General Hospital Hairpulling Severity Scale (MGH Scale) compared to 16 percent in the control group. In addition, 60.5 percent of participants in the memantine group reported a score of "very much improved" or "much improved" using the Clinical Global Impression-Improvement scale (CGI-I 1 or 2) compared with 8.3 percent in the control group. The findings of this study are encouraging when it comes to the search for beneficial pharmacological treatments for body focused repetitive behaviors (Greenberg & Geller, 2023).

There are no FDA approved medications for TTM in children. Two randomized controlled trials that pertained to the treatment of TTM in those younger than 18 years proved to be negative studies.

1. NAC vs. placebo: 39 children who were randomly assigned to receive either NAC or placebo were followed over 12 weeks. 25 percent of the NAC group and 21 percent of the placebo group were treatment responders with no significant differences between groups (Bloch et al., 2013).
2. Milk thistle vs. placebo: Silymarin is an antioxidant contained in the plant milk thistle. Symptom measures from four children/adolescents

with TTM who were a part of a larger trial (total n=20) that predominantly included adults were separately examined and showed no differences between silymarin and placebo in terms of treatment responders, reduction in TTM symptom severity, depressive symptoms, or functional impairment (Grant et al., 2019; Hoffman et al., 2021).

An open-label pilot study that examined the use of naltrexone (mean dose: 66.07 + − 22.23 mg) in 14 children with TTM showed promising results with positive response in 11 children as depicted by improvement in CGI scores, the frequency of hair pulling, and the intensity of the urge to pull. Naltrexone was well tolerated. There is no data from controlled trials including larger samples (De Sousa, 2008).

Single case reports have shown benefits from using or augmenting with olanzapine, valproate, and atomoxetine in the treatment of TTM in children and adolescents (Adewuya, Zinser, & Thomas, 2008; Pathak, Danielya, & Kowatch, 2004; Türkoğlu & Çetin, 2018).

Excoriation (Skin Picking) Disorder

Excoriation disorder is described as repetitive skin picking resulting in skin lesions that is accompanied by repeated attempts to decrease or stop hair pulling. This behavior causes clinically significant distress or impairment. Comorbidity with mood and anxiety disorders is common. Behavioral therapy with HRT is recommended as the initial approach to treatment. SSRI medication and lamotrigine have been studied in open-label and controlled trials in adults and though these agents have demonstrated benefit, a significant placebo response has been noted that impacts interpretation of the extent of benefit. A discontinuation trial of fluoxetine adds to evidence in support of this medication in adults with SPD (Selles et al., 2016). A randomized controlled trial in adults that utilized NAC showed substantially greater improvement in those who received NAC (Grant et al., 2016).

There is no controlled data on medication and no FDA approved treatments for this disorder in children. Case studies and open-label studies suggest that NAC could potentially be useful (Miller & Angulo, 2014; Percinel & Yazici, 2014). When behavioral therapy is inadequate or unsuccessful, combining it with an SSRI medication such as fluoxetine may be appropriate considering the limited adult data as well as typical comorbidity patterns.

Hoarding Disorder

Hoarding symptoms were initially considered a part of OCD. The current version of the DSM describes hoarding disorder as a separate and distinct disorder although featured under the OCRD section. This disorder is characterized by persistent difficulties with discarding possessions regardless of their value resulting in an accumulation of possessions that clutters the living space and leads to clinically significant distress and/or impairment in functioning. Hoarding symptoms were thought to represent a subset of those with poor insight, more severe illness, and poor response to treatment.

A naturalistic study of children with OCD (Masi et al., 2005) had noted an association between hoarding symptoms and a diminished response to medication. A meta-analysis by Bloch et al. (2014) suggested a 50 percent poorer response to treatment in those with OCD and hoarding as opposed to those without hoarding symptoms independent of treatment type and age, though there were only four included studies that pertained to children.

Efforts directed at the treatment of hoarding symptoms primarily rely on cognitive-behavioral strategies with case studies describing tailored approaches targeted at addressing hoarding including in children (McKay, 2016; Tolin et al., 2015). Recent literature notes no differences in response to CBT in those children with hoarding disorder (Højgaard et al., 2019; Rozenman et al., 2019).

Conclusion

Comorbidity is a common feature in pediatric OCD, necessitating careful consideration during treatment planning. CBT and SSRIs remain the primary treatment modalities for pediatric OCD even in the presence of comorbidity, although bipolar disorder may require a different treatment approach. The grouping of OCD, body-focused repetitive behavioral disorders, and hoarding disorders under the category of OCRDs reflects their clinical similarities and shared treatment approaches involving SSRIs and CBT, though the evidence base supporting these treatments is weaker relative to what is known regarding pediatric OCD. Glutamatergic medication represent an emerging class of treatment that holds promise in the treatment of body-focused repetitive behavior disorders.

References

Adewuya, E.C., Zinser, W., & Thomas, C. (2008). Trichotillomania: A case of response to valproic acid. *Journal of Child and Adolescent Psychopharmacology*, *18*(5), 533–536. https://doi.org/10.1089/cap.2008.076.

Albertini, R.S., & Phillips, K.A. (1999). Thirty-three cases of body dysmorphic disorder in children and adolescents. *Journal of the American Academy of Child & Adolescent Psychiatry*, *38*(4), 453–459. https://doi.org/10.1097/00004583-1999 04000-00019.

American Psychiatric Association. (2013). *Diagnostic and statistical manual of mental disorders* (5th ed.). https://doi.org/10.1176/appi.books.9780890425596.

Amerio, A., Maina, G., & Ghaemi, S.N. (2019). Updates in treating comorbid bipolar disorder and obsessive-compulsive disorder: A systematic review.

Journal of Affective Disorders, *256*, 433–440. https://doi.org/10.1016/j.jad. 2019.06.015.

Amerio, A., Tonna, M., Odone, A., Stubbs, B., & Ghaemi, S.N. (2016). Comorbid bipolar disorder and obsessive-compulsive disorder in children and adolescents: Treatment implications. *Australian & New Zealand Journal of Psychiatry*, *50*(6), 594–596. https://doi.org/10.1177/0004867415611235.

Angelakis, I., Gooding, P.A., & Panagioti, M. (2016). Suicidality in body dysmorphic disorder (BDD): A systematic review with meta-analysis. *Clinical Psychology Review*, *49*, 55–66. https://doi.org/10.1016/j.cpr.2016.08.002.

Bjornsson, A.S., Didie, E.R., Grant, J.E., Menard, W., Stalker, E., & Phillips, K.A. (2013). Age at onset and clinical correlates in body dysmorphic disorder. *Comprehensive Psychiatry*, *54*(7), 893–903. https://doi.org/10.1016/j.comppsy ch.2013.03.019.

Bloch, M.H., Bartley, C.A., Zipperer, L., Jakubovski, E., Landeros-Weisenberger, A., Pittenger, C., & Leckman, J.F. (2014). Meta-analysis: Hoarding symptoms associated with poor treatment outcome in obsessive-compulsive disorder. *Molecular Psychiatry*, *19*(9), 1025–1030. https://doi.org/10.1038/mp.2014.50.

Bloch, M.H., Landeros-Weisenberger, A., Dombrowski, P., Kelmendi, B., Wegner, R., Nudel, J., Pittenger, C., Leckman, J.F., & Coric, V. (2007). Systematic review: Pharmacological and behavioral treatment for trichotillomania. *Biological Psychiatry*, *62*(8), 839–846. https://doi.org/10.1016/j.biopsych.2007.05.019.

Bloch, M.H., Landeros-Weisenberger, A., Kelmendi, B., Coric, V., Bracken, M.B., & Leckman, J.F. (2006). A systematic review: Antipsychotic augmentation with treatment refractory obsessive-compulsive disorder. *Molecular Psychiatry*, *11*(7), 622–632. https://doi.org/10.1038/sj.mp.4001823.

Bloch, M.H., Panza, K.E., Grant, J.E., Pittenger, C., & Leckman, J.F. (2013). N-Acetylcysteine in the treatment of pediatric trichotillomania: A randomized, double-blind, placebo-controlled add-on trial. *Journal of the American Academy of Child & Adolescent Psychiatry*, *52*(3), 231–240. https://doi.org/10.1016/j. jaac.2012.12.020.

De Sousa, A. (2008). An open-label pilot study of naltrexone in childhood-onset trichotillomania. *Journal of Child and Adolescent Psychopharmacology*, *18*(1), 30–33. https://doi.org/10.1089/cap.2006.0111.

Duke, D.C., Keeley, M.L., Geffken, G.R., & Storch, E.A. (2010). Trichotillomania: A current review. *Clinical Psychology Review*, *30*(2), 181–193. https://doi. org/10.1016/j.cpr.2009.10.008.

Flessner, C., Penzel, F., & Keuthen, N. (2010). Current treatment practices for children and adults with trichotillomania: Consensus among experts. *Cognitive and Behavioral Practice*, *17*(3), 290–300. https://doi.org/10.1016/j.cbpra. 2009.10.006.

Geller, D.A., Biederman, J., Stewart, S.E., Mullin, B., Farrell, C., Wagner, K.D., Emslie, G., & Carpenter, D. (2003). Impact of comorbidity on treatment response to paroxetine in pediatric obsessive-compulsive disorder: Is the use of exclusion criteria empirically supported in randomized clinical trials? *Journal of Child & Adolescent Psychopharmacology*, *13*, S19–29. https://doi. org/10.1089/104454603322126313.

Grant, J.E., Chamberlain, S.R., Redden, S.A., Leppink, E.W., Odlaug, B.L., & Kim, S.W. (2016). N-acetylcysteine in the treatment of excoriation disorder: A randomized clinical trial. *Journal of the American Medical Association Psychiatry*, *73*(5), 490–496. https://doi.org/10.1001/jamapsychiatry.2016.0060.

Grant, J.E., Chesivoir, E., Valle, S., Ehsan, D., & Chamberlain, S.R. (2023). Double-blind placebo-controlled study of memantine in trichotillomania and skin-picking disorder. *The American Journal of Psychiatry, 180*(5), 348–356. https://doi.org/10.1176/appi.ajp.20220737.

Grant, J.E., Odlaug, B.L., & Kim, S.W. (2009). N-acetylcysteine, a glutamate modulator, in the treatment of trichotillomania: A double-blind, placebo-controlled study. *Archives of General Psychiatry, 66*(7), 756–763. https://doi.org/10.1001/archgenpsychiatry.2009.60.

Grant, J.E., Redden, S.A., & Chamberlain, S.R. (2019). Milk thistle treatment for children and adults with trichotillomania: A double-blind, placebo-controlled, crossover negative study. *Journal of Clinical Psychopharmacology, 39*(2), 129–134. https://doi.org/10.1097/jcp.0000000000001005.

Greenberg, E.L., & Geller, D.A. (2023). Cautious optimism for a new treatment option for body-focused repetitive behavior disorders. *The American Journal of Psychiatry, 180*(5), 325–327. https://doi.org/10.1176/appi.ajp.20230226.

Hanna, G.L., Piacentini, J., Cantwell, D.P., Fischer, D.J., Himle, J.A., & Van Etten, M. (2002). Obsessive-compulsive disorder with and without tics in a clinical sample of children and adolescents. *Depression and Anxiety, 16*(2), 59–63. https://doi.org/10.1002/da.10058.

Hartmann, A.S., Thomas, J.J., Wilson, A.C., & Wilhelm, S. (2013). Insight impairment in body image disorders: Delusionality and overvalued ideas in anorexia nervosa versus body dysmorphic disorder. *Psychiatry Research, 210*(3), 1129–1135. https://doi.org/10.1016/j.psychres.2013.08.010.

Hoffman, J., Williams, T., Rothbart, R., Ipser, J.C., Fineberg, N., Chamberlain, S.R., & Stein, D.J. (2021). Pharmacotherapy for trichotillomania. *Cochrane Database of Systematic Reviews, 9*(9), CD007662. https://doi.org/10.1002/14651858.CD007662.pub3.

Højgaard, D., Skarphedinsson, G., Ivarsson, T., Weidle, B., Nissen, J.B., Hybel, K.A., Torp, N.C., Melin, K., & Thomsen, P.H. (2019). Hoarding in children and adolescents with obsessive-compulsive disorder: Prevalence, clinical correlates, and cognitive behavioral therapy outcome. *European Child & Adolescent Psychiatry, 28*(8), 1097–1106. https://doi.org/10.1007/s00787-019-01276-x.

Hong, K., Nezgovorova, V., Uzunova, G., Schlussel, D., & Hollander, E. (2019). Pharmacological treatment of body dysmorphic disorder. *Current Neuropharmacology, 17*(8), 697–702. https://doi.org/10.2174/1570159x16666180426153940.

Ipser, J.C., Sander, C., & Stein, D.J. (2009). Pharmacotherapy and psychotherapy for body dysmorphic disorder. *Cochrane Database of Systematic Reviews, 2009*(1), CD005332. https://doi.org/10.1002/14651858.CD005332.pub2.

Joshi, G., Wozniak, J., Petty, C., Vivas, F., Yorks, D., Biederman, J., & Geller, D. (2010). Clinical characteristics of comorbid obsessive-compulsive disorder and bipolar disorder in children and adolescents. *Bipolar Disorders, 12*(2), 185–195. https://doi.org/10.1111/j.1399-5618.2010.00795.x.

King, J., Dowling, N., & Leow, F. (2017). Methylphenidate in the treatment of an adolescent female with obsessive-compulsive disorder and attention deficit hyperactivity disorder: A case report. *Australasian Psychiatry, 25*(2), 178–180. https://doi.org/10.1177/1039856216671664.

Krebs, G., Fernández de la Cruz, L., Monzani, B., Bowyer, L., Anson, M., Cadman, J., Heyman, I., Turner, C., Veale, D., & Mataix-Cols, D. (2017). Long-term outcomes of cognitive-behavioral therapy for adolescent body dysmorphic disorder. *Behavior Therapy, 48*(4), 462–473. https://doi.org/10.1016/j.beth.2017.01.001.

Leckman, J.F., Denys, D., Simpson, H.B., Mataix-Cols, D., Hollander, E., Saxena, S., Miguel, E.C., Rauch, S.L., Goodman, W.K., Phillips, K.A., & Stein, D.J.

(2010). Obsessive-compulsive disorder: A review of the diagnostic criteria and possible subtypes and dimensional specifiers for DSM-V. *Depression and Anxiety*, 27(6), 507–527. https://doi.org/10.1002/da.20669.

Leckman, J.F., Grice, D.E., Barr, L.C., de Vries, A.L., Martin, C., Cohen, D.J., McDougle, C.J., Goodman, W.K., & Rasmussen, S.A. (1994). Tic-related vs. non-tic-related obsessive compulsive disorder. *Anxiety*, 1(5), 208–215.

March, J.S., Franklin, M.E., Leonard, H., Garcia, A., Moore, P., Freeman, J., & Foa, E. (2007). Tics moderate treatment outcome with sertraline but not cognitive-behavior therapy in pediatric obsessive-compulsive disorder. *Biological Psychiatry*, 61(3), 344–347. https://doi.org/10.1016/j.biopsych.2006.09.035.

Martin, A.F., Jassi, A., Cullen, A.E., Broadbent, M., Downs, J., & Krebs, G. (2020). Co-occurring obsessive-compulsive disorder and autism spectrum disorder in young people: Prevalence, clinical characteristics and outcomes. *European Child & Adolescent Psychiatry*, 29(11), 1603–1611. https://doi.org/10.1007/s00787-020-01478-8.

Masi, G., Millepiedi, S., Mucci, M., Bertini, N., Milantoni, L., & Arcangeli, F. (2005). A naturalistic study of referred children and adolescents with obsessive-compulsive disorder. *Journal of the American Academy of Child and Adolescent Psychiatry*, 44(7), 673–681. https://doi.org/10.1097/01.chi.0000161648.82775.ee.

Masi, G., Millepiedi, S., Perugi, G., Pfanner, C., Berloffa, S., Pari, C., Mucci, M., & Akiskal, H.S. (2010). A naturalistic exploratory study of the impact of demographic, phenotypic and comorbid features in pediatric obsessive-compulsive disorder. *Psychopathology*, 43(2), 69–78. https://doi.org/10.1159/000274175.

Masi, G., Pfanner, C., & Brovedani, P. (2013). Antipsychotic augmentation of selective serotonin reuptake inhibitors in resistant tic-related obsessive-compulsive disorder in children and adolescents: A naturalistic comparative study. *Journal of Psychiatric Research*, 47(8), 1007–1012. https://doi.org/10.1016/j.jpsychires.2013.04.003.

McGuire, J.F., Ung, D., Selles, R.R., Rahman, O., Lewin, A.B., Murphy, T.K., & Storch, E.A. (2014). Treating trichotillomania: A meta-analysis of treatment effects and moderators for behavior therapy and serotonin reuptake inhibitors. *Journal of Psychiatric Research*, 58, 76–83. https://doi.org/10.1016/j.jpsychires.2014.07.015.

McGuire, J.F., Piacentini, J., Lewin, A.B., Brennan, E.A., Murphy, T.K., & Storch, E.A. (2015). A meta-analysis of cognitive behavior therapy and medication for child obsessive–compulsive disorder: Moderators of treatment efficacy, response, and remission. *Depression and anxiety*, 32(8), 580–593. https://doi.org/10.1002/da.22389.

McKay, D. (2016). Cognitive-behavioral treatment of hoarding in youth: A case illustration. *Journal of Clinical Psychology*, 72(11), 1209–1218. https://doi.org/10.1002/jclp.22400.

Miller, J.L., & Angulo, M. (2014). An open-label pilot study of N-acetylcysteine for skin-picking in Prader-Willi syndrome. *American Journal of Medical Genetics Part A*, 164a(2), 421–424. https://doi.org/10.1002/ajmg.a.36306.

Mufaddel, A., Osman, O.T., Almugaddam, F., & Jafferany, M. (2013). A review of body dysmorphic disorder and its presentation in different clinical settings. *Primary Care Companion for CNS Disorders*, 15(4). https://doi.org/10.4088/PCC.12r01464.

Owley, T., Owley, S., Leventhal, B., & Cook, E.H., Jr. (2002). Case series: Adderall augmentation of serotonin reuptake inhibitors in childhood-onset obsessive compulsive disorder. *Journal of Child and Adolescent Psychopharmacology*, 12(2), 165–171. https://doi.org/10.1089/104454602760219207.

Panza, K.E., Pittenger, C., & Bloch, M.H. (2013). Age and gender correlates of pulling in pediatric trichotillomania. *Journal of the American Academy of Child and Adolescent Psychiatry*, 52(3), 241–249. https://doi.org/10.1016/j.jaac.2012.12.019.

Pathak, S., Danielyan, A., & Kowatch, R.A. (2004). Successful treatment of trichotillomania with olanzapine augmentation in an adolescent. *Journal of Child and Adolescent Psychopharmacology*, 14(1), 153–154. https://doi.org/10.1089/104454604773840616.

Pellegrini, L., Maietti, E., Rucci, P., Casadei, G., Maina, G., Fineberg, N.A., & Albert, U. (2020). Suicide attempts and suicidal ideation in patients with obsessive-compulsive disorder: A systematic review and meta-analysis. *Journal of Affective Disorders*, 276, 1001–1021. https://doi.org/10.1016/j.jad.2020.07.115.

Percinel, I., & Yazici, K.U. (2014). Glutamatergic dysfunction in skin-picking disorder: Treatment of a pediatric patient with N-acetylcysteine. *Journal of Clinical Psychopharmacology*, 34(6), 772–774. https://doi.org/10.1097/jcp.0000000000000210.

Phillips, K.A. (2009). *Understanding body dysmorphic disorder: An essential guide.* Oxford University Press.

Phillips, K.A., Hart, A.S., Simpson, H.B., & Stein, D.J. (2014). Delusional versus nondelusional body dysmorphic disorder: Recommendations for DSM-5. *CNS Spectrums*, 19(1), 10–20. https://doi.org/10.1017/s1092852913000266.

Rashid, H., Khan, A.A., & Fineberg, N.A. (2015). Adjunctive antipsychotic in the treatment of body dysmorphic disorder: A retrospective naturalistic case note study. *International Journal of Psychiatry in Clinical Practice*, 19(2), 84–89. https://doi.org/10.3109/13651501.2014.981546.

Rautio, D., Jassi, A., Krebs, G., Andrén, P., Monzani, B., Gumpert, M., Lewis, A., Peile, L., Sevilla-Cermeño, L., Jansson-Fröjmark, M., Lundgren, T., Hillborg, M., Silverberg-Morse, M., Clark, B., Fernández de la Cruz, L., & Mataix-Cols, D. (2022). Clinical characteristics of 172 children and adolescents with body dysmorphic disorder. *European Child & Adolescent Psychiatry*, 31(1), 133–144. https://doi.org/10.1007/s00787-020-01677-3.

Reddihough, D.S., Marraffa, C., Mouti, A., O'Sullivan, M., Lee, K.J., Orsini, F., Hazell, P., Granich, J., Whitehouse, A.J.O., Wray, J., Dossetor, D., Santosh, P., Silove, N., & Kohn, M. (2019). Effect of fluoxetine on obsessive-compulsive behaviors in children and adolescents with autism spectrum disorders: A randomized clinical trial. *Journal of the American Medical Association Psychiatry*, 322(16), 1561–1569. https://doi.org/10.1001/jama.2019.14685.

Rozenman, M., McGuire, J., Wu, M., Ricketts, E., Peris, T., O'Neill, J., Bergman, R.L., Chang, S., & Piacentini, J. (2019). Hoarding symptoms in children and adolescents with obsessive-compulsive disorder: Clinical features and response to cognitive-behavioral therapy. *Journal of the American Academy of Child and Adolescent Psychiatry*, 58(8), 799–805. https://doi.org/10.1016/j.jaac.2019.01.017.

Selles, R.R., McGuire, J.F., Small, B.J., & Storch, E.A. (2016). A systematic review and meta-analysis of psychiatric treatments for excoriation (skin-picking) disorder. *General Hospital Psychiatry*, 41, 29–37. https://doi.org/10.1016/j.genhosppsych.2016.04.001.

Sobanski, E., & Schmidt, M.H. (2000). 'Everybody looks at my pubic bone'—a case report of an adolescent patient with body dysmorphic disorder. *Acta Psychiatrica*

Scandinavica, *101*(1), 80–82. https://doi.org/10.1034/j.1600-0447.2000.10100 1080.x.

Storch, E.A., Lewin, A.B., Larson, M.J., Geffken, G.R., Murphy, T.K., & Geller, D.A. (2012). Depression in youth with obsessive-compulsive disorder: Clinical phenomenology and correlates. *Psychiatry Research*, *196*(1), 83–89. https://doi.org/10.1016/j.psychres.2011.10.013.

Tolin, D.F., Frost, R.O., Steketee, G., & Muroff, J. (2015). Cognitive behavioral therapy for hoarding disorder: A meta-analysis. *Depression and anxiety*, *32*(3), 158–166. https://doi.org/10.1002/da.22327.

Türkoğlu, S., & Çetin, F.H. (2018). Atomoxetine in the treatment of adolescent with trichotillomania and attention-deficit/hyperactivity disorder. *Clinical Neuropharmacology*, *41*(2), 84–85. https://doi.org/10.1097/wnf.0000000000000273.

Van Ameringen, M., Mancini, C., Patterson, B., Bennett, M., & Oakman, J. (2010). A randomized, double-blind, placebo-controlled trial of olanzapine in the treatment of trichotillomania. *Journal of Clinical Psychiatry*, *71*(10), 1336–1343. https://doi.org/10.4088/JCP.09m05114gre.

Walther, M.R., Snorrason, I., Flessner, C.A., Franklin, M.E., Burkel, R., & Woods, D.W. (2014). The trichotillomania impact project in young children (TIP-YC): Clinical characteristics, comorbidity, functional impairment and treatment utilization. *Child Psychiatry & Human Development*, *45*(1), 24–31. https://doi.org/10.1007/s10578-013-0373-y.

Zheng, H., Jia, F., Han, H., Wang, S., Guo, G., Quan, D., Li, G., & Huang, H. (2019). Combined fluvoxamine and extended-release methylphenidate improved treatment response compared to fluvoxamine alone in patients with treatment-refractory obsessive-compulsive disorder: A randomized double-blind, placebo-controlled study. *European Neuropsychopharmacology*, *29*(3), 397–404. https://doi.org/10.1016/j.euroneuro.2018.12.010.

Zohar, A.H., Pauls, D.L., Ratzoni, G., Apter, A., Dycian, A., Binder, M., King, R., Leckman, J.F., Kron, S., & Cohen, D.J. (1997). Obsessive-compulsive disorder with and without tics in an epidemiological sample of adolescents. *American Journal of Psychiatry*, *154*(2), 274–276. https://doi.org/10.1176/ajp.154.2.274.

13 Advancing Dissemination and Implementation of Treatment for Obsessive-Compulsive and Related Disorders

Gudmundur Skarphedinsson,[1] *Orri Smárason*[1] *and Davíð R.M.A. Højgaard*[2]

[1] *Faculty of Psychology, University of Iceland, Reykjavik, Iceland*

[2] *Department of Child and Adolescent Psychiatry, Aarhus University Hospital Psychiatry, Denmark*

I. Introduction

Obsessive-compulsive and related disorders (OCRDs), tic disorders (TDs), and illness anxiety disorder represent a set of psychiatric conditions characterized by repetitive thoughts, behaviors, or impulses that significantly impact daily functioning. OCRDs include obsessive-compulsive disorder (OCD), body dysmorphic disorder (BDD), trichotillomania (hair-pulling disorder), excoriation disorder (skin-picking disorder), and hoarding disorder. While TDs involve involuntary muscle movements or vocalizations, illness anxiety disorder revolves around preoccupation with having a serious illness. Although they are distinct conditions, they often co-occur and share similarities in treatment approaches (American Psychiatric Association, 2022).

Although evidence-based treatments, including cognitive-behavioral therapy (CBT) and pharmacological interventions, are available, many young people suffering from these conditions do not receive adequate care. This is primarily due to barriers like a scarcity of specialized mental health professionals, limited availability of evidence-based treatment, and societal stigma surrounding mental health treatment. This necessitates the development of effective strategies for the dissemination and implementation of these evidence-based treatments (Geller & March, 2012).

Dissemination and implementation (DI) science aims at creating opportunities to develop, adapt, and evaluate mental health treatments within community settings (American Academy of Child and Adolescent Psychiatry, 2009; Proctor et al., 2009). Expanding access to CBT for OCD and related disorders through dissemination is crucial for public health (McHugh &

DOI: 10.4324/9781003386278-13

Barlow, 2010; Freeman et al., 2018) and consequently, has become a key funding priority (National Institute of Mental Health [NIMH], 2023).

This chapter provides a comprehensive overview of the current efforts to disseminate and implement evidence-based treatments of OCRDs for children and adolescents. We will discuss theoretical foundations, supporting evidence, and future directions for the field, covering various dissemination strategies such as professional training, public awareness campaigns, and advocacy and policy development. The chapter will also describe implementation strategies, including task-shifting and task-sharing approaches, the use of technology to deliver treatment, and culturally and contextually adapted interventions. By examining these strategies and their potential impact, this chapter aims to contribute to the ongoing efforts to improve access to care and outcomes for children and adolescents with OCRDs.

II. Evidence-Based Treatment for Obsessive-Compulsive and Related Disorders

Cognitive and Behavioral Approaches

CBT is the most efficacious and well-studied psychotherapy for OCD, BDD, health anxiety, and hoarding disorder (Cooper et al., 2017; David, Crone, & Norberg, 2022; Harrison et al., 2016; Skarphedinsson et al., 2015; Ost et al., 2016). Numerous studies have demonstrated the efficacy of CBT with exposure and response prevention (ERP) for OCD compared with pharmacotherapy alone, as well as other active control conditions (Ivarsson et al., 2015; Ferrando & Selai, 2021). CBT with ERP for BDD has also demonstrated efficacy, although most studies use waitlist and psychological placebo control conditions in adult populations (Harrison et al., 2016). For health anxiety, CBT has also been found to be effective compared to medication and active control conditions in adults (Cooper et al., 2017), but very few data are available for pediatric populations (Rask, 2019). For hoarding disorder, CBT is superior to waitlist control conditions in adults (David, Crone & Norberg, 2022), but minimal data exist for pediatric populations (Højgaard & Skarphedinsson, 2023). Although CBT with ERP is typically delivered in a face-to-face setting with weekly hour-long therapy sessions, it has also been found to be effective in intensive (Remmerswaal et al., 2021; Storch et al., 2010) and telehealth formats (Hiranandani et al., 2023; Orsolini et al., 2021)(Storch et al., 2011).

For TD and body-focused repetitive behaviors (BFRB), including trichotillomania and excoriation disorder, habit reversal training (HRT) is the most efficacious known psychotherapy (Liu, Li, & Cui, 2020; Skurya et al., 2020). HRT consists of training patients to become acutely aware of their premonitory urges to tic, or do other repetitive behaviors, and then implement a competing, incompatible response instead of performing the tic or repetitive behavior (Liu et al., 2020). HRT, as well as protocols primarily based on HRT – such as the Comprehensive Behavioral Intervention for Tics (CBIT; Franklin, Walther, & Woods, 2010; Piacentini et al., 2010) – have demonstrated efficacy in pediatric samples for TD compared to waitlist and active treatment control conditions (Liu et al., 2020; Yu et al., 2020). For BFRB, HRT has shown efficacy compared to waitlist and attentional control conditions (Farhat et al., 2020).

Pharmacotherapy

First-line medications for OCD in children and adolescents are selective serotonin reuptake inhibitors (SSRIs) due to their efficacy and tolerability (Weidle et al., 2021). SSRI's have also been found to be potentially effective in BDD, hoarding, and health anxiety, but have almost exclusively been studied in adult samples for those disorders (Asmundson et al., 2010; Bjornsson, Didie, & Phillips, 2010; Morris et al., 2016; Rask, 2019). Randomized controlled trials (RCTs) have demonstrated that serotonin reuptake inhibitors (SRIs) (both SSRIs and clomipramine) are superior to placebo in the treatment of OCD (Ivarsson et al., 2015).

For TD, the first-line medications are alpha agonists, which have demonstrated efficacy compared to placebo control conditions (Cothros, Medina, & Pringsheim, 2020). However, antipsychotics are the most effective pharmacotherapy for TD, but their use is limited by common and serious side effects, such as sedation, metabolic side effects, and drug-induced movement disorders (Cothros, Medina, & Pringsheim, 2020). For BFRB, a recent Cochrane review concluded that there was insufficient evidence to confirm or refute the efficacy of any agent or class of medication for the treatment of trichotillomania in adults, children, or adolescents (Hoffman et al., 2021). No pharmacotherapy studies were found for other OCRD subtypes.

Challenges in Accessing Evidence-Based Treatment

Following the onset of symptoms, obtaining a diagnosis for OCRD is frequently delayed, and getting access to evidence-based specialized treatment can be challenging (García-Soriano et al., 2014; Poyraz et al., 2015). Several common barriers to treatment have been identified in the literature. One such barrier is the limited availability of specialized providers. Treating OCRDs requires specialized training and finding mental health professionals with expertise in pediatric OCRD treatment may be difficult, especially in rural areas (Marques et al., 2010; Poyraz et al., 2015). Financial barriers also present a major challenge, as many OCRD patients cannot afford evidence-based treatment from private providers. Research indicates that patients from higher-income families are more likely to seek treatment (García-Soriano et al., 2014; Robertson, Paparo, & Wootton, 2020).

In addition to practical barriers, certain patient characteristics may impact treatment-seeking behavior. Studies consistently report that individuals who seek or are currently receiving treatment often experience higher symptom interference, lower quality of life, greater severity, greater insight, a higher number of symptoms, a higher number of aggressive or religious obsessions (for OCD), and more comorbidity (García-Soriano et al., 2014). Many OCRD patients feel ashamed of their thoughts and of needing help for their mental health problems, making fear of stigma a major barrier to treatment (Belloch et al., 2009; Weingarden et al., 2018; Williams et al., 2012). Lack of mental health literacy is also a treatment barrier. Patients with OCRD and their parents often believe they can manage their symptoms on their own, or that their symptoms are temporary and not serious, or do not require professional help (García-Soriano et al., 2014; Robertson, Paparo, & Wootton, 2020). Demographic factors also influence the ability to seek treatment: non-Hispanic White individuals are less likely to experience barriers related to transportation or scheduling of sessions, or choosing their provider, compared to other racial/ethnic groups (Glazier et al., 2015). African Americans are more likely than European Americans to report barriers related to cost, stigma, and transportation, especially when uninsured (Williams et al., 2012), and almost a quarter of the patients in an African-American sample reported fear of being treated unfairly because of their ethnicity (Williams et al., 2012). Inadequate or delayed intervention can result in chronic symptoms and an increased risk for further psychopathology (Fineberg et al., 2019). Consequently, it is crucial to minimize barriers to evidence-based treatment through dissemination and implementation efforts.

III.   Dissemination Strategies

Disseminating evidence-based interventions in community settings has historically been challenging, leading to a persistent "research-to-practice gap" (Schoenwald, Sheidow, & Letourneau, 2004; Weisz et al., 2013; Kazdin & Blase, 2011). For instance, many community providers have limited knowledge of exposure therapy, resulting in underutilization and inadequate treatment (Freiheit et al., 2004; Harned et al., 2014; Schwartz et al., 2013; Cook et al., 2010; Spencer et al., 2023). This knowledge gap can lead to negative beliefs about exposure therapy and suboptimal delivery (Olatunji, Deacon, & Abramowitz, 2009; Deacon et al., 2013). Therefore, it is crucial to disseminate accurate information on the assessment and treatment of OCRDs to enhance clinician competence and reduce misconceptions about exposure therapy and related techniques.

The dissemination of treatment strategies for OCRD can be understood within the Diffusion of Innovation theory (Rogers, 2003). According to this theory, the spread of new ideas and practices is influenced by the attributes of the intervention, the characteristics of individuals involved, the nature of organizational settings, and external factors such as social networks, policies, regulations, and incentives (Dearing, 2009). Organizations with stable staff, supportive leadership, open communication, and flexibility are generally more likely to effectively implement strategies (Damschroder et al., 2009; Dearing, 2009).

Implementation of treatments for OCRD is influenced by intervention characteristics, individual factors, and research literacy (Franklin et al., 2013; Dearing, 2009; Lehman, Greener, & Simpson, 2002). Therapists inclined towards CBT and trained in exposure therapy are more likely to use these treatments whereas older and more anxious therapists may be less likely to employ them (Langthorne, Beard, & Waller, 2023).

Addressing implementation barriers involves considering funding, infrastructure costs, and attitudes concerning potential effects on client-therapist relationships. Following this, external factors such as social networks, policies, regulations, and incentives also impact the adoption of OCRD treatments (Lehman, Greener, & Simpson, 2002). Strategies to encourage uptake might include expanding public-private partnerships, developing infrastructure, and implementing regulations for end-user privacy and security.

To enhance the dissemination of effective treatment strategies for OCRD, a multifaceted approach is necessary. This approach may include comprehensive professional training and development, public awareness and education campaigns, and leveraging external factors such as social networks, policies, and incentives. By examining each of these aspects in detail, a comprehensive understanding of the ways in which the field is working to promote the dissemination of evidence-based treatment approaches for OCRD can be achieved. This section of the paper on dissemination and implementation for OCDR focuses on the various strategies employed to promote the adoption and integration of evidence-based treatment approaches for OCDR. These strategies include three primary areas: professional training and development, public awareness and education campaigns, and advocacy and policy development. By examining each of these facets, we provide a comprehensive understanding of the ways in which the field is working to enhance the dissemination and implementation of effective treatment strategies for obsessive-compulsive and related disorders.

A. Professional Training and Development

To enhance professional training and development in the treatment of OCRDs, efforts should include organizing workshops and seminars, offering online training and certification programs, and expanding graduate and postgraduate curricula in psychology, psychiatry, and other mental health disciplines.

Training Workshops and Seminars

One way to disseminate evidence-based treatments is through organizing training workshops and seminars. These events should be led by experienced clinicians and researchers with expertise in OCRD. Workshops and seminars ought to provide participants with practical tools and resources, such as treatment manuals and case studies, to support the implementation of evidence-based treatments in their clinical practice.

The International OCD Foundations (IOCDF) Behavior Therapy Training Institute (BTTI) offers an interactive workshop for community clinicians seeking expertise in ERP for OCD (Reese et al., 2016). A study on BTTI outcomes reported increased use of BTTI skills and referrals for OCD patients (Reese et al., 2016). A major barrier to accessing training in CBT for OCD is the time commitment of workshops like BTTI, which requires three days of in-person attendance. Compounding the issue is the high demand for these workshops, resulting in rapid sell-outs and a large waitlist (Behavior Therapy Training Institute [BTTI], 2023). To address these issues, BTTI has implemented online workshops (Behavior Therapy Training Institute [BTTI], 2023). This adaptation not only provides a more convenient and flexible option for participants but also stands to dramatically expand the program's reach and reduce associated costs. Since only 37.5 percent of clinicians have access to CBT experts for anxiety disorders in their community (Hipol & Deacon, 2013), technology enables ongoing supervision through virtual conferencing and web-based discussion boards (Beidas et al., 2012; Harned et al., 2014).

The Progressive Cascading Model (PCM), an innovative training approach for teaching exposure-based techniques to novice therapists treating OCD, has been effectively employed in the University of Florida's OCD treatment and training program. The model leverages the idea of graduated learning, where knowledge and skills are accumulated and reinforced progressively. It allows trainees to master foundational components of treatment before moving on to more complex elements (Balkhi et al., 2016; Reid et al., 2017). After completing training within the PCM, therapists have demonstrated a more intense delivery of exposure therapy, employing less cautious behaviors and distress reduction tactics. They also exhibited reduced negative beliefs about exposure therapy and reported lower disgust sensitivity (Balkhi et al., 2016; Reid et al., 2017). The trainees expressed satisfaction with their experience, especially valuing the co-therapy approach, and felt competent in implementing exposure therapy upon program completion. Given the challenges in disseminating exposure therapy and the trend toward competency-based education, PCM warrants further research and is recommended for wider implementation in graduate training clinics (Balkhi et al., 2016; Reid et al., 2017).

Online Training and Certification Programs

Online training programs and certification courses can help disseminate evidence-based treatments to a wider audience of mental health professionals, particularly those in remote or underserved areas (McCarty et al., 2022; Ashbaugh, Cohen, & Dobson, 2021). These online programs can include a combination of self-paced learning modules, video demonstrations, live webinars, and supervised practice sessions. To ensure the quality of training, online certification programs should adhere to established standards and guidelines and require participants to complete a rigorous assessment of their skills and knowledge before granting certification.

Online training can improve therapists' knowledge and skills in the short term, particularly for CBT interventions (Dimeff et al., 2011; Kobak et al., 2013; Kobak et al., 2017). Studies have found comparable improvements in training outcomes for online and in-person formats (Stein et al., 2015; Mallonee et al., 2018). However, online training alone may not be sufficient to improve CBT competence in practice; consultation improves outcomes (Rakovshik et al., 2016; Ruzek et al., 2017). Enhancements to web-based training, such as brief support and online learning communities, may lead to better compliance with training requirements and improved proficiency (Harned et al., 2014).

A longitudinal study examined the effectiveness of disseminating CBT for OCD through two methods: (a) an online, low-intensity Psychiatry Academy for clinicians new to CBT for OCD, and (b) an in-person, intensive BTTI for experienced clinicians in OCD (Jacoby et al., 2019). Results showed that both types of training led to increased self-reported comfort in assessing and treating OCD, more positive beliefs about exposure, improved knowledge of CBT for OCD, and greater use of empirically supported principles. Online training like the Psychiatry Academy shows promise in making CBT for OCD more accessible; however, further research is needed to explore the benefits of progressing from introductory to advanced courses (Jacoby et al., 2019).

Intensive Training Approaches

Another option is intensive training approaches, which have demonstrated improvements in therapist knowledge, intervention use, and competence, with consultation being a key element (Karlin et al., 2012; Creed et al.,

2016; Stirman et al., 2017). While intensive training can be cost- and resource-intensive, some studies have found promising results with more resource-efficient models, such as web-based training with peer-led consultation (Kolko et al., 2012; German et al., 2018). However, web-based training may have lower completion rates compared to in-person training. Strategies to improve engagement in web-based training could include training with a cohort of trainees or offering salary increases for evidence-based intervention certification.

Expanding Graduate and Postgraduate Curricula

To promote the dissemination of evidence-based treatments for OCRD, it may be important to integrate specialized training into graduate and postgraduate curricula in psychology, psychiatry, and other mental health disciplines (McQuaid & Spirito, 2012). This can be achieved through the development of dedicated courses, clinical practicums, and research opportunities focused on these disorders (Hatcher et al., 2012; VanderVeen et al., 2012). By incorporating specialized training in evidence-based treatments into formal education programs, future generations of mental health professionals will be better prepared to identify and treat individuals with OCRD. This approach also promotes a culture of lifelong learning and professional development, as graduates will have a solid foundation on which to build their clinical skills and knowledge throughout their careers.

Another option might be to integrate research training into clinical internship. Doing so not only prepares mental health professionals for various career options but also enhances the scientific foundation of their practice. Potential strategies are involving interns in ongoing research projects, encouraging them to develop their own research projects, and providing exposure to the process of grantsmanship (McQuaid & Spirito, 2012).

Postdoctoral training is crucial in shaping career decisions for emerging clinical scientists. Advanced training introduces students to new research areas, collaborations, and methodologies. There is a growing focus on DI science, which leads to a call for "deployment-focused training" that prepares students for DI challenges early in their training (Weisz & Gray, 2008). Deployment-focused training aims to (a) integrate treatments into clinical practice early in their development and (b) view testing in practice settings as a sequential process rather than a single final phase. The primary goal is to adapt evidence-based treatments, which have shown efficacy, for testing and use in their intended practice contexts. The underlying premise is that a treatment's potential is most likely to be realized if adapted to practice conditions after initial efficacy trials (Weisz, 2015).

Collaboration with professional associations, academic institutions, and healthcare organizations is essential to provide ongoing education and training opportunities for mental health professionals. This collaboration can contribute to more widespread and effective implementation of evidence-based treatments in clinical practice.

In conclusion, comprehensive professional training and development are crucial for effective dissemination of evidence-based CBT for OCD. A combination of training workshops and seminars, online training and certification programs, and expanded graduate and postgraduate curricula can help achieve this goal. The PCM and other novel training approaches, along with the adoption of competency-based education models in graduate training programs, show promise in enhancing the knowledge and skills of mental health professionals in treating OCD. Further research is needed to refine these approaches and ensure their effectiveness in diverse settings and populations.

B. Public Awareness and Education Campaigns

Increasing public awareness and understanding of OCRDs is a crucial component of effective dissemination strategies. By raising awareness about these conditions, their symptoms, and available treatments, public education campaigns can help reduce stigma, encourage individuals to seek help, and foster a supportive environment for those affected by these disorders.

Use of Media and Social Platforms

Media outlets and social platforms can be instrumental in disseminating accurate and accessible information about mental health awareness (Latha et al., 2020; Chen & Wang, 2021). Collaborations with journalists, influencers, and online communities can help raise awareness and promote understanding of these conditions. Public service announcements, documentaries, and informative articles can be leveraged to provide accurate information about the symptoms, prevalence, and available treatments for these disorders (Chen & Wang, 2021). Social media platforms can be valuable for patient engagement, publicity, transparency, knowledge sharing, and implementing research findings in society (Chen & Wang, 2021).

Community Outreach and Engagement, Collaboration With Schools

Community-based outreach programs and events can be organized to educate the public about OCRDs. These can include workshops, support groups, and educational sessions held at local schools, community centers, and places of worship. By partnering with community leaders and organizations, mental health professionals can reach a broader audience and promote a more inclusive approach to mental health education. These outreach initiatives can also provide opportunities for individuals with OCRDs and their families to connect with others who share similar experiences, fostering a sense of belonging and support within the community (McDavitt et al., 2016).

It may also be important to share research findings with community members and engage them in the dissemination process. Key strategies include creating a flexible dissemination plan, tailoring presentations to various community groups, establishing a community liaison, and continuing dialogue with community members after presentations. Building trust is crucial and can be achieved by engaging community members at every step, allowing ample time for discussion, sharing personal experiences, being receptive to criticism, and implementing community input. This approach can lead to a better understanding of research findings, strengthen community-academic partnerships, and promote culturally relevant interventions and public policy (McDavitt et al., 2016).

One key resource in the awareness and education efforts for pediatric OCD is the website www.ocdinkids.org, which offers up-to-date information for various stakeholders. The website's content is developed by leading pediatric OCD experts from the Scientific and Clinical Advisory Board. A new resource, the Anxiety in the Classroom website, https://anxietyinthe classroom.org, will offer a digital educational tool for understanding anxiety and OCD in school settings. Additionally, informational brochures, fact sheets, and FAQs about pediatric OCD and pediatric autoimmune neuropsychiatric disorder associated with streptococcus/pediatric acute neuropsychiatric syndrome (PANDAS/PANS) are available. The Annual OCD Conference is another platform for learning and support, providing programming for various age groups, families, and professionals. Personal accounts from individuals dealing with pediatric OCD are also shared on their website, blog, and newsletter to reduce stigma and raise awareness.

C. *Advocacy and Policy Development*

Advocacy and policy development play a vital role in the dissemination and implementation of evidence-based treatments for obsessive-compulsive and related disorders. By influencing legislation, funding priorities, and healthcare practices, advocacy efforts can help ensure that individuals with these disorders have access to high-quality care and support.

The International OCD Foundation (IOCDF) advocates for public policy that positively impacts individuals with OCRDs, their families, and professionals. Their strategic goals aim to improve access to effective treatment and support in communities and enhance clinicians' capacity to provide effective care. This means making treatment for OCD and related disorders affordable, widely available, and effective, and ensuring community support. To achieve these goals, the IOCDF collaborates with mental health organizations, raises awareness of policy issues, engages in lobbying and grassroots activism, involves stakeholders, and provides training and capacity-building (International OCD Foundation, 2023).

Lobbying for Increased Funding for Research and Treatment

Advocacy efforts should focus on securing increased funding for research and treatment of OCRDs. This can include lobbying for more government and private sector funding for basic and clinical research (Hegde & Sampat, 2015), as well as advocating for expanded insurance coverage and reimbursement for evidence-based treatments. Increased funding can help support the development of new treatment approaches, facilitate the evaluation and refinement of existing interventions, and ultimately improve access to care for individuals with these disorders.

Integrating Mental Health Services Into Primary Care Settings

Policy development should aim to integrate mental health services into primary care settings, which can help reduce barriers to treatment and promote early identification and intervention for individuals with OCRDs. By incorporating mental health screenings and referrals into routine primary care visits, healthcare professionals can better identify patients who may be struggling with these disorders and facilitate their access to specialized care. Advocacy efforts should also focus on promoting collaboration and communication between primary care providers and mental health specialists. This can include the development of shared care models, referral networks, and collaborative treatment planning processes that ensure individuals with OCRDs receive comprehensive and coordinated care (Raphel & Fry-Bowers, 2021; Funk et al., 2008).

Developing Guidelines and Best Practices

To ensure the consistent and effective dissemination and implementation of evidence-based treatments for OCRDs, it is crucial to develop guidelines and best practices that can be adopted by mental health professionals and healthcare organizations (Geller & March, 2012; National Institute for Health and Clinical Excellence, 2005).

Professional associations, in collaboration with researchers and clinicians, should develop evidence-based guidelines that outline the recommended assessment, diagnosis, and treatment approaches for these disorders. These guidelines should be regularly updated to reflect advances in research and clinical practice (Geller & March, 2012). Additionally, advocacy efforts should focus on promoting the adoption of these guidelines and best practices by healthcare organizations and providers. This can include developing resources and training materials to support the implementation of evidence-based treatments, as well as advocating for the inclusion of these guidelines in accreditation and quality assurance processes.

IV. Implementation Strategies

Implementation

While effective treatment options for OCRDs exist, their utilization in clinical practice remains surprisingly low. This discrepancy emphasizes a significant issue known as the "research-to-practice-gap" (Kazdin & Blase, 2011), a persistent delay in the application of research-derived methods in actual clinical settings. Indeed, studies indicate that nearly half of new clinical developments fail to become routine practice (Balas & Boren, 2000).

Primary among evidence-based psychological treatment for OCRDs is CBT with ERP. However, research from the US has shown that exposure-based therapy is rarely used in routine care outside universities. A majority of mental health professionals report that they never or rarely use this form of therapy (Cook et al., 2010; Whiteside et al., 2016). When asked directly, only 29.3 percent indicated that they were treated with exposure-based interventions during treatment (Böhm et al., 2008).

In this context, proper implementation becomes another factor that affects treatment outcomes. A recent review identified 23 contextual factors potentially influencing implementation (Durlak & DuPre, 2008). Implementing evidence-based psychological treatments for OCDRs in community and hospital settings has specific challenges. The subsequent discussion aims to briefly outline these obstacles and suggest potential strategies to overcome them.

Available Resources, Training, and Task-Shifting

The foremost challenge in implementing evidence-based psychological treatments for OCRDs is that they are very resource demanding. In most scenarios, the availability of trained specialists is limited, with trained therapists often entirely absent, particularly in rural areas and low-income countries (Raj et al., 2022).

One way to overcome this is to increase the availability of training opportunities for already available therapists to make them meet the current requirements of expertise. However, it is important to raise the awareness of clinicians about the effectiveness of these treatment programs. Since training programs can be time-consuming and expensive, their introduction would require government investment in mental healthcare. One way to overcome this and meet demand is by task shifting (also known as task sharing), which involves the shifting of tasks from highly trained therapists to less trained individuals, including non-specialist healthcare providers, allowing for more efficient use of resources (Hoeft et al., 2018). Task shifting would, in many cases, change the role of the specialist therapist to a supervisor or consultant, instead of an actual therapist.

Digitally Administered Interventions and Training Programs

Another barrier to accessing evidence-based treatment for OCDRs is geographical distance, in addition to economic constraints and limited availability. Digitally administered treatments and videoconferencing, preferably with therapist guidance via text or video conversations, can help to overcome the geographical distance barrier (Lundström et al., 2022).

Digitally applied CBT programs can also increase the availability of evidence-based therapy. These programs are cost-effective and not location-dependent, requiring minimal therapist contact during the treatment (Aspvall et al., 2021). Despite their effectiveness, more programs specific to OCRDs other than OCD are needed. Regarding digitally applied CBT for pediatric OCD, there is valuable information to be gained from the implementation of a program developed in Sweden (Aspvall et al., 2020). Based on their program called BIP OCD, which had previously been shown to be effective in the initial studies in clinical-academic settings, they aimed to evaluate the implementation of the program in different settings, including three different clinics in Sweden, the United Kingdom, and Australia. To do this they measured the acceptability, feasibility, and preliminary effectiveness of BIP OCD implementation. They found the implementation to be successful as the program was transferrable to outpatient clinics. However, it is important to continuously revise the intervention as well as gather data from completers as well as non-completers. Additionally, they concluded that the implementation was dependent on specific healthcare contexts as well as the training of therapists (Aspvall et al., 2020). Future work should evaluate if digitally administrated CBT programs for OCRDs are efficacious when assisted by non-specialists who have been properly trained and are supervised during treatment.

Digitally administered training to therapists may be advantageous in several ways as it permits audio and visual examples of implementing therapeutic strategies that match the needs of the therapist. It can also be fitted to the therapists' time schedule and can be easily accessed.

To be able to implement digitally administered therapy, there are some prerequisites that need to be fulfilled, including internet access, computer access, and the required minimum knowledge to use this technology. In low-income countries where internet access is not readily available, a solution could be to establish centers where users could be offered the required equipment and guidance to use it. Another aspect of this is that privacy needs to be ensured, both technology-wise and at the user end. In some cases, the clinic has provided patients with equipment during the length of the treatment, and in this way also ensured hardware compatibility as well as sound and video quality (Khanna, Kerns, & Carper, 2014).

Assessment and monitoring of patients with OCRDs can also be done by administrating psychological questionnaires via webpages, phone apps, or videoconferencing systems. However, to ensure proper implementation more validation of these tools is needed as they are not as well examined as some of the treatment tools (Ferreri et al., 2019).

Stigma and Cultural Aspects of Implementation

Stigma is unfortunately still a major concern regarding treatment of OCRDs and many individuals may be reluctant to seek treatment due to societal prejudice. This issue varies considerably across countries and is influenced by culture and traditions. This may even manifest in such a way that the one affected is unaware that his or her symptoms are related to a specific disorder, and that effective treatments exist. When this is the case, it is important to increase public awareness of OCRDs with educational campaigns that also talk about the availability of treatment.

A specific issue with the implementation of exposure-based interventions is the stigma surrounding exposure in therapy. A survey from 2019 showed that among therapists, between 23 percent and 52 percent agreed with negative beliefs that either exposure caused too much distress for the patient or that the effects were superficial only. In the same survey, 24.8 percent of therapists believed that sessions outside the office would endanger patient confidentiality, but according to research the effect of exposure is optimized when it is performed in the patient's usual settings. These beliefs are problematic as they may lead to a less than optimal treatment and outcome, and the implementation of exposure-based CBT should therefore take these views into account (Pittig, Kotter, & Hoyer, 2019).

Digitally delivered CBT may also mitigate the stigma sometimes associated with mental health services by offering more privacy than visiting a clinic or hospital in person (Gega, Marks, & Mataix-Cols, 2004).

In the adaptation of treatment programs, cultural considerations often play a significant role. In fact, a recent review revealed that 64.3 percent of the adaptations were made due to cultural factors (Escoffery et al., 2018).

Before implementation, it is therefore important to evaluate any mismatch between the original treatment protocol and the characteristics of the population. Several elements of the treatment may need to be adapted, including program components, content, provider, and means of delivery (Smith & Caldwell, 2007). An example of adaptation in digitally administered programs for OCRDs could be remaking videos and illustrations to reflect the culture and setting, rather than just translating the language. This could also be as simple as adding a moment of silence to the beginning of therapy each session to acknowledge the spiritual practices of participants (Escoffery et al., 2018).

In conclusion, implementing evidence-based treatments for OCDRs in community settings can be challenging, but these challenges can be partially overcome by using the right strategies. Increasing the availability of training programs for therapists, task-shifting, developing digital treatment programs, making cultural adaptations, and increasing awareness of OCDRs and the available treatment options are important to achieve this goal.

V. Measuring Success and Outcomes

Evaluating Dissemination and Implementation Strategies

Dissemination and implementation ultimately aim to improve the adoption, delivery, and sustainment of effective interventions. Several frameworks have been developed to assess the outcomes and relative success of dissemination and implementation efforts (Brown et al., 2017). However, studies have used widely varying approaches to measure how well a new treatment or program is disseminated and/or implemented. Debates about research designs for this emerging field are often predicated on conflicting views of dissemination and implementation research and practice, such as whether the evaluation is intended to produce generalizable knowledge, support local quality improvement, or both (Cheung & Duan, 2014), as well as debates about how much emphasis to place on internal validity compared with external validity (Brown et al., 2017; Green & Glasgow, 2006). Despite these debates and differing frameworks, there are certain well-established outcomes of dissemination and implementation research, namely, adoption, fidelity, sustainability, and cost (Dopp et al., 2019; Proctor et al., 2011; Shelton et al., 2020). Adoption, also referred to as uptake, is the intention or initial decision to try or employ an innovation or therapy in clinical practice (Lewis, Proctor, & Brownson, 2017). Fidelity is the degree to which an intervention is implemented as prescribed in a treatment protocol or manual designed by treatment developers (Proctor et al., 2011). Fidelity consists of at least three components: (1) *treatment adherence* (i.e., the degree to which a clinician delivers the treatment as designed), (2) *treatment differentiation* (i.e., the degree to which a treatment differs from other treatments in specific ways as specified in a treatment manual), and (3) *competence* (i.e., the skill and responsiveness of the clinician in delivering the technical and relational components of the treatment) (McLeod, Southam-Gerow, & Weisz, 2009). Sustainability is defined as the extent to which a newly implemented treatment is maintained within a service setting's ongoing operations (Proctor, Powell, & Feely, 2014). Assessing the costs, as well as benefits, associated with an evidence-based intervention and the implementation strategies that are necessary for implementing it, is essential to provide meaningful guidance to decision-makers in real-world service contexts (Proctor, Powell, & Feely, 2014). Several measurement tools and assessment protocols exist for these outcomes and should be used when implementing new interventions (Proctor, Powell, & Feely, 2014).

VI.   Future Directions

With increasing demand for psychiatric services and limited human resources, even in the most developed countries, there is a need for a shift in how these resources are allocated. CBT for OCRDs is, and will continue to be, the recommended treatment for the foreseeable future, at least until a breakthrough in our understanding of the etiology of these disorders has occurred. Until then, the utilization of technology in assessment and treatment seems to be the most effective strategy for increasing the cost-effectiveness of treatment, as examples from OCD treatments have shown (Aspvall et al., 2021).

The implementation of evidence-based CBT programs in communities where they are broadly accessible, along with training of therapists that can support them, should be a high priority. However, the development of these programs needs to go hand in hand with technological development, evaluation, and implementation (Marsch et al., 2015). Also, future studies should examine digitally delivered CBT in the context of stepped-care models, where the level of therapist contact is carefully evaluated in each step. Furthermore, as implementation is highly dependent on the local healthcare structure and culture, future studies need to be performed in the actual settings where the programs will be implemented.

Technology advances at a high speed, and when new technologies emerge that may hold the potential to improve the delivery of CBT, they should be explored. Artificial intelligence (AI) is an inevitable part of future digital interventions for psychiatric disorders, including OCDRs. A possible benefit of AI supplementing internet-delivered CBT could be active monitoring of treatment assignments, saving some of the therapists' time, as well as potentially reduced attrition as the interaction becomes more "human-like". Furthermore, AI could be used to tailor treatment according to individual needs. Currently, there is not much research available in the field of OCRDs, but AI in the form of chatbots has been shown to be more effective in RCTs than psychoeducation alone in treating symptoms of depression and anxiety in young adults (Fitzpatrick et al., 2017; Fulmer et al., 2018; Klos et al., 2021). One study has demonstrated the feasibility of using an AI chatbot to deliver CBT to adolescents suffering from moderate depression during the COVID-19 pandemic (Nicol et al., 2022). Future research should therefore examine the advantages and possible drawbacks of implementing AI into digitally delivered CBT for OCRDs.

The importance of implementing evidence-based digitally delivered CBT cannot be overstated, but future studies should also focus on developing new treatments for OCRDs as well as strengthening our research methods (Geller & Hosker, 2020). This is important as many do not benefit sufficiently from CBT alone. Currently, there are limited means to predict who will benefit from CBT and psychopharmacological treatment, and therefore research should strive to examine possible predictors of treatment outcome. Expanding interdisciplinary collaborations with various somatic fields of medicine is critical to further advancement in the field. Already, studies of genetics and immunology have shown promise for the future of OCD treatment (Grassi & Pallanti, 2018; International Obsessive Compulsive Disorder Foundation Genetics & Studies, 2017), and strengthening the research collaboration with these fields will be necessary for further progress. Several second-line medications have proven to be effective in OCRDs, but many only seem to work for a small subpopulation of patients. This indicates a certain heterogeneity amongst patients within each disorder. For example, both anti-glutamatergic and pro-glutamatergic agents have been shown to be effective in treatment-resistant OCD patients, and to answer what works for whom, research should look at this from a precision-medicine perspective (Grassi & Pallanti, 2018) that would lead to more individualized treatments for OCRDs. However, achieving these advancements requires the commitment and support of local policymakers for further research funding. Thus, it is important for researchers and clinicians to engage actively with policymakers, advocating for the significance and potential impact of their work.

VII. Conclusion

To conclude, the advancement of treatments for OCRDs hinges on the effective dissemination and implementation of evidence-based treatments. In this chapter, we discussed strategies to increase the accessibility and effectiveness of these treatments, such as professional training and development, public education campaigns, and policy development.

An exploration into the current landscape of OCRDs research and treatment underscores the significance of our prevailing treatments. It became apparent that expanding the reach of these treatments relies heavily on professional training. Task-shifting strategies show promise in optimizing resource use by empowering non-specialists to deliver treatment under the supervision of specialists.

In addressing the geographical and economic barriers to treatment, we highlighted the role of digitally administered interventions and training programs. These offer cost-effective solutions to improve treatment availability across geographical locations. Furthermore, the need for continuous evaluation and development of digital interventions cannot be understated.

Stigma emerged as a substantial barrier to treatment. Thus, advocating for increased public awareness about OCRDs and the available treatments is vital. Digitally delivered interventions can potentially reduce the stigma associated with mental health services by offering a more private, accessible treatment mode.

The significance of evaluating implementation strategies, including measures of adoption, fidelity, sustainability, and cost outcomes, was also explored. The role of technology is important for the future of treatments for OCRDS, particularly AI, which may enhance the delivery of CBT and make it more interactive and efficient.

As the field progresses, anticipation surrounds the emergence of new treatments and a deepened understanding of these disorders. This reinforces the importance of research seeking to uncover potential predictors of treatment outcomes. Interdisciplinary collaboration for a more comprehensive approach is also important. Increased commitment and support from policymakers for further research funding is necessary.

Despite the challenges faced by individuals with OCRDs, looking back at the past 20 years provides a reason for hope and optimism. Notably, we have seen significant advancements in research and the use of task-shifting strategies, which have empowered non-specialists to deliver treatment under specialist supervision, transforming service provision. Over the past decade, progress has further quickened, with digital interventions breaking down geographical and economic barriers to treatment access. These improvements over the past two decades reaffirm our optimism; they highlight the promise of continued innovation and commitment, and suggest that the future holds great hope for the treatment of these conditions.

References

American Academy of Child and Adolescent Psychiatry. (2009). Improving mental health services in primary care: Reducing administrative and financial barriers to access and collaboration. *Pediatrics*, *123*(4), 1248–1251. https://doi.org/10.1542/peds.2009-0048.

American Psychiatric Association. (2022). *Diagnostic and Statistical Manual of Mental Disorders, Text Revision (DSM-5-TR)* (5th ed.). American Psychiatric Publishing.

Ashbaugh, A.R., Cohen, J.N., & Dobson, K.S. (2021). Training in cognitive behavioural therapy (CBT): National training guidelines from the Canadian Association of Cognitive and Behavioural Therapies. *Canadian Psychology/Psychologie canadienne, 62*(3), 239–251. https://doi.org/10.1037/cap0000224.

Asmundson, G.J., Abramowitz, J.S., Richter, A.A., & Whedon, M. (2010). Health anxiety: current perspectives and future directions. *Curr Psychiatry Rep, 12*(4), 306–312. https://doi.org/10.1007/s11920-010-0123-9.

Aspvall, K., Lenhard, F., Melin, K., Krebs, G., Norlin, L., Näsström, K., Jassi, A., Turner, C., Knoetze, E., Serlachius, E., Andersson, E., & Mataix-Cols, D. (2020). Implementation of internet-delivered cognitive behaviour therapy for pediatric obsessive-compulsive disorder: Lessons from clinics in Sweden, United Kingdom and Australia. *Internet Interv, 20*, 100308. *https://doi.org/10.1016/j.invent.2020.100308.*

Aspvall, K., Sampaio, F., Lenhard, F., Melin, K., Norlin, L., Serlachius, E., Mataix-Cols, D., & Andersson, E. (2021). Cost-effectiveness of internet-delivered vs in-person cognitive behavioral therapy for children and adolescents with obsessive-compulsive disorder. *JAMA Netw Open, 4*(7), e2118516. https://doi.org/10.1001/jamanetworkopen.2021.18516.

Balas, E.A., & Boren, S.A. (2000). Managing clinical knowledge for health care improvement. *Yearb Med Inform*, (1), 65–70. https://pubmed.ncbi.nlm.nih.gov/27699347.

Balkhi, A.M., Reid, A.M., Guzick, A.G., Geffken, G.R., & McNamara, J.P.H. (2016). The progress cascading model: A scalable model for teaching and mentoring graduate trainees in exposure therapy. *Journal of Obsessive-Compulsive and Related Disorders, 9*, 36–42. https://doi.org/10.1016/j.jocrd.2016.02.005.

Behavior Therapy Training Institute [BTTI]. (2023). *Behavior Therapy Training Institute (BTTI)*. https://iocdf.org/professionals/training-institute/btti/.

Beidas, R.S., Edmunds, J.M., Marcus, S.C., & Kendall, P.C. (2012). Training and consultation to promote implementation of an empirically supported treatment: A randomized trial. *Psychiatr Serv, 63*(7), 660–665. https://doi.org/10.1176/appi.ps.201100401.

Belloch, A., Del Valle, G., Morillo, C., Carrió, C., & Cabedo, E. (2009). To seek advice or not to seek advice about the problem: The help-seeking dilemma for obsessive-compulsive disorder. *Soc Psychiatry Psychiatr Epidemiol, 44*(4), 257–264. https://doi.org/10.1007/s00127-008-0423-0.

Bjornsson, A.S., Didie, E.R., & Phillips, K.A. (2010). Body dysmorphic disorder. *Dialogues Clin Neurosci, 12*(2), 221–232. https://doi.org/10.31887/DCNS.2010.12.2/abjornsson.

Böhm, K., Förstner, U., Kulz, A., & Voderholzer, U. (2008). Versorgungsrealität der Zwangsstörungen: Werden Expositionsverfahren eingesetzt? *Verhaltenstherapie, 18*(1), 18–24. *https://doi.org/10.1159/000115956.*

Brown, C.H., Curran, G., Palinkas, L.A., Aarons, G.A., Wells, K.B., Jones, L., Collins, L.M., Duan, N., Mittman, B.S., Wallace, A., Tabak, R.G., Ducharme, L., Chambers, D.A., Neta, G., Wiley, T., Landsverk, J., Cheung, K., & Cruden, G. (2017). An overview of research and evaluation designs for dissemination and implementation. *Annu Rev Public Health, 38*, 1–22. https://doi.org/10.1146/annurev-publhealth-031816-044215.

Chen, J., & Wang, Y. (2021). Social media use for health purposes: Systematic review. *J Med Internet Res, 23*(5), e17917. https://doi.org/10.2196/17917.

Cheung, K., & Duan, N. (2014). Design of implementation studies for quality improvement programs: An effectiveness-cost-effectiveness framework. *Am J Public Health*, *104*(1), e23–30. https://doi.org/10.2105/AJPH.2013.301579.

Cook, J.M., Biyanova, T., Elhai, J., Schnurr, P.P., & Coyne, J.C. (2010). What do psychotherapists really do in practice? An internet study of over 2,000 practitioners. *Psychotherapy (Chic)*, *47*(2), 260–267. https://doi.org/10.1037/a0019788

Cooper, K., Gregory, J.D., Walker, I., Lambe, S., & Salkovskis, P.M. (2017). Cognitive behaviour therapy for health anxiety: A systematic review and meta-analysis. *Behav Cogn Psychother*, *45*(2), 110–123. https://doi.org/10.1017/S1352465816000527.

Cothros, N., Medina, A., & Pringsheim, T. (2020). Current pharmacotherapy for tic disorders. *Expert Opin Pharmacother*, *21*(5), 567–580. https://doi.org/10.1080/14656566.2020.1721465.

Creed, T.A., Wolk, C.B., Feinberg, B., Evans, A.C., & Beck, A.T. (2016). Beyond the label: Relationship between community therapists' self-report of a cognitive behavioral therapy orientation and observed Skills. *Adm Policy Ment Health*, *43*(1), 36–43. https://doi.org/10.1007/s10488-014-0618-5.

Damschroder, L.J., Aron, D.C., Keith, R.E., Kirsh, S.R., Alexander, J.A., & Lowery, J.C. (2009). Fostering implementation of health services research findings into practice: A consolidated framework for advancing implementation science. *Implement Sci*, *4*, 50. https://doi.org/10.1186/1748-5908-4-50.

David, J., Crone, C., & Norberg, M.M. (2022). A critical review of cognitive behavioural therapy for hoarding disorder: How can we improve outcomes. *Clin Psychol Psychother*, *29*(2), 469–488. https://doi.org/10.1002/cpp.2660.

Deacon, B.J., Lickel, J.J., Farrell, N.R., Kemp, J.J., & Hipol, L.J. (2013). Therapist perceptions and delivery of interoceptive exposure for panic disorder. *Journal of Anxiety Disorders*, *27*(2), 259–264. https://doi.org/https://doi.org/10.1016/j.janxdis.2013.02.004.

Dearing, J.W. (2009). Applying diffusion of innovation theory to intervention development. *Res Soc Work Pract*, *19*(5), 503–518. *https://doi.org/10.1177/1049731509335569.*

Dimeff, L.A., Woodcock, E.A., Harned, M.S., & Beadnell, B. (2011). Can dialectical behavior therapy be learned in highly structured learning environments? Results from a randomized controlled dissemination trial. *Behav Ther*, *42*(2), 263–275. https://doi.org/10.1016/j.beth.2010.06.004.

Dopp, A.R., Mundey, P., Beasley, L.O., Silovsky, J.F., & Eisenberg, D. (2019). Mixed-method approaches to strengthen economic evaluations in implementation research. *Implement Sci*, *14*(1), 2. https://doi.org/10.1186/s13012-018-0850-6.

Durlak, J.A., & DuPre, E.P. (2008). Implementation matters: A review of research on the influence of implementation on program outcomes and the factors affecting implementation. *Am J Community Psychol*, *41*(3–4), 327–350. https://doi.org/10.1007/s10464-008-9165-0.

Escoffery, C., Lebow-Skelley, E., Haardoerfer, R., Boing, E., Udelson, H., Wood, R., Hartman, M., Fernandez, M.E., & Mullen, P.D. (2018). A systematic review of adaptations of evidence-based public health interventions globally. *Implement Sci*, *13*(1), 125. https://doi.org/10.1186/s13012-018-0815-9.

Farhat, L.C., Olfson, E., Nasir, M., Levine, J.L.S., Li, F., Miguel, E.C., & Bloch, M.H. (2020). Pharmacological and behavioral treatment for trichotillomania: An updated systematic review with meta-analysis. *Depress Anxiety*, *37*(8), 715–727. https://doi.org/10.1002/da.23028.

Ferrando, C., & Selai, C. (2021). A systematic review and meta-analysis on the effectiveness of exposure and response prevention therapy in the treatment of Obsessive-Compulsive Disorder. *Journal of Obsessive-Compulsive and Related Disorders, 31*, 100684. https://doi.org/10.1016/j.jocrd.2021.100684.

Ferreri, F., Bourla, A., Peretti, C.S., Segawa, T., Jaafari, N., & Mouchabac, S. (2019). How new technologies can improve prediction, assessment, and intervention in Obsessive-Compulsive Disorder (e-OCD): Review. *JMIR Ment Health, 6*(12), e11643. https://doi.org/10.2196/11643.

Fineberg, N.A., Dell'Osso, B., Albert, U., Maina, G., Geller, D., Carmi, L., Sireau, N., Walitza, S., Grassi, G., Pallanti, S., Hollander, E., Brakoulias, V., Menchon, J.M., Marazziti, D., Ioannidis, K., Apergis-Schoute, A., Stein, D.J., Cath, D.C., Veltman, D.J., . . . Zohar, J. (2019). Early intervention for obsessive compulsive disorder: An expert consensus statement. *Eur Neuropsychopharmacol, 29*(4), 549–565. *https://doi.org/10.1016/j.euroneuro.2019.02.002.*

Fitzpatrick, K.K., Darcy, A., & Vierhile, M. (2017). Delivering cognitive behavior therapy to young adults with symptoms of depression and anxiety using a fully automated conversational agent (Woebot): A randomized controlled trial. *JMIR Ment Health, 4*(2), e19. https://doi.org/10.2196/mental.7785.

Franklin, M.E., Dingfelder, H.E., Coogan, C.G., Garcia, A.M., Sapyta, J.J., & Freeman, J.L. (2013). Cognitive behavioral therapy for pediatric obsessive-compulsive disorder: Development of expert-level competence and implications for dissemination. *Journal of Anxiety Disorders, 27*(8), 745–753. https://doi.org/http://dx.doi.org/10.1016/j.janxdis.2013.09.007.

Franklin, S.A., Walther, M.R., & Woods, D.W. (2010). Behavioral interventions for tic disorders. *Psychiatr Clin North Am, 33*(3), 641–655. https://doi.org/10.1016/j.psc.2010.04.013.

Freeman, J., Benito, K., Herren, J., Kemp, J., Sung, J., Georgiadis, C., Arora, A., Walther, M., & Garcia, A. (2018). Evidence base update of psychosocial treatments for pediatric obsessive-compulsive disorder: Evaluating, improving, and transporting what works. *J Clin Child Adolesc Psychol, 47*(5), 669–698. https://doi.org/10.1080/15374416.2018.1496443.

Freiheit, S.R., Vye, C., Swan, R., & Cady, M. (2004). Cognitive-behavioral therapy for anxiety: Is dissemination working? *The Behavior Therapist, 27*(2), 25–32.

Fulmer, R., Joerin, A., Gentile, B., Lakerink, L., & Rauws, M. (2018). Using psychological artificial intelligence (Tess) to relieve symptoms of depression and anxiety: Randomized controlled Trial. *JMIR Ment Health, 5*(4), e64. https://doi.org/10.2196/mental.9782.

Funk, M., Saraceno, B., Drew, N., & Faydi, E. (2008). Integrating mental health into primary healthcare. *Ment Health Fam Med, 5*(1), 5–8.

García-Soriano, G., Rufer, M., Delsignore, A., & Weidt, S. (2014). Factors associated with non-treatment or delayed treatment seeking in OCD sufferers: A review of the literature. *Psychiatry Res, 220*(1–2), 1–10. https://doi.org/10.1016/j.psychres.2014.07.009.

Gega, L., Marks, I., & Mataix-Cols, D. (2004). Computer-aided CBT self-help for anxiety and depressive disorders: Experience of a London clinic and future directions. *J Clin Psychol, 60*(2), 147–157. https://doi.org/10.1002/jclp.10241.

Geller, D.A., & Hosker, D. (2020). When science challenges our long-held assumptions about the robustness of evidence for standard of care. *Journal of the American Academy of Child & Adolescent Psychiatry, 59*(7), 792–793. https://doi.org/10.1016/j.jaac.2020.05.003.

Geller, D., & March, J. (2012). Practice parameter for the assessment and treatment of children and adolescents with obsessive-compulsive disorder. *Journal of the American Academy of Child and Adolescent Psychiatry, 51*(1), 98–113. https://doi.org/10.1016/j.jaac.2011.09.019.

German, R.E., Adler, A., Frankel, S.A., Stirman, S.W., Pinedo, P., Evans, A.C., Beck, A.T., & Creed, T.A. (2018). Testing a web-based, trained-peer model to build capacity for evidence-based practices in community mental health systems. *Psychiatr Serv, 69*(3), 286–292. https://doi.org/10.1176/appi.ps.201700029.

Glazier, K., Wetterneck, C.T., Singh, S., & Williams, M. (2015). Stigma and shame as barriers to treatment for obsessive-compulsive and related disorders. *Journal of Depression and Anxiety, 4*, 3. http://doi.org/10.4191/2167-1044.1000191.

Grassi, G., & Pallanti, S. (2018). Current and up-and-coming pharmacotherapy for obsessive-compulsive disorder in adults. *Expert Opin Pharmacother, 19*(14), 1541–1550. https://doi.org/10.1080/14656566.2018.1528230.

Green, L.W., & Glasgow, R.E. (2006). Evaluating the relevance, generalization, and applicability of research: Issues in external validation and translation methodology. *Eval Health Prof, 29*(1), 126–153. https://doi.org/10.1177/0163278705284445.

Harned, M.S., Dimeff, L.A., Woodcock, E.A., Kelly, T., Zavertnik, J., Contreras, I., & Danner, S.M. (2014). Exposing clinicians to exposure: A randomized controlled dissemination trial of exposure therapy for anxiety disorders. *Behav Ther, 45*(6), 731–744. https://doi.org/10.1016/j.beth.2014.04.005.

Harrison, A., Fernández de la Cruz, L., Enander, J., Radua, J., & Mataix-Cols, D. (2016). Cognitive-behavioral therapy for body dysmorphic disorder: A systematic review and meta-analysis of randomized controlled trials. *Clin Psychol Rev, 48*, 43–51. https://doi.org/10.1016/j.cpr.2016.05.007.

Hatcher, R.L., Wise, E.H., Grus, C.L., Mangione, L., & Emmons, L. (2012). Inside the practicum in professional psychology: A survey of practicum site coordinators. *Training and Education in Professional Psychology, 6*(4), 220–228. https://doi.org/10.1037/a0029542.

Hegde, D., & Sampat, B. (2015). Can private money buy public science? Disease group lobbying and federal funding for biomedical research. *Management Science, 61*(10), 2281–2298. https://doi.org/10.1287/mnsc.2014.2107.

Hipol, L.J., & Deacon, B.J. (2013). Dissemination of evidence-based practices for anxiety disorders in Wyoming: A survey of practicing psychotherapists. *Behavior Modification, 37*(2), 170–188. https://doi.org/10.1177/0145445512458794.

Hiranandani, S., Ipek, S.I., Wilhelm, S., & Greenberg, J.L. (2023). Digital mental health interventions for obsessive compulsive and related disorders: A brief review of evidence-based interventions and future directions. *Journal of Obsessive-Compulsive and Related Disorders, 36*, 100765. https://doi.org/10.1016/j.jocrd.2022.100765.

Hoeft, T.J., Fortney, J.C., Patel, V., & Unützer, J. (2018). Task-sharing approaches to improve mental health care in rural and other low-resource settings: A systematic review. *J Rural Health, 34*(1), 48–62. https://doi.org/10.1111/jrh.12229.

Hoffman, J., Williams, T., Rothbart, R., Ipser, J.C., Fineberg, N., Chamberlain, S.R., & Stein, D.J. (2021). Pharmacotherapy for trichotillomania. *Cochrane Database Syst Rev, 9*(9), CD007662. https://doi.org/10.1002/14651858.CD007662.pub3.

Højgaard, D.R.M.A., & Skarphedinsson, G. (2023). Cognitive behavioral therapy for child and adolescent hoarding disorder. In C.R. Marin, V.B. Patel, & V.R. Preedy (Eds.), *Handbook of Lifespan Cognitive Behavioral Therapy* (pp. 109–121). Elsevier. https://doi.org/10.1016/b978-0-323-85757-4.00037-7.

International Obsessive Compulsive Disorder Foundation Genetics, C., & Studies, O.C.D.C.G.A. (2017). Revealing the complex genetic architecture of obsessive-compulsive disorder using meta-analysis. *Molecular Psychiatry*. https://doi.org/10.1038/mp.2017.154.

International OCD Foundation. (2023). *Public Policy Advocacy*. https://iocdf.org/public-policy/.

Ivarsson, T., Skarphedinsson, G., Kornør, H., Axelsdottir, B., Biedilæ, S., Heyman, I., Asbahr, F., Thomsen, P.H., Fineberg, N., March, J., & Accreditation, T.F.O.T.C.I.F.O.C.D. (2015). The place of and evidence for serotonin reuptake inhibitors (SRIs) for obsessive compulsive disorder (OCD) in children and adolescents: Views based on a systematic review and meta-analysis. *Psychiatry Res*, 227(1), 93–103. https://doi.org/10.1016/j.psychres.2015.01.015.

Jacoby, R.J., Berman, N.C., Reese, H.E., Shin, J., Sprich, S., Szymanski, J., Pollard, C.A., & Wilhelm, S. (2019). Disseminating Cognitive-Behavioral Therapy for obsessive compulsive disorder: Comparing in person vs. online training modalities. *Journal of Obsessive-Compulsive and Related Disorders*, 23, 100485. https://doi.org/10.1016/j.jocrd.2019.100485.

Karlin, B.E., Brown, G.K., Trockel, M., Cunning, D., Zeiss, A.M., & Taylor, C.B. (2012). National dissemination of cognitive behavioral therapy for depression in the department of veterans affairs health care system: Therapist and patient-level outcomes. *Journal of Consulting and Clinical Psychology*, 80(5), 707–718. https://doi.org/10.1037/a0029328.

Kazdin, A.E., & Blase, S.L. (2011). Rebooting psychotherapy research and practice to reduce the burden of mental illness. *Perspect Psychol Sci*, 6(1), 21–37. https://doi.org/10.1177/1745691610393527.

Khanna, M., Kerns, C.M., & Carper, M. (2014). Internet-based dissemination and implementation of cognitive behavioral therapy for child anxiety. In R. S. Beidas & P. C. Kendall (Eds.), *Dissemination and Implementation of Evidence-Based Practices in Child and Adolescent Mental Health* (pp. 313–335). Oxford University Press.

Klos, M.C., Escoredo, M., Joerin, A., Lemos, V.N., Rauws, M., & Bunge, E.L. (2021). Artificial intelligence-based chatbot for anxiety and depression in university students: Pilot randomized controlled trial. *JMIR Form Res*, 5(8), e20678. https://doi.org/10.2196/20678.

Kobak, K.A., Craske, M.G., Rose, R.D., & Wolitsky-Taylor, K. (2013). Web-based therapist training on cognitive behavior therapy for anxiety disorders: A pilot study. *Psychotherapy (Chic)*, 50(2), 235–247. https://doi.org/10.1037/a0030568.

Kobak, K.A., Wolitzky-Taylor, K., Craske, M.G., & Rose, R.D. (2017). Therapist training on cognitive behavior therapy for anxiety disorders using internet-based technologies. *Cognit Ther Res*, 41(2), 252–265. https://doi.org/10.1007/s10608-016-9819-4.

Kolko, D.J., Baumann, B.L., Herschell, A.D., Hart, J.A., Holden, E.A., & Wisniewski, S.R. (2012). Implementation of AF-CBT by community practitioners serving child welfare and mental health: A randomized trial. *Child Maltreat*, 17(1), 32–46. https://doi.org/10.1177/1077559511427346.

Langthorne, D., Beard, J., & Waller, G. (2023). Therapist factors associated with intent to use exposure therapy: A systematic review and meta-analysis. *Cogn Behav Ther*, 1–33. https://doi.org/10.1080/16506073.2023.2191824.

Latha, K., Meena, K.S., Pravitha, M.R., Dasgupta, M., & Chaturvedi, S.K. (2020). Effective use of social media platforms for promotion of mental health awareness. *J Educ Health Promot*, 9, 124. https://doi.org/10.4103/jehp.jehp_90_20.

Lehman, W.E., Greener, J.M., & Simpson, D.D. (2002). Assessing organizational readiness for change. *J Subst Abuse Treat*, 22(4), 197–209. https://doi.org/10.1016/s0740-5472(02)00233-7.

Lewis, C.C., Proctor, E.K., & Brownson, R.C. (2017). *Measurement Issues in Dissemination and Implementation Research.* Oxford University Press. https://doi.org/10.1093/oso/9780190683214.003.0014.

Liu, S., Li, Y., & Cui, Y. (2020). Review of habit reversal training for tic disorders. *Pediatr Investig*, 4(2), 127–132. https://doi.org/10.1002/ped4.12190.

Lundström, L., Flygare, O., Andersson, E., Enander, J., Bottai, M., Ivanov, V.Z., Boberg, J., Pascal, D., Mataix-Cols, D., & Rück, C. (2022). Effect of internet-based vs face-to-face cognitive behavioral therapy for adults With obsessive-compulsive disorder: A randomized clinical trial. *JAMA Netw Open*, 5(3), e221967. https://doi.org/10.1001/jamanetworkopen.2022.1967.

Mallonee, S., Phillips, J., Holloway, K., & Riggs, D. (2018). Training providers in the use of evidence-based treatments: A comparison of in-person and online delivery modes. *Psychology Learning & Teaching*, 17(1), 6–72. https://doi.org/10.1177/1475725717744678.

Marques, L., LeBlanc, N.J., Weingarden, H.M., Timpano, K.R., Jenike, M., & Wilhelm, S. (2010). Barriers to treatment and service utilization in an internet sample of individuals with obsessive-compulsive symptoms. *Depress Anxiety*, 27(5), 470–475. https://doi.org/10.1002/da.20694.

Marsch, L.A., Lord, S.E., & Dallery, J. (2015). *Behavioral healthcare and technology: Using science-based innovations to transform practice.* Oxford University Press.

McCarty, R.J., Cooke, D.L., Lazaroe, L.M., Guzick, A.G., Guastello, A.D., Budd, S.M., Downing, S.T., Ordway, A.R., Mathews, C.A., & McNamara, J.P.H. (2022). The effects of an exposure therapy training program for pre-professionals in an intensive exposure-based summer camp. *The Cognitive Behaviour Therapist*, 15. https://doi.org/10.1017/s1754470x22000010.

McDavitt, B., Bogart, L.M., Mutchler, M.G., Wagner, G.J., Green, H.D., Lawrence, S.J., Mutepfa, K.D., & Nogg, K.A. (2016). Dissemination as dialogue: Building trust and sharing research findings through community engagement. *Prev Chronic Dis*, 13, E38. https://doi.org/10.5888/pcd13.150473.

McHugh, R.K., & Barlow, D.H. (2010). The dissemination and implementation of evidence-based psychological treatments: A review of current efforts. *Am Psychol*, 65(2), 73–84. https://doi.org/10.1037/a0018121.

McLeod, B.D., Southam-Gerow, M.A., & Weisz, J.R. (2009). Conceptual and methodological issues in treatment integrity measurement. *School Psychology Review*, 38, 541–546.

McQuaid, E.L., & Spirito, A. (2012). Integrating research into clinical internship training bridging the science/practice gap in pediatric psychology. *J Pediatr Psychol*, 37(2), 149–157. https://doi.org/10.1093/jpepsy/jsr114.

Morris, S.H., Jaffee, S.R., Goodwin, G.P., & Franklin, M.E. (2016). Hoarding in children and adolescents: A Review. *Child Psychiatry & Human Development*, 47(5), 740–750. https://doi.org/10.1007/s10578-015-0607-2.

National Institute for Health and Clinical Excellence. (2005). Obsessive compulsive disorder (OCD) and body dysmorphic disorder (BDD). http://guidance.nice.org.uk/CG31.

National Institute of Mental Health [NIMH]. (2023). *The National Institute of Mental Health strategic plan.* https://www.nimh.nih.gov/sites/default/files/documents/

about/strategic-planning-reports/NIMH_Strategic_Plan_for_Research_2023_Update.pdf

Nicol, G., Wang, R., Graham, S., Dodd, S., & Garbutt, J. (2022). Chatbot-delivered cognitive behavioral therapy in adolescents with depression and anxiety during the COVID-19 pandemic: Feasibility and acceptability study. *JMIR Form Res*, 6(11), e40242. https://doi.org/10.2196/40242.

Olatunji, B.O., Deacon, B.J., & Abramowitz, J.S. (2009). Is hypochondriasis an anxiety disorder? *Br J Psychiatry*, 194(6), 481–482. https://doi.org/10.1192/bjp.bp.108.061085.

Orsolini, L., Pompili, S., Salvi, V., & Volpe, U. (2021). A systematic review on telemental health in youth mental health: Focus on anxiety, depression and obsessive-compulsive disorder. *Medicina (Kaunas)*, 57(8), 793. https://doi.org/10.3390/medicina57080793.

Ost, L.-G., Riise, E.N., Wergeland, G.J., Hansen, B., & Kvale, G. (2016). Cognitive behavioral and pharmacological treatments of OCD in children: A systematic review and meta-analysis. *Journal of Anxiety Disorders*, 43, 58–69. https://doi.org/10.1016/j.janxdis.2016.08.003.

Piacentini, J., Woods, D.W., Scahill, L., Wilhelm, S., Peterson, A.L., Chang, S., Ginsburg, G.S., Deckersbach, T., Dziura, J., Levi-Pearl, S., & Walkup, J.T. (2010). Behavior therapy for children with Tourette disorder: A randomized controlled trial. *JAMA*, 303(19), 1929–1937. https://doi.org/10.1001/jama.2010.607.

Pittig, A., Kotter, R., & Hoyer, J. (2019). The struggle of behavioral therapists with exposure: Self-reported practicability, negative beliefs, and therapist distress about exposure-based interventions. *Behav Ther*, 50(2), 353–366. https://doi.org/10.1016/j.beth.2018.07.003.

Poyraz, C.A., Turan, Ş., Sağlam, N.G., Batun, G.Ç., Yassa, A., & Duran, A. (2015). Factors associated with the duration of untreated illness among patients with obsessive compulsive disorder. *Compr Psychiatry*, 58, 88–93. https://doi.org/10.1016/j.comppsych.2014.12.019.

Proctor, E., Powell, B.J., & Feely, M.A. (2014). Measurement in dissemination and implementation science. In R.S. Beidas & P.C. Kendall (Eds.), *Dissemination and implementation of evidence-based practices in child and adolescent mental health* (pp. 22–43). Oxford University Press.

Proctor, E., Silmere, H., Raghavan, R., Hovmand, P., Aarons, G., Bunger, A., Griffey, R., & Hensley, M. (2011). Outcomes for implementation research: Conceptual distinctions, measurement challenges, and research agenda. *Adm Policy Ment Health*, 38(2), 65–76. https://doi.org/10.1007/s10488-010-0319-7.

Proctor, E.K., Landsverk, J., Aarons, G., Chambers, D., Glisson, C., & Mittman, B. (2009). Implementation research in mental health services: An emerging science with conceptual, methodological, and training challenges. *Adm Policy Ment Health*, 36(1), 24–34. https://doi.org/10.1007/s10488-008-0197-4.

Raj, V., Raykar, V., Robinson, A.M., & Islam, M.R. (2022). Child and adolescent mental health training programs for non-specialist mental health professionals in low and middle income countries: A scoping review of literature. *Community Mental Health Journal*, 58(1), 154–165. https://doi.org/10.1007/s10597-021-00805-w.

Rakovshik, S.G., McManus, F., Vazquez-Montes, M., Muse, K., & Ougrin, D. (2016). Is supervision necessary? Examining the effects of internet-based CBT training with and without supervision. *J Consult Clin Psychol*, 84(3), 191–199. https://doi.org/10.1037/ccp0000079.

Raphel, S., & Fry-Bowers, E.K. (2021). Child and Adolescent Mental Health Policy. In E.L. Yearwood, G.S. Pearson, & J.A. Newland (Eds.), *Child and Adolescent Behavioral Health: A Resource for Advanced Practice Psychiatric and Primary Care Practitioners in Nursing* (pp. 555–569). Wiley. https://doi.org/10.1002/9781119487593.ch33.

Rask, C.U. (2019). Health anxiety in children and adolescents. In E. Hedman-Lagerlöf (Ed.), *The Clinician's Guide to Treating Health Anxiety* (pp. 165–176). Elsevier. https://doi.org/10.1016/b978-0-12-811806-1.00010-x.

Reese, H.E., Pollard, C.A., Szymanski, J., Berman, N., Crowe, K., Rosenfield, E., & Wilhelm, S. (2016). The behavior therapy training institute for OCD: A preliminary report. *Journal of Obsessive-Compulsive and Related Disorders, 8,* 79–85. https://doi.org/10.1016/j.jocrd.2015.12.005.

Reid, A.M., Guzick, A.G., Balkhi, A.M., McBride, M., Geffken, G.R., & McNamara, J.P.H. (2017). The progressive cascading model improves exposure delivery in trainee therapists learning exposure therapy for obsessive-compulsive disorder. *Training and Education in Professional Psychology, 11*(4), 260–265. https://doi.org/10.1037/tep0000159.

Remmerswaal, K.C.P., Lans, L., Seldenrijk, A., Hoogendoorn, A.W., van Balkom, A.J.L.M., & Batelaan, N.M. (2021). Effectiveness and feasibility of intensive versus regular cognitive behaviour therapy in patients with anxiety and obsessive-compulsive disorders: A meta-analysis. *Journal of Affective Disorders Reports, 6,* 100267. https://doi.org/10.1016/j.jadr.2021.100267.

Robertson, L., Paparo, J., & Wootton, B.M. (2020). Understanding barriers to treatment and treatment delivery preferences for individuals with symptoms of hoarding disorder: A preliminary study. *Journal of Obsessive-Compulsive and Related Disorders, 26,* 100560. https://doi.org/10.1016/j.jocrd.2020.100560.

Rogers, E.M. (2003). *Diffusion of Innovations* (5th ed.). Free Press.

Ruzek, J.I., Eftekhari, A., Crowley, J., Kuhn, E., Karlin, B.E., & Rosen, C.S. (2017). Post-training beliefs, intentions, and use of prolonged exposure therapy by clinicians in the veterans health administration. *Adm Policy Ment Health, 44*(1), 123–132. https://doi.org/10.1007/s10488-015-0689-y.

Schoenwald, S.K., Sheidow, A.J., & Letourneau, E.J. (2004). Toward effective quality assurance in evidence-based practice: Links between expert consultation, therapist fidelity, and child outcomes. *J Clin Child Adolesc Psychol, 33*(1), 94–104. https://doi.org/10.1207/S15374424JCCP3301_10.

Schwartz, C., Schlegl, S., Kuelz, A.K., & Voderholzer, U. (2013). Treatment-seeking in OCD community cases and psychological treatment actually provided to treatment-seeking patients: A systematic review. *Journal of Obsessive-Compulsive and Related Disorders, 2*(4), 448–456. https://doi.org/10.1016/j.jocrd.2013.10.006.

Shelton, R.C., Lee, M., Brotzman, L.E., Wolfenden, L., Nathan, N., & Wainberg, M.L. (2020). What is dissemination and implementation science?: An introduction and opportunities to advance behavioral medicine and public health globally. *Int J Behav Med, 27*(1), 3–20. https://doi.org/10.1007/s12529-020-09848-x.

Skarphedinsson, G., Hanssen-Bauer, K., Kornør, H., Heiervang, E.R., Landrø, N.I., Axelsdottir, B., Biedilæ, S., & Ivarsson, T. (2015). Standard individual cognitive behaviour therapy for paediatric obsessive-compulsive disorder: A systematic review of effect estimates across comparisons. *Nord J Psychiatry, 69*(2), 81–92. https://doi.org/10.3109/08039488.2014.941395.

Skurya, J., Jafferany, M., & Everett, G.J. (2020). Habit reversal therapy in the management of body focused repetitive behavior disorders. *Dermatol Ther*, *33*(6), e13811. https://doi.org/10.1111/dth.13811.

Smith, E., & Caldwell, L. (2007). Adapting evidence-based programs to new contexts: What needs to be changed. *The Journal of Rural Health*, *23*(s1), 37–41. https://doi.org/10.1111/j.1748-0361.2007.00122.x.

Spencer, S.D., Stiede, J.T., Wiese, A.D., Guzick, A.G., Cervin, M., McKay, D., & Storch, E.A. (2023). Things that make you go Hmm: Myths and misconceptions within cognitive-behavioral treatment of obsessive-compulsive disorder. *Journal of Obsessive-Compulsive and Related Disorders*, *37*, 100805. https://doi.org/10.1016/j.jocrd.2023.100805.

Stein, B.D., Celedonia, K.L., Swartz, H.A., DeRosier, M.E., Sorbero, M.J., Brindley, R.A., Burns, R.M., Dick, A.W., & Frank, E. (2015). Implementing a web-based intervention to train community clinicians in an evidence-based psychotherapy: A pilot study. *Psychiatr Serv*, *66*(9), 988–991. https://doi.org/10.1176/appi.ps.201400318.

Stirman, S.W., Pontoski, K., Creed, T., Xhezo, R., Evans, A.C., Beck, A.T., & Crits-Christoph, P. (2017). A non-randomized comparison of strategies for consultation in a community-academic training program to implement an evidence-based psychotherapy. *Adm Policy Ment Health*, *44*(1), 55–66. https://doi.org/10.1007/s10488-015-0700-7.

Storch, E.A., Caporino, N.E., Morgan, J.R., Lewin, A.B., Rojas, A., Brauer, L., Larson, M.J., & Murphy, T.K. (2011). Preliminary investigation of web-camera delivered cognitive-behavioral therapy for youth with obsessive-compulsive disorder. *Psychiatry Research*, *189*(3), 407–412. https://doi.org/10.1016/j.psychres.2011.05.047.

Storch, E.A., Lehmkuhl, H.D., Ricketts, E., Geffken, G.R., Marien, W., & Murphy, T.K. (2010). An open trial of intensive family based cognitive-behavioral therapy in youth with obsessive-compulsive disorder who are medication partial responders or nonresponders. *Journal of Clinical Child and Adolescent Psychology*, *39*(2), 260–268. http://ovidsp.ovid.com/ovidweb.cgi?T=JS&CSC=Y&NEW S=N&PAGE=fulltext&D=medl&AN=20390817.

VanderVeen, J.W., Reddy, L.F., Veilleux, J.C., January, A.M., & DiLillo, D. (2012). Clinical PhD graduate student views of their scientist-practitioner training. *J Clin Psychol*, *68*(9), 1048–1057. https://doi.org/10.1002/jclp.21883.

Weidle, B., Ivarsson, T., Asbahr, F.R., Calvo, R., Mataix-Cols, D., Rynn, M.A., & Storch, E.A. (2021). Specialty knowledge and competency standards for pharmacotherapy for pediatric obsessive-compulsive disorder. *Psychiatry Res*, *299*, 113858. https://doi.org/10.1016/j.psychres.2021.113858.

Weingarden, H., Shaw, A.M., Phillips, K.A., & Wilhelm, S. (2018). Shame and defectiveness beliefs in treatment seeking patients with body dysmorphic disorder. *J Nerv Ment Dis*, *206*(6), 417–422. https://doi.org/10.1097/NMD.0000000000000808.

Weisz, J.R. (2015). Bridging the research-practice divide in youth Ppychotherapy: The deployment-focused model and transdiagnostic treatment. *Verhaltenstherapie*, *25*(2), 129–132. https://doi.org/10.1159/000430432.

Weisz, J.R., & Gray, J.S. (2008). Evidence-based psychotherapy for children and adolescents: Data from the present and a model for the future. *Child Adolesc Ment Health*, *13*(2), 54–65. https://doi.org/10.1111/j.1475-3588.2007.00475.x.

Weisz, J.R., Ugueto, A.M., Cheron, D.M., & Herren, J. (2013). Evidence-based youth psychotherapy in the mental health ecosystem. *J Clin Child Adolesc Psychol*, 42(2), 274–286. https://doi.org/10.1080/15374416.2013.764824.

Whiteside, S.P.H., Deacon, B.J., Benito, K., & Stewart, E. (2016). Factors associated with practitioners' use of exposure therapy for childhood anxiety disorders. *Journal of Anxiety Disorders*, 40, 29–36. https://doi.org/https://dx.doi.org/10.1016/j.janxdis.2016.04.001.

Williams, M.T., Domanico, J., Marques, L., Leblanc, N.J., & Turkheimer, E. (2012). Barriers to treatment among African Americans with obsessive-compulsive disorder. *J Anxiety Disord*, 26(4), 555–563. https://doi.org/10.1016/j.janxdis.2012.02.009.

Yu, L., Li, Y., Zhang, J., Yan, C., Wen, F., Yan, J., Wang, F., Liu, J., & Cui, Y. (2020). The therapeutic effect of habit reversal training for Tourette syndrome: A meta-analysis of randomized control trials. *Expert Rev Neurother*, 20(11), 1189–1196. https://doi.org/10.1080/14737175.2020.1826933.

14 Improving Diversity in Childhood Obsessive-Compulsive and Related Disorders Research

Andreas Bezahler,[1] *Elizabeth S. Bocanegra,*[2]
Katie H. Mangen,[3] *and Caitlin M. Pinciotti*[3]

[1] *Department of Psychology, Fordham University, Bronx, NY*

[2] *University of California, Los Angeles, Division of Life Sciences, Los Angeles, CA*

[3] *Menninger Department of Psychiatry and Behavioral Sciences, Baylor College of Medicine, Houston, TX*

Introduction

It is well documented that research published in psychological sciences has primarily focused on non-minoritized populations (i.e., White, non-Latin/x, cisgender, heterosexual, medium to high socioeconomic status, Christian, etc.), and a myriad of other societally privileged identities in the United States and abroad. This crisis in psychology research has led to the National Institutes of Health (NIHs) to require that researchers include and document minority participation in research studies to address broad gaps in the inclusivity of research participants. Strikingly, of the 100 studies in the Reproducibility Project, results demonstrated that context and specific identities were predominantly privileged identities, and intersectional identities were rarely, if ever, documented (Sabik et al., 2021). Moreover, intersectionality (i.e., the role of intersecting identities) among counseling psychology research was represented in fewer than 1 percent of studies in 2016 (Shin et al., 2017). This lack of characterization of a sample leaves readers, reviewers, and clinical scientists unable to identify the efficacy of treatments and/or proposed mechanisms among diverse populations. The bias in research towards socially dominant characteristics translates to research on obsessive-compulsive and related disorders (OCRDs).

The lack of minority inclusion and consideration in OCRD research is problematic for multiple reasons. First, without diverse representation in OCRD research, it is unclear how the findings or effects translate beyond

DOI: 10.4324/9781003386278-14

the demographic sample of the proposed study. Second, it reinforces the notion that diverse identities are not welcomed or worth including alongside their non-minoritized peers. Third, there are unique experiences of those with a minority identity(ies) that may impact the development, presentation, or maintenance of these conditions that would not be otherwise captured in a mainly non-minoritized sample (e.g., the impact of heterosexism on coping strategies of sexual minority men). Fourth, the impact of social determinants of health on mental health cannot be examined, and neither can these inequities be addressed in an empirically informed manner without minority participation and consideration. Last, clinical science should be a service provided for an entire population, including all the diverse identities that make up that population; systematic exclusion of minoritized identities only serves those who do not hold a minoritized identity(ies) and neglects the unique needs of minoritized groups. Thus, there is a dire need to both identify significant gaps of representation in OCRD research and provide practical next steps for how to address these gaps to promote research that accounts for and benefits everyone. This chapter reviews the available literature and offers suggestions for improving diversity in OCRD research.

Obsessive-Compulsive Disorder

Obsessive-compulsive disorder (OCD), characterized by repetitive, disturbing intrusive thoughts (obsessions) and engagement in physical or mental actions in order to suppress, neutralize, or avoid obsessions and the distress they cause (compulsions), impacts 1–2 percent of children and adolescents (Nazeer et al., 2020). Over the past five decades, there has been increased attention to pediatric OCD, its onset, course, treatment outcomes, and assessment, however, the diversity of these research samples is unclear and often unreported.

Problematically, most meta-analyses on OCD treatment, assessment, and prognostics among youth only report sex assigned at birth (i.e., male or female) (McKay et al., 2006) or do not report any sample characteristics at all (Mataix-Cols et al., 2008; Stewart et al., 2004; Stewart et al., 2007). For example, sex assigned at birth only was reported in pediatric OCD treatment meta-analyses spanning 1970 to 2007 (Abramowitz, Whiteside, & Deacon, 2005; Ginsburg et al., 2008; Watson & Rees, 2008), and one-quarter of OCD treatment efficacy randomized control trials including adults and youth between 1998 to 2008 did not report any information regarding the racial composition of the sample (Williams, M.T. et al., 2010). When information about race and ethnicity is made available, it is clear that OCD treatment studies are largely homogenous. Across 28 North American studies, the samples were found to be overwhelmingly White (>90 percent) (Williams, M.T. et al., 2010), and across 90 American and Canadian studies spanning 1977 to 2010, only 12.2 percent included Latin/x people (Wetterneck et al., 2012).

Unfortunately, this lack of minority representation in research extends to racial/ethnic minority representation in OCD treatment centers among African American/Black and Latin/x people, highlighting gaps in access to these resources (Fernández de la Cruz et al., 2015). These documented exclusion rates in OCD research may be due to barriers unique to minoritized racial/ethnic identities, which include not knowing where to receive treatment, fear of experiencing inequity within the treatment context, and language barriers (Wetterneck et al., 2012; Williams, M.T. et al., 2012a). These barriers were similarly found among African American/Black youth with OCD, with additional factors related to family (e.g., parenting styles) (Williams, M.T. & Jahn, 2017). Moreover, in a large (N > 3,500) sample of African American/Black adults with OCD, notable demographic correlates were identified among those who reported obsessions and compulsions, namely fewer years of education and increased material hardships (e.g., inability to secure housing, food, medical care) (Williams, M.T. et al., 2017).

Beyond the need from a broader equity standpoint to make OCD research more equitable and accessible to marginalized and minoritized youth, emerging research suggesting possible unique symptom presentations and treatment outcomes indicates that these gaps are even more important to address. Racial/ethnic, sexual minority (e.g., gay, lesbian, bisexual+), and gender minority (e.g., transgender and gender diverse) adults report unique OCD symptom profiles and clinical presentations (Pinciotti et al., 2022; Pinciotti & Orcutt, 2021; Pinciotti et al., 2024; Williams, M.T. et al., 2012b). Sexual minority undergraduate students were more likely to report obsessions related to unacceptable thoughts (e.g., violence, sex) compared to their heterosexual peers, which the authors suggest may be due to a propensity to respond more strongly to intrusive thoughts that may compound the stigma they have already experienced due to their sexual orientation (Pinciotti & Orcutt, 2021), though this finding did not replicate to a clinical sample (Pinciotti et al., 2024). Similarly, more severe contamination symptoms in gender minority adults with OCD compared to their cisgender male peers may reflect responses to identity-related sexual, physical, and emotional violations more likely to give rise to mental contamination (Pinciotti et al., 2022). Unique symptom presentations were also highlighted among African American/Black adults, who were more likely to report contamination-related obsessions and concerns related to animals compared to their White peers, which the authors attribute to potential overcompensation for stereotypes regarding cleanliness, (Williams et al., 2008).

There is also the potential that the unique, identity-based stressors experienced by sexual, gender, and racial minority individuals may impact responding to self-report measures, such that, in the absence of measurement invariance research, it is not clear whether these measures are appropriately normed for individuals with non-majority identities. Of note, despite endorsing more contamination-related obsessions and concerns related to animals, African American/Black adults were not more distressed by these symptoms, suggesting these response differences may instead be an artifact of measurement variance rather than true differences in OCD (Williams, M.T. et al., 2012b).

When in treatment, individuals with marginalized identities also appear to experience challenges in treatment relative to their peers who do not hold marginalized identities. At admission to a partial hospital/residential treatment program for OCD, sexual minority adults report marginally more severe OCD symptoms, less capacity for emotion regulation and distress tolerance, and higher depression severity (Bezahler et al., 2022; Bezahler et al., 2024b), and multi-attracted (bi+; e.g., bisexual, pansexual) individuals report more severe underlying dysfunctional beliefs related to perfectionism and fear of harm/threat compared to their heterosexual peers (Bezahler et al., 2024a). In another study, individuals with more than one marginalized identity reported more severe OCD and depression symptoms and obsessive beliefs, as well as a lower quality of life (Wadsworth et al., 2020). Additionally, adults with racial/ethnic identities and those with gender minority identities required longer lengths of stay in intensive treatment for OCD compared to their non-minoritized peers, emphasizing the need for these programs to be equipped to understand and address the unique needs of these minoritized populations (Pinciotti et al., 2022; Williams, M.T. et al., 2015).

Unfortunately, as noted above, there is a relative dearth of research examining the unique experiences of marginalized and minoritized people with OCD, and these studies have focused exclusively on adult samples. Research is needed to examine if these patterns among racially/ethnically minoritized adults and sexual and gender minority adults are found among youth with OCD, while also diversifying the range of identity characteristics being reported and examined. Normal developmental tasks among youth (e.g., identity formation during adolescence) may intersect with many of these minoritized identities, further complicating clinical presentations, underscoring the need for further research and clinical services for these populations. For example, it is not uncommon for adolescents with OCD to present to clinicians with obsessions related to gender or sexual identity; since personally held identities are still often developing at this time, this can create additional challenges that should be considered in this research.

Body Dysmorphic Disorder

Body dysmorphic disorder (BDD) is a condition characterized by excessive preoccupation with a "defect" or "flaw" in one's appearance that is not noticeable to others, but which leads to significant distress and associated compulsive behaviors in the individual (American Psychological Association (APA), 2022). It has an estimated prevalence rate of 1.9 percent in the general population, with slightly higher rates of 2.2 percent in adolescents and 3.3 percent in university and college students (mean age = 21.1 years) (Veale et al., 2016).

There is a growing body of literature examining differences in prevalence rates of BDD among adults of diverse backgrounds. Sexual minority women have demonstrated a particularly high prevalence rate of BDD at 7.7 percent (Boroughs, Krawczyk, & Thompson, 2010). Likewise, a study of sexual minority men found an overall prevalence rate of 5.4 percent for BDD, with higher prevalence among younger adults (aged 18–34 years) compared to older adults (Fabris et al., 2020). The prevalence rate of BDD varies across racial/ethnic groups, with higher estimated prevalence rates among White American university students than in Latin/x American, Asian American, and African American students (Boroughs, Krawczyk, & Thompson, 2010). Although research is more limited in youth samples, one study of BDD symptoms in high school students found that African Americans had significantly more positive body image scores than other groups (Mayville et al., 1998) (though it is worth noting this is an older study that may not translate to the present day).

Specific associations between BDD symptoms and minority stress factors have been identified in the adult-focused literature. For example, a history of experiencing "racial teasing" has been shown to predict greater BDD symptoms among ethnic minorities in Singapore (Pillai & Sündermann, 2019). Furthermore, in one sample of gay men, sexual orientation-related rejection sensitivity (i.e., anticipation of and propensity to perceive rejection) and identity concealment were associated with more severe BDD symptoms (Oshana, Klimek, & Blashill, 2020). Separate research has also shown an association between body image concerns and (1) internalized homophobia, (2) sexual orientation concealment, and (3) heterosexist discrimination, with some indication that involvement in sexual minority communities does not serve as a buffer against these minority stressors (Convertino et al., 2021). Compounding minority stress factors may also explain findings that, among sexual minorities, Hispanic/Latin/x individuals show higher rates of BDD symptoms (Gonzales & Blashill, 2021).

Among the most significant limitations of the BDD literature as it relates to diversity is the lack of studies of pediatric and adolescent samples. In their review of developments in BDD research over the past 25 years, Jassi and Krebs (2021) identify a need for increased awareness of pediatric BDD and improvements in diagnostic methods for youth in order to bolster a greater understanding of BDD presentations across diverse groups. The adult literature may offer some insight into means by which clinicians and researchers can improve the ability to detect BDD in youth of diverse backgrounds. At least one measure, the Dysmorphic Concern Questionnaire

(DCM) (Oosthuizen, Lambert, & Castle, 1998), has demonstrated measurement invariance across gender, race, and Hispanic/Latin/x ethnicity in sexual minority adults, suggesting that it is a valid tool for these populations (Rozzell et al., 2020). More such research examining the reliability and validity of BDD symptom measures for individuals of diverse backgrounds, especially for youth, is needed. Additionally, methods of measuring BDD must be sensitive to cultural differences in body image and body-related concerns. One study has demonstrated that cultural body dissatisfaction concerns significantly predict BDD symptoms in women of color (Sotiriou, 2021). Specifically, differences in body-related concerns (e.g., which body parts are the focus of concern, most common compulsions) have been identified between White and Asian individuals (Marques et al., 2011a).

An additional limitation to note in the BDD literature is the exclusion of transgender individuals (e.g., Rautio et al., 2020). Although not studied directly, transgender and gender diverse individuals with BDD may be more likely to develop concerns regarding body types or parts that are traditionally considered masculine or feminine that may not fit with their desired gender presentation. For example, transmasculine individuals may experience muscle dysmorphia, or a pervasive fear of insufficient muscularity (Nagata et al., 2022). Although caution is required to appropriately differentiate BDD from gender dysphoria, it is possible in some cases that body concerns associated with gender dysphoria could become so exaggerated that they could overlap with BDD (e.g., perceiving that one's chest or genitals are much larger and more observable than is actually true). Despite these unique concerns, no research has studied the prevalence or presentation of BDD in transgender and gender diverse samples, a gap that is even more glaring in youth considering the physiological changes that occur during puberty that may give rise to gender dysphoria and BDD. This gap also translates to a lack of research on best clinical practices for treating transgender individuals with BDD, including how best to address these body concerns without compounding existing gender dysphoria.

Furthermore, there is a need for BDD treatments that are culturally sensitive. There is evidence to suggest that barriers to BDD treatment differentially affect members of various racial/ethnic groups; for example, after controlling for income, Latin/x individuals endorse more barriers related to finances, stigma, and treatment satisfaction than do Whites, while Asians report significantly fewer barriers across all three categories (Marques et al., 2011b). Although these barriers are numerous and complex, further research may help to yield solutions. For instance, research with adults has shown that modifications can be made to cognitive behavioral therapy for BDD to improve the cultural sensitivity of this treatment approach (Weingarden et al., 2011). Such modifications might be expected to improve treatment satisfaction, which may be one avenue for ensuring that diverse individuals – adults and youth alike – are able to obtain equitable treatment for BDD.

Finally, the BDD literature would benefit from examining a broader range of diversity variables, both in adult and pediatric samples. As discussed, much of the existing research in this area is focused on broadly defined categories of race and on sexual minorities. A more thorough investigation of cultural variables, as well as the use of more inclusive samples, is needed in order to form a more culturally responsive understanding of BDD across all age groups.

Body-Focused Repetitive Behaviors

Body-focused repetitive behaviors (BFRBs) are iterative, ritualistic actions that primarily target the body, characterized by the compulsive engagement in activities that result in the physical damage of one's appearance or infliction of physical harm. These behaviors encompass a spectrum of behaviors, including excoriation disorder (skin-picking), trichotillomania (hair-pulling), onychophagia (nail-biting), as well as lip- and cheek-biting or chewing. Estimates suggest that as many as 5–29 percent of youth experience BFRB symptoms (Duke et al., 2009; Garde et al., 2014; Hayes, Storch, & Berlanga, 2009), with nail-biting being the most prevalent behavior (Garde et al., 2014). Several studies have explored various aspects of BFRBs, shedding light on their prevalence and potential contributing factors, however, the research on BFRBs in diverse groups is limited, especially in diverse youth.

Some research has begun to examine the differential impact of BFRB on ethnic/racial minority youth. Regarding prevalence, Moreno-Amador and colleagues (2023) conducted a study among a Spanish adolescent population, finding a notable prevalence of hair-pulling and skin-picking symptoms in this group. Notably, this prevalence in youth was consistent with rates reported among adult samples, highlighting the potential pervasiveness of these symptoms across different age groups in this Spanish sample. In a study of Salvadorian youth, Selles and colleagues (2015) found that a significant proportion of individuals engaged in BFRBs, yet only a fraction of them met the criteria for a clinical diagnosis. This suggests that, despite a high frequency of engaging in BFRBs, not all individuals who engage in BFRBs experience enough distress or interference to warrant clinical attention. Of note, this study used parent-report data, which could have influenced responses. Cultural factors have played a role in the parents' reporting of their child's BFRBs – stigma, lack of psychoeducation, and social desirability could have influenced how parents responded, perhaps minimizing their ratings on impact and distress experienced from BFRBs (Solley & Turner, 2018).

Indeed, other studies using self-report data have reported conflicting evidence on impairment and distress. Neal-Barnett and colleagues (2010) found that Black and Latin/x individuals were more likely to report impairment in their home life due to trichotillomania. Similarly, recent data has suggested that Black, Asian, and Latin/x individuals experience more distressing and longer lasting BFRB symptoms than their White counterparts (Grant et al., 2021). Both studies also found that individuals from these groups were less likely to seek treatment for BFRBs. Though not empirically tested, some researchers have suggested that Black individuals may be more likely to seek help for trichotillomania symptoms from haircare professionals, or may not seek out clinical care as they are better able to hide their symptoms (Mansueto, Thomas, & Brice, 2007). These findings suggest that the expression and impairment of BFRBs could be influenced by sociocultural factors.

BFRBs represent a significant challenge for affected individuals, and research is ongoing to better understand their prevalence and potential contributing factors. Cultural factors may play a role in the expression and treatment-seeking of BFRBs, and further research is needed to better understand these complex phenomena, especially in children and adolescents.

Illness Anxiety Disorder

Illness anxiety disorder (IAD) is a disorder characterized by excessive concern about having or developing a serious medical condition despite a lack of evidence indicating a need for this concern (American Psychiatric Association, 2022). As IAD and the related somatic symptom disorder (SSD) are newly defined diagnoses, replacing hypochondriasis as of the publication of the *Diagnostic and Statistical Manual of Mental Disorders* (5th edition, 2022) (DSM-5TR; American Psychiatric Association, 2022), studies of prevalence are relatively limited. One study has shown an estimated prevalence rate of 3.28 per cent for combined IAD and SSD among medical and graduate students (Manore et al., 2021). IAD is common in adolescents, with an average age of onset of 20 years and tends to worsen with age (Newby et al., 2017).

To date, research investigating diversity-related issues in IAD is limited. Inconsistent associations have been observed between health anxiety and various demographic variables, and cultural factors remain understudied (Looper & Dickinson, 2014). However, some research conducted with adult samples has demonstrated that factors linked with inequities in healthcare are also relevant to IAD. For example, individuals with higher socioeconomic status are less likely to experience health anxiety symptoms (Barbek et al., 2022b). Additionally, one systematic review and meta-analysis demonstrated that migrants and members of minoritized ethnic groups are at higher risk for experiencing health anxiety (Barbek et al., 2022a).

One uniquely important diversity factor that must be considered in relation to IAD is chronic illness. People who are chronically ill often experience normative and appropriate concern about the possibility of their chronic illness worsening, and, as of now, there is no clear method for identifying the point at which these fears become "excessive" (Lebel et al., 2020). It is important that this distinction be more clearly defined in order to avoid either (1) underdiagnosing IAD or (2) over-pathologizing normal health anxiety in these populations (Lebel et al., 2020).

Currently, research on diversity factors in youth with IAD is extremely limited. Much more work is needed to explore cultural variables that may be of specific significance to IAD presentations across individuals of diverse backgrounds. For example, the apparent association between health care inequities and health anxiety in certain minoritized groups is an area for further focus in both adult and pediatric samples.

Hoarding Disorder

Hoarding disorder (HD) is defined as a persistent difficulty in discarding possessions, leading to a progressive accumulation of belongings that generate excessive clutter and impede the free use of living spaces, resulting in significant distress and impairment in functioning. The prevalence rate of HD in children has not been established, however, HD has been found to affect roughly 2 percent of adolescents (Ivanov et al., 2013). Although hoarding is generally believed to be a widespread occurrence with consistent clinical characteristics that are similar across cultures and settings (Mataix-Cols et al., 2010), our current understanding of this phenomenon is still quite limited. A large barrier to our understanding of HD is that most of the existing literature on this disorder, including nosological, epidemiological, and clinical studies, has been conducted mainly with adult European or Euro-American samples (Fernández de la Cruz, Nordsletten, & Mataix-Cols, 2016). However, a small body of literature suggests that conceptualizations of HD and its related symptoms (e.g., saving and acquiring items, clutter) may differ between cultures. Of note, most of the existing literature has focused on adult samples. Still, given that cultural factors impact the presentation and development of psychopathology (Hwang et al., 2008), the literature is relevant to our understanding of HD in children and adolescents.

Timpano and colleagues (2015) conducted a study comparing hoarding symptoms among college students in China and the United States and found significantly more HD symptoms within the Chinese sample. The authors hypothesized that cultural beliefs regarding saving, self-control, and wastefulness could be attributed to this discrepancy, highlighting the role that cultural values and norms could play in influencing hoarding symptoms. However, HD might present differently within Asian cultures, as a sample of participants from Singapore found a lower prevalence of HD compared to German and American samples (Subramaniam et al., 2014) – these disparities in findings can be theorized as stemming from differences in cultural values. For example, it could be that, because saving and "being thrifty" are considered virtues in some Asian communities, an individual presenting with hoarding symptoms may not be as distressed by their symptoms, or perhaps may not view their symptoms as a clinical issue to be concerned about (Li et al., 2009; Subramaniam et al., 2014). While these findings come from Asian samples, it is reasonable to assume that other ethnic/racial groups' cultural values could influence the etiology of HD.

Indeed, a common theme across a few cultural groups and HD research is the difficulty in conceptualizing clutter. Studies have found that, despite high levels of HD symptoms, ethnic/racial minority groups often report a lower amount of clutter in their homes. For example, a study conducted by Ong and colleagues (2016) reported that 30 percent of outpatient adult individuals seeking treatment in Singapore exhibited high severity of HD symptoms but with significantly lower levels of reported clutter on the Clutter Image Rating (CIR) measure (Frost et al., 2008), a widely used pictorial scale that assesses the extent of clutter in the home, compared to Western sample populations. Similarly, Nordsletten and colleagues (2018) reported that Brazilian adults endorsed lower levels of clutter on the CIR compared to individuals in Spain and England. Likewise, Stamatis and colleagues (2021) found that Latin/x, Spanish-speaking respondents with the same level of hoarding symptoms as their counterparts were slightly less likely to endorse clutter on the CIR. Based on these findings, it could be hypothesized that conceptualizations of clutter and what clutter looks like are likely to be shaped by cultural and environmental factors such as collectivism, familism, stigma, living arrangements, and space availability. Considering clutter is a key facet of HD, thus, acknowledging sociocultural influences on how clutter is conceptualized by individuals from diverse groups is necessary.

Despite this progress regarding our understanding of HD across different populations and cultures, there are still wide gaps in our knowledge which must be addressed. To better validate hoarding measures and ensure that treatments are effective and acceptable across cultural groups, it is crucial that future research is more inclusive. As such, sociocultural factors, such as ethnic and racial identity, should be further explored to better understand their impact on symptom development, presentation, trajectory, and treatment of HD. Another limitation in the HD literature is that the assessment tools we use to improve our understanding of HD have primarily been normed with individuals of European or Euro-American descent. This limits the generalizability of research findings, as previous studies have demonstrated that clinical cut-off scores and clinical presentation of OCD can vary among ethnic groups. This will help to ensure that assessment tools are not only accurate but also culturally sensitive and appropriate. As noted, most of the literature on HD has examined adult samples, limiting our understanding of the development of HD and the potential differential impact it can have on youth in comparison to adults. Further research with child and adolescent samples is warranted.

Tic Disorder/Tourette's Syndrome (TS)

Tic disorder (including Tourette's syndrome, TS) is a condition marked by uncontrollable movements (motor) and/or verbalizations (vocal), which impacts 1 percent of youth (i.e., 0.77 percent) (Knight et al., 2012). The prevalence of TS diagnosis appears lower among communities in Sub-Saharan Africa. However, this finding may be due to cultural differences among psychological health care access, stigma, and the multi-dimensional nature of TS, which makes identification and assessment challenging (Robertson & Cavanna, 2008). A recent characterization of tic disorder/TS in China highlighted that relevant cultural factors may impact the treatment and assessment of the condition (e.g., incorporating "non-Western" medical practices into treatment, the unique stigma associated with tics, and a low rate of pediatric psychiatrists) (Liu et al., 2020). In America, a study of youth, ranging from pre-school, elementary, and secondary school students, identified that African American pre-school and elementary students were more likely to receive behavioral tic ratings compared to White students. Additionally, belonging to a lower socioeconomic status (i.e., being enrolled in a head-start program) predicted increased tic ratings across all groups (Gadow et al., 2002).

Indeed, research examining the assessment and treatment of tic disorder is sparse, and its inclusion of demographic characteristics is equally undocumented. A meta-analysis examining the prognosis of TS from 1990 to 2010, including seven studies that represented both adults and youth, reported no demographic characteristics beyond sex assigned at birth (Hassan & Cavanna, 2012). Moreover, a recent clinical guideline to treatment for TS among youth examined data from 1965 to 2013, including a large number of studies (N = 174) and participants (N > 1,000), but provided no demographic data on the samples included (Murphy, T.K. et al., 2013b). Of the limited youth research that has characterized their sample beyond sex assigned at birth, most participants were White (86 percent, 85 percent, and 76 per cent, respectively) (Conelea et al., 2011; Garcia-Delgar et al., 2022; Hanks et al., 2016), while adult/parent samples reported mid-education level (i.e., graduated high school and had at least an associate's degree) (Garcia-Delgar et al., 2022), earning over 60,000 USD annually (73 percent) (Johnco et al., 2016). The overarching theme of missing demographic data from the past 50+ years suggests a systematic issue in primarily collecting and reporting sample demographics, regardless of NIH-specific guidelines. Thus, decades of past work examining TS may not be able to identify for which participant demographics the prognosis and treatment of TS were effective.

Pediatric Autoimmune Neuropsychiatric Disorder Associated with Streptococcus and Pediatric Acute-Onset Neuropsychiatric Syndrome

Pediatric acute-onset neuropsychiatric syndrome (PANS), refers to the sudden and dramatic development of OCD, tic disorders, or other major psychiatric or behavioral changes, which are often associated with autoimmune infections (Allen, Leonard, & Swedo, 1995; Swedo et al., 1998). Although definitive research regarding the prevalence of pediatric autoimmune neuropsychiatric disorder associated with streptococcus (PANDAS)/ PANS is lacking, one study found that approximately 5 percent of children presenting to a pediatric OCD clinic had OCD due to PANDAS/PANS (Jaspers-Fayer et al., 2017).

Unfortunately, research into PANDAS/PANS studies and treatment outcomes rarely reports on demographic information, and when it does, only age or sex assigned at birth is reported (Esposito et al., 2014; Leon et al., 2018; Macerollo & Martino, 2013; Murphy, T.K. et al., 2013a; Murphy, M.L. & Pichichero, 2002; Orefici et al., 2016; Shulman, 2009; Sigra, Hesselmark, & Bejerot, 2018). This lack of demographic reporting further complicates the ability to examine potential differences in prevalence rates across different racial, ethnic, and gender identity groups. Because PANDAS/PANS stems from infection, youth who have marginalized identities may have less access to timely, necessary treatment to prevent the development of these conditions and may therefore be more vulnerable to experiencing severe symptoms following infection. The lack of reporting of important demographic information also interferes with researchers' ability to ensure that PANDAS/PANS treatments are as effective for youth with marginalized identities as those without.

Of the PANDAS/PANS studies that directly report racial identification, samples were mostly White (80.1–92 percent) (Gabbay et al., 2008; Murphy, T.K. et al., 2004; Williams, K.A. et al., 2016), further limiting generalizability to non-White samples who may experience unique symptoms or challenges in treatment. As such, future research on PANDAS/PANS that both reports and analyzes potential group differences across varying gender identities, sexual orientations, and racial and ethnic identities is necessary.

Recommendations for Improving Diversity

Recently, literature and institutions have attempted to promote diversity, equity, and inclusion (DEI) within research efforts, however, these terms and their applications are often not well defined or vary in meaning across contexts. The DEI model framework is one that aims to promote and include all voices in research, especially those who have been historically marginalized based on any demographic characteristic(s). Equity refers to the equitable distribution of resources, with the aim of enabling all communities to thrive. Diversity denotes the representation of individuals from various backgrounds and identities. Inclusion pertains to an environment that not only tolerates differences but also actively affirms and celebrates them (APA, 2021). Throughout the current chapter, major themes related to improving DEI among OCRD research have been suggested, and we use these principles to highlight recommendations for future research here. Importantly, while specific recommendations may pertain to one identification group (e.g., African American/Black youth), we urge researchers to approach research from an intersectional lens. This includes thoughtfully incorporating the ways multiple identifications may interact to improve the quality of research findings by recognizing that sociocultural identities do not exist in a vacuum.

With respect to equity, it is crucial that researchers conducting research into clinical outcomes ensure that these trials are available to individuals with marginalized or minoritized identities, so that their experiences can be captured in the outcomes data and so that they can personally benefit from treatment that may otherwise be unavailable to them. We emphasize the need for assessment measurements that are culturally sensitive and adapted to specific youth communities. It should not be assumed that a tool utilized to assess OCD amongst a majority, privileged sample will extend to other populations. For example, in the adult OCD literature, the Yale-Brown Obsessive Compulsive Scale (Y-BOCS) (Goodman et al., 1989) is considered the "gold-standard" assessment tool for measuring OCD symptom severity. However, prior to 2015, its psychometric properties in African American/Black adult samples remained unexamined (Williams, M.T. et al., 2013b). Both the Y-BOCS and the Obsessive-Compulsive Inventory – Revised (OCI-R) (Foa et al., 2002; Abramowitz & Deacon, 2006) appear psychometrically sound among

African American/Black adults compared to predominantly White samples (Williams, M.T. et al., 2013b; Williams, M.T. et al., 2013a). However, psychometrics of youth measures of OCD across different communities must be examined in a similar way to ensure they perform consistently across groups. In addition, to address limitations in the national/global use of psychometric tools related to OCRDs, future research should work to translate and validate assessment tools to non-English languages, with appropriate cultural considerations.

With respect to diversity, research can be improved both by collecting data from more representatively diverse samples and by reporting comprehensively on the demographics of said samples. A major theme noted in this chapter is a lack of demographic characteristics collected or reported by studies. For most samples, there were virtually no other demographic characteristics reported in these studies beyond sex assigned at birth and age. Approximately 20 percent of individuals from younger generations (e.g., "Generation Z") identify with a sexual orientation other than heterosexual, a notable leap from prevalence rates of sexual minority identification across all ages (3.5–7.1 percent) (Gates, 2011; Jones, 2022). However, research studies are not capturing this phenomenon nor reporting these characteristics, which limits our ability to understand empirically how identity-related stigma may impact OCRD prevalence and presentation. For guidelines on how to assess sexual identity, see The National Academies of Sciences, Engineering, and Medicine (NASEM) recently published recommendations (NASEM, 2022).

While not the fault of any individual researcher or team, this lack of demographic reporting reflects the low priority of including individuals from a wide range of backgrounds, perhaps due to a misconception that findings can be generalized and treatments do not require any adaptations or considerations for different communities. Therefore, our first recommendation for improving the diversity of OCRD research is to encourage research groups to both collect and report demographics beyond age and sex assigned at birth. This is especially important in light of recent findings that suggest minoritized adult populations report unique OCD symptoms, and mixed findings suggest that they may, in some cases, have required a larger dose of evidence-based treatment to achieve the same outcomes as their non-minoritized peers (Bezahler et al., 2022; Pinciotti et al., 2024; Pinciotti et al., 2022; Pinciotti & Orcutt, 2021; Williams, M.T. et al., 2015).

Among the few research studies that did include race or ethnicity, samples were found to be overwhelmingly non-Latin/x White, and the lack of racial and ethnic minority representation in OCRD research spans decades. Suggestions for improving racial and ethnic representation in OCRD research may include pre-selecting recruitment targets that are consistent with census data to ensure representativeness of samples and implementing research-based recruitment strategies to incorporate diverse perspectives (e.g., the use of radio advertisements and Craig's list advertisements for recruiting African American/Black adults) (Williams, M.T. et al., 2012c). Specific recruitment methods for Latin/x populations include reaching out to community organizations (e.g., churches, clinics, schools) to reduce stigma and increase the visibility of OCD treatment, utilizing Spanish for recruitment and intervention materials, and informing medical professionals about OCD treatment so that appropriate referrals can be made (Wetterneck et al., 2012).

Lastly, with respect to inclusion, more consideration should be made regarding the unique ways that OCRDs may develop, present, or be maintained in individuals with marginalized or minoritized identities (e.g., symptoms that stem from or are impacted by minority stress experiences), including how these experiences may differ from individuals who hold majority identities. For example, Latin/x individuals often present with more somatic psychological symptoms compared to their White counterparts (Escovar et al., 2018), though research is limited on how this somatization could impact the presentation of obsessive-compulsive and related disorders in this population. The work of bridging this gap could begin by descriptively examining differences between minority and non-minority groups, though longer-term research should not use minority group identity as a proxy for other factors that could be relevant to the etiology and expression of obsessive-compulsive disorders, such as discrimination, related racial trauma, and acculturation. Instead, future work should consider how these more nuanced factors, which have been shown to impact psychological health broadly (Hwang et al., 2008), specifically affect the heterogeneity of obsessive-compulsive symptoms. Of note, the field especially lacks this data in youth struggling with these disorders. Enhanced comprehension of these disorders within marginalized groups has the potential to facilitate the creation of assessments and treatments that are culturally suitable.

Resilience factors across unique cultures and identities are important to consider in research examining onset and maintenance of OCRDs. As a result of their marginalization, many marginalized and minoritized communities develop a deep sense of community connectedness that may, along with other resilience factors such as pride in one's identity, serve as a buffer against the development of OCRDs and other psychopathology (Gray, Mendelsohn, & Omoto, 2015). It is important to understand and celebrate the positive features and experiences of these groups, despite being subjected to pervasive and systemic oppression.

Conclusion

OCRD research largely lacks diversity of samples. This represents a crucial gap because unique differences have been observed in OCRD research that has considered minoritized identities, suggesting that OCRDs may be experienced differentially, or our assessment tools and interventions may not be culturally adapted to identifying and treating symptomology in individuals with non-privileged identities. Future research examining OCRDs with youth would benefit significantly from more intentional recruitment of diverse samples, more thorough reporting on a variety of demographic characteristics, and continued examination into whether differences exist across measure assessment tools, diagnostic rates, and interventions.

References

Abramowitz, J.S., & Deacon, B.J. (2006). Psychometric properties and construct validity of the Obsessive–Compulsive Inventory – Revised: Replication and extension with a clinical sample. *Journal of Anxiety Disorders*, 20(8), 1016–1035. https://doi.org/10.1016/j.janxdis.2006.03.001.

Abramowitz, J.S., Whiteside, S.P., & Deacon, B.J. (2005). The effectiveness of treatment for pediatric obsessive-compulsive disorder: A meta-analysis. *Behavior Therapy*, 36(1), 55–63. https://doi.org/10.1016/S0005-7894(05)80054-1.

Allen, A.J., Leonard, H.L., & Swedo, S.E. (1995). Case study: A new infection-triggered, autoimmune subtype of pediatric OCD and Tourette's syndrome. *Journal of the American Academy of Child & Adolescent Psychiatry*, 34(3), 307–311. https://doi.org/10.1097/00004583-199503000-00015.

American Psychiatric Association. (2022). *Diagnostic and statistical manual of mental disorders* (5th ed., text rev.). https://doi.org/10.1176/appi.books.978 0890425787.

American Psychological Association. (2021, April 8). Equity, diversity, and inclusion. *American Psychological Association*. Retrieved from https://www.apa.org/about/apa/equitydiversity-inclusion.

Barbek, R., Henning, S., Ludwig, J., & von dem Knesebeck, O. (2022a). Ethnic and migration-related inequalities in health anxiety: A systematic review and meta-analysis. *Frontiers in Psychology*, 13. https://doi.org/10.3389/fpsyg.2022.960256.

Barbek, R.M., Makowski, A.C., & von dem Knesebeck, O. (2022b). Social inequalities in health anxiety: A systematic review and meta-analysis. *Journal of Psychosomatic Research*, 153, 110706. https://doi.org/10.1016/j.jpsychores.2021.110706.

Bezahler, A., Falkenstein, M. J., & Kuckertz, J. M. (2024a). What Do You Believe? Differentiating Obsessive Beliefs between Bi+, Gay/Lesbian and Heterosexual Adults with OCD. Journal of Obsessive-Compulsive and Related Disorders, 100898. https://doi.org/10.1016/j.jocrd.2024.100898

Bezahler, A., Kuckertz, J. M., McKay, D., Falkenstein, M. J., & Feinstein, B. A. (2024b). Emotion regulation and OCD among sexual minority people: Identifying treatment targets. Journal of Anxiety Disorders, 101, 102807. https://doi.org/10.1016/j.janxdis.2023.102807

Bezahler, A., Kuckertz, J.M., Schreck, M., Narine, K., Dattolico, D., & Falkenstein, M.J. (2022). Examination of outcomes among sexual minorities in treatment for obsessive-compulsive and related disorders. *Journal of Obsessive-Compulsive and Related Disorders*, 33, 100724. https://doi.org/10.1016/j.jocrd.2022.100724.

Boroughs, M.S., Krawczyk, R., & Thompson, J.K. (2010). Body dysmorphic disorder among diverse racial/ethnic and sexual orientation groups: Prevalence estimates and associated factors. *Sex Roles: A Journal of Research, 63*(9–10), 725–737. https://doi.org/10.1007/s11199-010-9831-1.

Conelea, C.A., Woods, D.W., Zinner, S.H., Budman, C., Murphy, T.K, Scahill, L.D., . . . & Walkup, J. (2011). Exploring the impact of chronic tic disorders on youth: Results from the Tourette Syndrome Impact Survey. *Child Psychiatry & Human Development, 42,* 219–242. https://doi.org/10.1007/s10578-010-0211-4.

Convertino, A.D., Brady, J.P., Albright, C.A., Gonzales IV, M., & Blashill, A.J. (2021). The role of sexual minority stress and community involvement on disordered eating, dysmorphic concerns and appearance- and performance-enhancing drug misuse. *Body Image, 36,* 53–63. https://doi.org/10.1016/j.bodyim.2020.10.006.

Duke, D.C., Bodzin, D.K., Tavares, P., Geffken, G.R., & Storch, E.A. (2009). The phenomenology of hairpulling in a community sample. *Journal of Anxiety Disorders, 23*(8), 1118–1125.

Escovar, E.L., Craske, M., Roy-Byrne, P., Stein, M.B., Sullivan, G., Sherbourne, C.D., . . . & Chavira, D.A. (2018). Cultural influences on mental health symptoms in a primary care sample of Latinx patients. *Journal of Anxiety Disorders, 55,* 39–47.

Esposito, S., Bianchini, S., Baggi, E., Fattizzo, M., & Rigante, D. (2014). Pediatric autoimmune neuropsychiatric disorders associated with streptococcal infections: An overview. *European Journal of Clinical Microbiology & Infectious Diseases, 33,* 2105–2109. https://doi.org/10.1007/s10096-014-2185-9.

Fabris, M.A., Longobardi, C., Badenes-Ribera, L., & Settanni, M. (2020). Prevalence and co-occurrence of different types of body dysmorphic disorder among men having sex with men. *Journal of Homosexuality, 69*(1), 132–144.

Fernández de la Cruz, L., Llorens, M., Jassi, A., Krebs, G., Vidal-Ribas, P., Radua, J., . . . Mataix-Cols, D. (2015). Ethnic inequalities in the use of secondary and tertiary mental health services among patients with obsessive–compulsive disorder. *The British Journal of Psychiatry, 207*(6), 530–535. doi:10.1192/bjp.bp.114.154062.

Fernández de la Cruz, L., Nordsletten, A.E., & Mataix-Cols, D. (2016). Ethnocultural aspects of hoarding disorder. *Current Psychiatry Reviews, 12*(2), 115–123.

Foa, E.B., Huppert, J.D., Leiberg, S., Langner, R., Kichic, R., Hajcak, G., & Salkovskis, P.M. (2002). The Obsessive-Compulsive Inventory: Development and validation of a short version. *Psychological Assessment, 14*(4), 485. https://doi.org/10.1037/1040-3590.14.4.485.

Frost, R.O., Steketee, G., Tolin, D.F., & Renaud, S. (2008). Development and validation of the clutter image rating. *Journal of Psychopathology and Behavioral Assessment, 30,* 193–203. https://doi.org/10.1007/s10862-007-9068-7.

Gabbay, V., Coffey, B.J., Babb, J.S., Meyer, L., Wachtel, C., Anam, S., & Rabinovitz, B. (2008). Pediatric autoimmune neuropsychiatric disorders associated with streptococcus: Comparison of diagnosis and treatment in the community and at a specialty clinic. *Pediatrics, 122*(2), 273–278. https://doi.org/10.1542/peds.2007-1307.

Gadow, K., Nolan, E., Sprafkin, J., & Schwartz, J. (2002). Tics and psychiatric comorbidity in children and adolescents. *Developmental Medicine and Child Neurology, 44*(5), 330–338. doi:10.1017/S001216220100216X.

Garcia-Delgar, B., Servera, M., Coffey, B.J., Lázaro, L., Openneer, T., Benaroya-Milshtein, N., . . . & Morer, A. (2022). Tic disorders in children and adolescents: Does the clinical presentation differ in males and females? A report by the EMTICS group. *European Child & Adolescent Psychiatry, 31*(10), 1539–1548. https://doi.org/10.1007/s00787-021-01751-4.

Garde, J.B., Suryavanshi, R.K., Jawale, B.A., Deshmukh, V., Dadhe, D.P., & Suryavanshi, M.K. (2014). An epidemiological study to know the prevalence of deleterious oral habits among 6 to 12 year old children. *Journal of International Oral Health: JIOH, 6*(1), 39.

Gates, G.J. (2011). *How many people are lesbian, gay, bisexual, and transgender?* UCLA School of Law Williams Institute. Retrieved from: https://williamsinsti tute.law.ucla.edu/publications/how-many-people-lgbt/.

Ginsburg, G.S., Kingery, J.N., Drake, K.L., & Grados, M.A. (2008). Predictors of treatment response in pediatric obsessive-compulsive disorder. *Journal of the American Academy of Child & Adolescent Psychiatry, 47*(8), 868–878. https://doi.org/10.1097/CHI.0b013e3181799ebd.

Gonzales IV, M., & Blashill, A.J. (2021). Ethnic/racial and gender differences in body image disorders among a diverse sample of sexual minority US adults. *Body Image, 36*, 64–73. https://doi.org/10.1016/j.bodyim.2020.10.007.

Goodman, W.K., Price, L.H., Rasmussen, S.A., Mazure, C., Fleischmann, R.L., Hill, C.L., . . . & Charney, D.S. (1989). The Yale-Brown Obsessive Compulsive Scale: I. Development, use, and reliability. *Archives of General Psychiatry, 46*(11), 1006–1011. doi:10.1001/archpsyc.1989.01810110048007.

Grant, J.E., Valle, S., Aslan, I.H., & Chamberlain, S.R. (2021). Clinical presentation of body-focused repetitive behaviors in minority ethnic groups. *Comprehensive Psychiatry, 111*, 152272. https://doi.org/10.1007/s10464-014-9697-4.

Gray, N.N., Mendelsohn, D.M., & Omoto, A.M. (2015). Community connect-edness, challenges, and resilience among gay Latino immigrants. *American Journal of Community Psychology, 55*, 202–214. DOI: 10.1007/s10464-014-9697-4.

Hanks, C.E., McGuire, J.F., Lewin, A.B., Storch, E.A., & Murphy, T.K. (2016). Clinical correlates and mediators of self-concept in youth with chronic tic disorders. *Child Psychiatry & Human Development, 47*, 64–74. https://doi.org/10.1007/s10578-015-0544-0.

Hassan, N., & Cavanna, A. E. (2012). The prognosis of Tourette syndrome: implications for clinical practice. *Functional Neurology, 27*(1), 23. PMCID: PMC3812751.

Hayes, S.L., Storch, E.A., & Berlanga, L. (2009). Skin picking behaviors: An exam-ination of the prevalence and severity in a community sample. *Journal of Anxiety Disorders, 23*(3), 314–319. DOI: 10.1016/j.janxdis.2009.01.008.

Hwang, W.C., Myers, H.F., Abe-Kim, J., & Ting, J.Y. (2008). A conceptual para-digm for understanding culture's impact on mental health: The cultural influences on mental health (CIMH) model. *Clinical Psychology Review, 28*(2), 211–227. DOI: 10.1016/j.cpr.2007.05.001.

Ivanov, V.Z., Mataix-Cols, D., Serlachius, E., Lichtenstein, P., Ankarsäter, H., Chang, Z., . . . & Rück, C. (2013). Prevalence, comorbidity and heritability of hoarding symptoms in adolescence: A population-based twin study in 15-year olds. *Plos one, 8*(7), e69140. DOI: 10.1371/journal.pone.0069140.

Jaspers-Fayer, F., Han, S.H.J., Chan, E., McKenney, K., Simpson, A., Boyle, A., Ellwyn, R., & Stewart, S.E. (2017). Prevalence of acute-onset subtypes in pediat-ric obsessive-compulsive disorder. *Journal of Child and Adolescent Psychophar-macology, 27*(4), 332–341. https://doi.org/10.1089/cap.2016.0031.

Jassi, A., & Krebs, G. (2021). Body dysmorphic disorder: Reflections on the last 25 years. *Clinical Child Psychology and Psychiatry*, 26(1), 3–7. https://doi.org/10.1177/1359104520984818.

Johnco, C., McGuire, J.F., McBride, N.M., Murphy, T.K., Lewin, A.B., & Storch, E.A. (2016). Suicidal ideation in youth with tic disorders. *Journal of Affective Disorders*, 200, 204–211. https://doi.org/10.1016/j.jad.2016.04.027.

Jones, J.M. (2022). "LGBT identification in U.S. tics up to 7.1%." Gallup.com, Gallup, 10 June 2022. https://news.gallup.com/poll/389792/lgbt-identification-ticks-up.aspx.

Knight, T., Steeves, T., Day, L., Lowerison, M., Jette, N., & Pringsheim, T. (2012). Prevalence of tic disorders: A systematic review and meta-analysis. *Pediatric Neurology*, 47(2), 77–90. https://doi.org/10.1016/j.pediatrneurol.2012.05.002.

Lebel, S., Mutsaers, B., Tomei, C., Leclair, C.S., Jones, G., Petricone-Westwood, D., . . . & Dinkel, A. (2020). Health anxiety and illness-related fears across diverse chronic illnesses: A systematic review on conceptualization, measurement, prevalence, course, and correlates. *Plos One*, 15(7), e0234124. https://doi.org/10.1371/journal.pone.0234124.

Leon, J., Hommer, R., Grant, P., Farmer, C., D'Souza, P., Kessler, R., . . . & Swedo, S. (2018). Longitudinal outcomes of children with pediatric autoimmune neuropsychiatric disorder associated with streptococcal infections (PANDAS). *European Child & Adolescent Psychiatry*, 27, 637–643. https://doi.org/10.1007/s00787-017-1077-9.

Li, Y., Marques, L., Hinton, D.E., Wang, Y., & Xiao, Z.P. (2009). Symptom dimensions in Chinese patients with obsessive-compulsive disorder. *CNS Neuroscience & Therapeutics*, 15(3), 276–282. doi: 10.1111/j.1755-5949.2009.00099.x.

Liu, Z.S., Cui, Y.H., Sun, D., Lu, Q., Jiang, Y.W., Jiang, L., . . . & Qin, J. (2020). Current status, diagnosis, and treatment recommendation for tic disorders in China. *Frontiers in Psychiatry*, 11, 774. https://doi.org/10.3389/fpsyt.2020.00774.

Looper, K., & Dickinson, P. (2014). Epidemiological and economic aspects of hypochondriasis and health anxiety. *Hypochondriasis and health anxiety: A guide for clinicians*, 85–112. DOI: 10.1093/med/9780199996865.003.0006.

Macerollo, A., & Martino, D. (2013). Pediatric autoimmune neuropsychiatric disorders associated with streptococcal infections (PANDAS): An evolving concept. https://doi.org/10.7916/D8HD85TP.

Manore, S., Sahare, K., Bhawnani, D., & Umate, L. (2021). Prevalence of Illness Anxiety Disorder (IAD) and Somatic Symptom Disorder (SSD) among medical and non-medical students: A cross sectional study. *Highlights on Medicine and Medical Science*, 11, 146–151. https://dx.doi.org/10.18535/jmscr/v6i3.53.

Mansueto, C.S., Thomas, A.M., & Brice, A.L. (2007). Hair pulling and its affective correlates in an African-American university sample. *Journal of Anxiety Disorders*, 21(4), 590–599. https://doi.org/10.1016/j.janxdis.2006.08.004.

Marques, L., LeBlanc, N., Weingarden, H., Greenberg, J.L., Traeger, L.N., Keshaviah, A., & Wilhelm, S. (2011a). Body dysmorphic symptoms: Phenomenology and ethnicity. *Body Image*, 8(2), 163–167. https://doi.org/10.1016/j.bodyim.2010.12.006.

Marques, L., Weingarden, H.M., LeBlanc, N.J., & Wilhelm, S. (2011b). Treatment utilization and barriers to treatment engagement among people with body dysmorphic symptoms. *Journal of Psychosomatic Research*, *70*(3), 286–293. https://doi.org/10.1016/j.jpsychores.2010.10.002.

Mataix-Cols, D., Frost, R.O., Pertusa, A., Clark, L.A., Saxena, S., Leckman, J.F., Stein, D.J., Matsunaga, H., & Wilhelm, S. (2010). Hoarding disorder: A new diagnosis for DSM-V? *Depression and Anxiety*, *27*(6), 556–572. DOI: 10.1002/da.20693.

Mataix-Cols, D., Nakatani, E., Micali, N., & Heyman, I. (2008). Structure of obsessive-compulsive symptoms in pediatric OCD. *Journal of the American Academy of Child & Adolescent Psychiatry*, *47*(7), 773–778. https://doi.org/10.1097/CHI.0b013e31816b73c0.

Mayville, S., Katz, R.C., Gipson, M.T., & Cabral, K. (1998). Assessing the prevalence of body dysmorphic disorder in an ethnically diverse group of adolescents. *Journal of Child and Family Studies*, *8*, 357–362.

McKay, D., Piacentini, J., Greisberg, S., Graae, F., Jaffer, M., & Miller, J. (2006). The structure of childhood obsessions and compulsions: Dimensions in an outpatient sample. *Behaviour Research and Therapy*, *44*(1), 137–146. https://doi.org/10.1016/j.brat.2005.02.001.

Moreno-Amador, B., Cervin, M., Falcó, R., Marzo, J.C., & Piqueras, J.A. (2023). Body-dysmorphic, hoarding, hair-pulling, and skin-picking symptoms in a large sample of adolescents. *Current Psychology*, *42*(28), 24542–24553. https://doi.org/10.1007/s12144-022-03477-1.

Murphy, M.L., & Pichichero, M.E. (2002). Prospective identification and treatment of children with pediatric autoimmune neuropsychiatric disorder associated with group A streptococcal infection (PANDAS). *Archives of Pediatrics & Adolescent Medicine*, *156*(4), 356–361. doi:10.1001/archpedi.156.4.356.

Murphy, T.K., Lewin, A.B., Parker-Athill, E.C., Storch, E.A., & Mutch, P.J. (2013a). Tonsillectomies and adenoidectomies do not prevent the onset of pediatric autoimmune neuropsychiatric disorder associated with group A streptococcus. *The Pediatric Infectious Disease Journal*, *32*(8), 834. PMCID: PMC3740796.

Murphy, T.K., Lewin, A.B., Storch, E.A., & Stock, S. (2013b). Practice parameter for the assessment and treatment of children and adolescents with tic disorders. *Journal of the American Academy of Child & Adolescent Psychiatry*, *52*(12), 1341–1359. https://doi.org/10.1016/j.jaac.2013.09.015.

Murphy, T.K., Sajid, M., Soto, O., Shapira, N., Edge, P., Yang, M., . . . & Goodman, W.K. (2004). Detecting pediatric autoimmune neuropsychiatric disorders associated with streptococcus in children with obsessive-compulsive disorder and tics. *Biological Psychiatry*, *55*(1), 61–68. https://doi.org/10.1016/S0006-3223(03)00704-2.

Nagata, J.M., Compte, E.J., McGuire, F.H., Lavender, J.M., Murray, S.B., Brown, T.A., Capriotti, M.R., Flentje, A., Lubensky, M.E., Obedin-Maliver, J., & Lunn, M.R. (2022). Psychometric validation of the Muscle Dysmorphic Disorder Inventory (MDDI) among US transgender men. *Body Image*, *42*, 43–49. https://doi.org/10.1016/j.bodyim.2022.05.001.

NASEM (National Academies of Sciences, Engineering, and Medicine). Division of Behavioral and Social Sciences and Education; Committee on National Statistics; Committee on Measuring Sex, Gender Identity, and Sexual Orientation; Becker, T., Chin, M., & Bates, N. (Eds.). (2022, Mar 9). *Measuring sex, gender identity, and sexual orientation*. National Academies Press (US). Available from: https://www.ncbi.nlm.nih.gov/books/NBK578625/doi: 10.17226/26424.

Nazeer, A., Latif, F., Mondal, A., Azeem, M.W., & Greydanus, D.E. (2020). Obsessive-compulsive disorder in children and adolescents: Epidemiology, diagnosis and management. *Translational Pediatrics*, 9(Suppl 1), S76–S93. https://doi.org/10.21037/tp.2019.10.02.

Neal-Barnett, A., Flessner, C., Franklin, M.E., Woods, D.W., Keuthen, N.J., & Stein, D.J. (2010). Ethnic differences in trichotillomania: Phenomenology, interference, impairment, and treatment efficacy. *Journal of anxiety disorders*, 24(6), 553–558. https://doi.org/10.1016/j.janxdis.2010.03.014.

Newby, J.M., Hobbs, M.J., Mahoney, A.E., Wong, S.K., & Andrews, G. (2017). DSM-5 illness anxiety disorder and somatic symptom disorder: Comorbidity, correlates, and overlap with DSM-IV hypochondriasis. *Journal of Psychosomatic Research*, 101, 31–37. https://doi.org/10.1016/j.jpsychores.2017.07.010.

Nordsletten, A.E., Fernández de la Cruz, L., Aluco, E., Alonso, P., López-Solà, C., Menchón, J.M., Nakao, T., Kuwano, M., Yamada, S., & Fontenelle, L.F. (2018). A transcultural study of hoarding disorder: Insights from the United Kingdom, Spain, Japan, and Brazil. *Transcultural Psychiatry*, 55(2), 261–285. DOI: 10.1177/1363461518759203.

Ong, C., Sagayadevan, V., Lee, S.P., Ong, R., Chong, S.A., Frost, R.O., & Subramaniam, M. (2016). Hoarding among outpatients seeking treatment at a psychiatric hospital in Singapore. *Journal of Obsessive-Compulsive and Related Disorders*, 8, 56–63. 10.1016/j.jocrd.2015.12.002.

Oosthuizen, P., Lambert, T., & Castle, D.J. (1998). Dysmorphic concern: Prevalence and associations with clinical variables. *Australian and New Zealand Journal of Psychiatry*, 32(1), 129–132.

Orefici, G., Cardona, F., Cox, C.J., & Cunningham, M.W. (2016). Pediatric autoimmune neuropsychiatric disorders associated with streptococcal infections (PANDAS). *Streptococcus Pyogenes: Basic Biology to Clinical Manifestations*. Available from: https://www.ncbi.nlm.nih.gov/books/NBK333433/.

Oshana, A., Klimek, P., & Blashill, A.J. (2020). Minority stress and body dysmorphic disorder symptoms among sexual minority adolescents and adult men. *Body Image*, 34, 167–174. https://doi.org/10.1016/j.bodyim.2020.06.001.

Pillai, V.T., & Sündermann, O. (2019). Racial teasing and body dysmorphic disorder symptoms – A cross-sectional study of Asian ethnic groups in Singapore. *Asia Pacific Journal of Counseling and Psychotherapy*, 11(1), 47–59. https://doi.org/1 0.1080/21507686.2019.1708425.

Pinciotti, C. M., Feinstein, B. A., & Williams, M. T. (2024). Symptom profiles and intensive treatment outcomes in sexual minority and heterosexual patients with obsessive-compulsive disorder. Behavior Therapy. Advance online publication. https://doi.org/10.1016/j.beth.2024.06.006

Pinciotti, C.M., Nuñez, M., Riemann, B.C., & Bailey, B.E. (2022). Clinical presentation and treatment trajectory of gender minority patients with obsessive-compulsive disorder. *Journal of Cognitive Psychotherapy*, 36(1), 42–59. https://doi.org/10. 1891/jcpsy-d-20-00022.

Pinciotti, C.M., & Orcutt, H.K. (2021). Obsessive-compulsive symptoms in sexual minorities. *Psychology of Sexual Orientation and Gender Diversity*, 8(4), 487–495. https://doi.org/10.1037/sgd0000437.

Rautio, D., Jassi, A., Krebs, G., Andrén, P., Monzani, B., Gumpert, M., Lewis, A., Peile, L., Sevilla-Cermeño, L., Jansson-Fröjmark, M., Lundgren, T., Hillborg, M., Silverberg-Morse, M., Clark, B., Fernández de la Cruz, L., & Mataix-Cols, D. (2020). Clinical characteristics of 172 children and adolescents with body dysmorphic disorder. *European Child & Adolescent Psychiatry*, 31, 133–144. https://doi.org/10.1007/s00787-020-01677-3.

Robertson, M., & Cavanna, A. (2008). *Tourette syndrome*. Oxford University Press.

Rozzell, K.N., Carter, C., Convertino, A.D., Gonzales IV, M., & Blashill, A.J. (2020). The Dysmorphic Concern Questionnaire: Measurement invariance by gender and race/ethnicity among sexual minority adults. *Body Image, 35,* 201–206. https://doi.org/10.1016/j.bodyim.2020.08.010.

Sabik, N.J., Matsick, J.L., McCormick-Huhn, K., & Cole, E.R. (2021). Bringing an intersectional lens to "open" science: An analysis of representation in the reproducibility project. *Psychology of Women Quarterly, 45*(4), 475–492. https://doi.org/10.1177/03616843211035678.

Selles, R.R., Nelson, R., Zepeda, R., Dane, B.F., Wu, M.S., Novoa, J.C., Guttfreund, D., & Storch, E.A. (2015). Body focused repetitive behaviors among Salvadorian youth: Incidence and clinical correlates. *Journal of Obsessive-Compulsive and Related Disorders, 5,* 49–54. https://doi.org/10.1016/j.jocrd.2015.01.008.

Sigra, S., Hesselmark, E., & Bejerot, S. (2018). Treatment of PANDAS and PANS: A systematic review. *Neuroscience & Biobehavioral Reviews, 86,* 51–65. https://doi.org/10.1016/j.neubiorev.2018.01.001.

Shin, R.Q., Welch, J.C., Kaya, A.E., Yeung, J.G., Obana, C., Sharma, R., Vernay, C.N., & Yee, S. (2017). The intersectionality framework and identity intersections in the Journal of Counseling Psychology and The Counseling Psychologist: A content analysis. *Journal of Counseling Psychology, 64*(5), 458–474. https://doi.org/10.1037/cou0000204.

Shulman, S.T. (2009). Pediatric autoimmune neuropsychiatric disorders associated with streptococci (PANDAS): Update. *Current Opinion in Pediatrics, 21*(1), 127–130. DOI: 10.1097/MOP.0b013e32831db2c4.

Solley, K., & Turner, C. (2018). Prevalence and correlates of clinically significant body-focused repetitive behaviors in a non-clinical sample. *Comprehensive Psychiatry, 86,* 9–18.

Sotiriou, E.G. (2021). *Cultural components of body dissatisfaction in ethnically diverse women: Moving beyond weight focused body image.* (Unpublished doctoral dissertation.)

Stamatis, C.A., Muroff, J., Bocanegra, E.S., Rodriguez, C.I., & Timpano, K.R. (2021). A Spanish translation of the Hoarding Rating Scale: Differential item functioning and convergent validity. *Journal of Psychopathology and Behavioral Assessment, 43*(4), 946–959.

Stewart, S.E., Geller, D.A., Jenike, M., Pauls, D., Shaw, D., Mullin, B., & Faraone, S.V. (2004). Long-term outcome of pediatric obsessive–compulsive disorder: A meta-analysis and qualitative review of the literature. *Acta Psychiatrica Scandinavica, 110*(1), 4–13. https://doi.org/10.1111/j.1600-0447.2004.00302.x.

Stewart, S.E., Rosario, M.C., Brown, T.A., Carter, A.S., Leckman, J.F., Sukhodolsky, D., . . . & Pauls, D.L. (2007). Principal components analysis of obsessive–compulsive disorder symptoms in children and adolescents. *Biological Psychiatry, 61*(3), 285–291. https://doi.org/10.1016/j.biopsych.2006.08.040.

Subramaniam, M., Abdin, E., Vaingankar, J.A., Picco, L., & Chong, S.A. (2014). Hoarding in an Asian population: Prevalence, correlates, disability and quality of life. *Annals Academy of Medicine, Singapore, 43*(11), 535–543.

Swedo, S.E., Leonard, H.L., Garvey, M., Mittleman, B., Allen, A.J., Perlmutter, S., . . . & Lougee, L. (1998). Pediatric autoimmune neuropsychiatric disorders associated with streptococcal infections: Clinical description of the first 50 cases. *American Journal of Psychiatry, 155*(2), 264–271. https://doi.org/10.1176/ajp.155.2.264.

Timpano, K.R., Çek, D., Fu, Z.-F., Tang, T., Wang, J.-P., & Chasson, G.S. (2015). A consideration of hoarding disorder symptoms in China. *Comprehensive Psychiatry*, *57*, 36–45. https://doi.org/10.1016/j.comppsych.2014.11.006.

Veale, D., Gledhill, L.J., Christodoulou, P., & Hodsoll, J. (2016). Body dysmorphic disorder in different settings: A systematic review and estimated weighted prevalence. *Body Image*, *18*, 168–186. https://doi.org/10.1016/j.bodyim.2016.07.003.

Wadsworth, L.P., Potluri, S., Schreck, M., & Hernandez-Vallant, A. (2020). Measurement and impacts of intersectionality on obsessive-compulsive disorder symptoms across intensive treatment. *American Journal of Orthopsychiatry*, *90*(4), 445–457. https://doi.org/10.1037/ort0000447.

Watson, H.J., & Rees, C.S. (2008). Meta-analysis of randomized, controlled treatment trials for pediatric obsessive-compulsive disorder. *Journal of Child Psychology and Psychiatry*, *49*(5), 489–498. https://doi.org/10.1111/j.1469-7610.2007.01875.x.

Weingarden, H., Marques, L., Fang, A., LeBlanc, N., Buhlmann, U., Phillips, K.A., & Wilhelm, S. (2011). Culturally adapted cognitive behavioral therapy for body dysmorphic disorder: Case examples. *International Journal of Cognitive Therapy*, *4*(4), 381–396. https://doi.org/10.1521/ijct.2011.4.4.381.

Wetterneck, C.T., Little, T.E., Rinehart, K.L., Cervantes, M.E., Hyde, E., & Williams, M.T (2012). Latinos with obsessive-compulsive disorder: Mental healthcare utilization and inclusion in clinical trials. *Journal of Obsessive-Compulsive and Related Disorders*, *1*(2), 85–97. doi: 10.1016/j.jocrd.2011.12.001.

Williams, K.A., Swedo, S.E., Farmer, C.A., Grantz, H., Grant, P.J., D'Souza, P., . . . & Leckman, J.F. (2016). Randomized, controlled trial of intravenous immunoglobulin for pediatric autoimmune neuropsychiatric disorders associated with streptococcal infections. *Journal of the American Academy of Child & Adolescent Psychiatry*, *55*(10), 860–867. https://doi.org/10.1016/j.jaac.2016.06.017.

Williams, M.T, Davis, D.M., Thibodeau, M.A., & Bach, N. (2013a). Psychometric properties of the Obsessive-Compulsive Inventory revised in African Americans with and without obsessive-compulsive disorder. *Journal of Obsessive-Compulsive and Related Disorders*, *2*(4), 399–405. https://doi.org/10.1016/j.jocrd.2013.07.003.

Williams, M.T., Domanico, J., Marques, L., Leblanc, N.J., & Turkheimer, E. (2012a). Barriers to treatment among African Americans with obsessive-compulsive disorder. *Journal of Anxiety Disorders*, *26*(4), 555–563. https://doi.org/10.1016/j.janxdis.2012.02.009.

Williams, M.T., Elstein, J., Buckner, E., Abelson, J.M., & Himle, J.A. (2012b). Symptom dimensions in two samples of African Americans with obsessive-compulsive disorder. *Journal of Obsessive-Compulsive and Related Disorders*, *1*(3), 145–152. https://doi.org/10.1016/j.jocrd.2012.03.004.

Williams, M.T., & Jahn, M.E. (2017). Obsessive–compulsive disorder in African American children and adolescents: Risks, resiliency, and barriers to treatment. *American Journal of Orthopsychiatry*, *87*(3), 291. https://doi.org/10.1037/ort0000188.

Williams, M.T, Powers, M., Yun, Y.G., & Foa, E. (2010). Minority participation in randomized controlled trials for obsessive–compulsive disorder. *Journal of Anxiety Disorders*, *24*(2), 171. doi: 10.1016/j.janxdis.2009.11.004.

Williams, M.T., Proetto, D., Casiano, D., & Franklin, M.E. (2012c). Recruitment of a hidden population: African Americans with obsessive-compulsive disorder. *Contemporary Clinical Trials*, *33*(1), 67–75. https://doi.org/10.1016/j.cct.2011.09.001.

Williams, M.T., Sawyer, B., Leonard, R.C., Ellsworth, M., Simms, J., & Riemann, B.C. (2015). Minority participation in a major residential and intensive outpatient program for obsessive-compulsive disorder. *Journal of Obsessive-Compulsive and Related Disorders*, *5*, 67–75. https://doi.org/10.1016/j.jocrd.2015.02.004.

Williams, M.T., Taylor, R.J., Mouzon, D.M., Oshin, L.A., Himle, J.A., & Chatters, L.M. (2017). Discrimination and symptoms of obsessive-compulsive disorder among African Americans. *American Journal of Orthopsychiatry*, *87*(6), 636–645. https://doi.org/10.1037/ort0000285.

Williams, M.T., Turkheimer, E., Magee, E., & Guterbock, T. (2008). The effects of race and racial priming on self-report of contamination anxiety. *Personality and Individual Differences*, *44*(3), 746–757.

Williams, M.T., Wetterneck, C.T., Thibodeau, M.A., & Duque, G. (2013b). Validation of the Yale-Brown Obsessive-Compulsive Severity Scale in African Americans with obsessive-compulsive disorder. *Psychiatry Research*, *209*(2), 214–221. https://doi.org/10.1016/j.psychres.2013.04.007.

15 Pediatric Obsessive-Compulsive and Related Disorders

The Long and Winding Road

Eric A. Storch[1] *and Andrew G. Guzick*[2]

[1] *Baylor College of Medicine, Menninger Department of Psychiatry & Behavioral Sciences, Houston, TX*

[2] *Department of Psychiatry, University of Pennsylvania, Philadelphia, PA*

Disclosure Statement

Eric Storch reports receiving research funding to his institution from the Ream Foundation, International OCD Foundation, and NIH. He was a consultant for Brainsway and Biohaven Pharmaceuticals. He owns stock less than 5000 USD in NView. He receives book royalties from Elsevier, Wiley, Oxford, American Psychological Association, Guilford Press, Springer, and Jessica Kingsley. Dr Andrew Guzick receives research funding from the Ream Foundation.

As the present text illustrates, obsessive-compulsive and related disorders (OCRDs) among children represent a series of heterogeneous conditions that often onset during childhood and confer significant disability for the affected individual as well as their loved ones. Without treatment, these conditions tend to persist and increase risk for other co-occurring problems. Fortunately, significant progress has been made over the past several decades in terms of classification, recognition, and treatment of OCRDs. Despite these advances, much more remains to be done on this long and winding road of maximizing outcomes and wellness among those affected, particularly for youth. The purpose of this concluding chapter is to highlight several areas for future work.

Approximately 25 years ago, the state of the literature in childhood OCRDs consisted of open trials supporting cognitive behavioral therapy (CBT) for obsessive-compulsive disorder (OCD), strong controlled trials for various antidepressants for OCD, and case series-level data for other types of intervention for other OCRDs. A significant amount has changed since that time point. There are rigorous randomized controlled trials

DOI: 10.4324/9781003386278-15

published for OCD, body dysmorphic disorder, trichotillomania, and Tourette syndrome, as well as a solid empirical basis to guide treatment for related OCRDs (e.g., avoidant restrictive food intake disorder (ARFID)). However, more needs to be done in the efficacy space. In some cases, only a single trial has been conducted requiring replication or extension. In other cases, alternative treatment approaches need to be examined to ensure adequate options are available to meet stakeholder needs. Excellent examples of this include the introduction of parent-led and intensive interventions. While standard care CBT with exposure and response prevention has demonstrated robust and consistent efficacy across trials, having alternative approaches – including guiding the parent to provide intervention for their affected child or treating more intensively – allows for more tools in the toolkit to meet heterogeneous clinical and psychosocial needs. Promising interventions such as acceptance and commitment therapy have demonstrated utility across a number of small trials and case reports in childhood OCRDs, but they must meet efficacy standards in order to be considered a frontline treatment.

Treatment personalization is another important area of growth. While skilled therapists can typically successfully adapt interventions to meet the clinical needs of affected youth, it is critical to appreciate the role of other factors, including culture, sexual identity, and gender identity, to optimally meet clinical needs. Another way of personalizing intervention includes matching the dose with clinical severity and complexity. Staged interventions hold particular promise in which the level of clinical complexity is matched to the intensity of the intervention such that milder cases receive less intensive intervention (e.g., bibliotherapy, internet guided CBT) and more severe cases are treated more robustly (Farrell et al., 2023). Considering different dosages of treatment can be one way of personalizing care while concurrently saving resources. Work in adults with OCD (Tolin et al., 2005) as well as children with anxiety and post-traumatic stress (Rapee et al., 2017; Salloum et al., 2016) has illustrated this nicely in the form of stepped-care models, but this needs to be more conclusively studied in youth with OCRDs, particularly those with higher base rates (e.g., OCD, Tourette).

Dissemination studies are also critically needed. A tremendous amount of work has taken place in clinical settings and more recently real-world settings (Benito et al., 2021; Torp et al., 2015). However, dramatic variation in care persists throughout the world – even more so in less resourced areas. This is simply unacceptable. The field has come to a point where it is clear what interventions work for most childhood OCRDs (and emerging ones have the opportunity to demonstrate efficacy). It is now time to ensure that clinicians and trainees are uniformly educated in the application of these approaches, as well as being able to utilize such approaches.

It may be that generalist models of training should no longer be the norm; instead, educational models that train specialists in certain domains should be employed in order to develop skilled clinicians able to address these common presentations. This is comparable to medicine: while there are primary care providers who handle many front-line problems, providers thereafter are trained to provide specialist care in a particular domain. In the case of OCRDs – for children and adults alike – moving to a specialist model has key advantages to improve treatment quality and fidelity. Furthermore, while the workforce has expanded in applied psychology, it has not expanded sufficiently; and in many cases this expansion has not been coupled with robust training in evidence-based interventions for OCRDs. We highlight the need to develop uniformity in training models such that interventions that have established efficacy are systematically and consistently taught to the next generation of clinician scholars.

While established treatments exist for core OCRDs (i.e., OCD, body dysmorphic disorder (BDD), Tourette, trichotillomania), and emerging interventions have also been reported, there are newer conditions for which robust interventions do not exist. One such condition is *misophonia* which is thoughtfully described in this volume. Efforts have been made to explore interventions and a number of case reports have been published supporting various approaches (Dover & McGuire, 2021; McGuire, Wu, & Storch, 2015; Schneider & Arch, 2017) However, methodologically rigorous controlled studies have either not achieved efficacy (Lewin et al., 2021) or have room for improvement in terms of treatment effects (Jager et al., 2021) Utilizing a stakeholder-informed approach to develop a robust treatment model to address the clinical needs of this population may have the benefit of maximizing outcomes.

Finally, we highlight the need to consider the remaining questions in the field. Several come to mind. First, pharmacological interventions have demonstrated efficacy for childhood and adult OCD. However, it remains unclear how one might discontinue pharmacotherapy in children with OCD or other related conditions when these interventions are no longer needed. Evidence among adults suggest that treating someone to remission with CBT may be one approach (Foa et al., 2022) but this needs to be extended to youth with OCD as well as other conditions. Second, studies are needed to understand the core components of interventions as well as mechanisms of action. It remains surprising that certain core treatment elements are not maximally applied in the context of interventions. For example, in the case of childhood OCD treatment, it is unclear why some CBT protocols do not maximize the dose of exposure therapy nor do they provide a robust element of parent-led treatment. This is problematic given that exposure has been documented as the most salient component in this intervention approach (Guzick et al., 2022; Whiteside et al., 2020) and that parent involvement effectively targets one of the mechanisms underlying OCD pathology, namely family accommodation (Merlo et al., 2009). By understanding these factors, more robust interventions can be introduced and personalized for the affected child to maximize treatment outcomes.

It is our hope that the present text continues and extends the conversation about the nature, assessment, and treatment of childhood OCRDs. While it has been a long and windy road over the past three decades, more remains to be done. We hope that the present text engenders thought and discussion about these topics with the goal of furthering scholarship in this space, disseminating information to improve access and reduce treatment variation, and ultimately improving child and family outcomes.

References

Benito, K.G., Herren, J., Freeman, J.B., Garcia, A.M., Block, P., Cantor, E., Chorpita, B.F., Wellen, B., Stewart, E., Georgiadis, C., Frank, H., & Machan, J. (2021). Improving delivery behaviors during exposure for pediatric OCD: A multiple baseline training trial with community therapists. *Behavior Therapy*, 52(4), 806–820. https://doi.org/10.1016/j.beth.2020.10.003.

Dover, N., & McGuire, J.F. (2021). Family-based cognitive behavioral therapy for youth with misophonia: A case report. *Cognitive and Behavioral Practice*. https://doi.org/10.1016/j.cbpra.2021.05.005.

Farrell, L.J., Waters, A.M., Storch, E.A., Simcock, G., Perkes, I.E., Grisham, J.R., Dyason, K.M., & Ollendick, T.H. (2023). Closing the gap for children with OCD: A staged-care model of cognitive behavioural therapy with exposure and response prevention. *Clinical Child and Family Psychology Review*, 26(3), 642–664. https://doi.org/10.1007/s10567-023-00439-2.

Foa, E.B., Simpson, H.B., Gallagher, T., Wheaton, M.G., Gershkovich, M., Schmidt, A.B., Huppert, J.D., Imms, P., Campeas, R.B., Cahill, S., DiChiara, C., Tsao, S.D., Puliafico, A., Chazin, D., Asnaani, A., Moore, K., Tyler, J., Steinman, S.A., Sanches-LaCay, A., . . . Rosenfield, D. (2022). Maintenance of wellness in patients with obsessive-compulsive disorder who discontinue medication after exposure/response prevention augmentation: A randomized clinical trial. *JAMA Psychiatry*, 79(3), 193–200. https://doi.org/10.1001/jamapsychiatry.2021.3997.

Guzick, A.G., Schneider, S.C., Kendall, P.C., Wood, J.J., Kerns, C.M., Small, B.J., Park, Y.E., Cepeda, S.L., & Storch, E.A. (2022). Change during cognitive and exposure phases of cognitive-behavioral therapy for autistic youth with anxiety disorders. *Journal of Consulting and Clinical Psychology*, 90(9), 709–714. https://doi.org/10.1037/ccp0000755.

Jager, I.J., Vulink, N.C.C., Bergfeld, I.O., van Loon, A.J.J.M., & Denys, D.A.J.P. (2021). Cognitive behavioral therapy for misophonia: A randomized clinical trial. *Depression and Anxiety*, 38(7), 708–718. https://doi.org/10.1002/da.23127.

Lewin, A.B., Dickinson, S., Kudryk, K., Karlovich, A.R., Harmon, S.L., Phillips, D.A., Tonarely, N.A., Gruen, R., Small, B., & Ehrenreich-May, J. (2021). Transdiagnostic cognitive behavioral therapy for misophonia in youth: Methods for a clinical trial and four pilot cases. *Journal of Affective Disorders*, 291, 400–408. https://doi.org/10.1016/j.jad.2021.04.027.

McGuire, J.F., Wu, M.S., & Storch, E.A. (2015). Cognitive-behavioral therapy for 2 youths with misophonia. *The Journal of Clinical Psychiatry*, 76(5), 3143. https://doi.org/10.4088/JCP.14cr09343.

Merlo, L.J., Lehmkuhl, H.D., Geffken, G.R., & Storch, E.A. (2009). Decreased family accommodation associated with improved therapy outcome in pediatric obsessive-compulsive disorder. *Journal of Consulting and Clinical Psychology*, 77(2), 355–360. https://doi.org/10.1037/a0012652.

Rapee, R.M., Lyneham, H.J., Wuthrich, V., Chatterton, M.L., Hudson, J.L., Kangas, M., & Mihalopoulos, C. (2017). Comparison of stepped care delivery against a single, empirically validated cognitive-behavioral therapy program for youth with anxiety: A randomized clinical trial. *Journal of the American Academy of Child & Adolescent Psychiatry*, 56(10), 841–848. https://doi.org/10.1016/j.jaac.2017.08.001.

Salloum, A., Wang, W., Robst, J., Murphy, T.K., Scheeringa, M.S., Cohen, J.A., & Storch, E.A. (2016). Stepped care versus standard trauma-focused cognitive behavioral therapy for young children. *Journal of Child Psychology and Psychiatry*, 57(5), 614–622. https://doi.org/10.1111/jcpp.12471.

Schneider, R.L., & Arch, J.J. (2017). Case study: A novel application of mindfulness- and acceptance-based components to treat misophonia. *Journal of Contextual Behavioral Science*, 6(2), 221–225. https://doi.org/10.1016/j.jcbs.2017.04.003.

Tolin, D.F., Diefenbach, G.J., Maltby, N., & Hannan, S. (2005). Stepped care for obsessive-compulsive disorder: A pilot study. *Cognitive and Behavioral Practice*, 12(4), 403–414. https://doi.org/10.1016/S1077-7229(05)80068-9.

Torp, N.C., Dahl, K., Skarphedinsson, G., Thomsen, P.H., Valderhaug, R., Weidle, B., Melin, K.H., Hybel, K., Nissen, J.B., Lenhard, F., Wentzel-Larsen, T., Franklin, M.E., & Ivarsson, T. (2015). Effectiveness of cognitive behavior treatment for pediatric obsessive-compulsive disorder: Acute outcomes from the Nordic Long-term OCD Treatment Study (NordLOTS). *Behaviour Research and Therapy*, 64, 15–23. https://doi.org/10.1016/j.brat.2014.11.005.

Whiteside, S.P.H., Sim, L.A., Morrow, A.S., Farah, W.H., Hilliker, D.R., Murad, M.H., & Wang, Z. (2020). A meta-analysis to guide the enhancement of cbt for childhood anxiety: Exposure over anxiety management. *Clinical Child and Family Psychology Review*, 23(1), 102–121. https://doi.org/10.1007/s10567-019-00303-2.

Index

Page numbers in **bold** refer to tables.